W9-BTD-273

HUMAN DISEASES

A Systemic Approach

Fourth Edition

WITHDRAWN

WITHDRAWN

HUMAN DISEASES
A Systemic Approach

F o u r t h   E d i t i o n

Mary Lou Mulvihill, PhD
Professor Emeritus
William Rainey Harper College
Palatine, Illinois

CUMBERLAND COUNTY COLLEGE LIBRARY
3322 COLLEGE DRIVE
VINELAND, NJ 08360

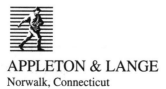

APPLETON & LANGE
Norwalk, Connecticut

RB
111
M83
1995

Notice: The author and the publisher of this volume have taken care to make certain that the doses of drugs and schedules of treatment are correct and compatible with the standards generally accepted at the time of publication. Nevertheless, as new information becomes available, changes in treatment and in the use of drugs become necessary. The reader is advised to carefully consult the instruction and information material included in the package insert of each drug or therapeutic agent before administration. This advice is especially important when using new or infrequently used drugs. The publisher disclaims any liability, loss, injury, or damage incurred as a consequence, directly or indirectly, of the use and application of any of the contents of this volume.

Copyright © 1995 by Appleton & Lange
A Simon & Schuster Company
Copyright © 1987, 1991 by Appleton & Lange
Copyright © 1980 by Robert J. Brady Co.

All rights reserved. This book, or any parts thereof, may not be used or reproduced in any manner without written permission. For information, address Appleton & Lange, 25 Van Zant Street, East Norwalk, Connecticut 06855.

95 96 97 98 99 / 10 9 8 7 6 5 4 3 2 1

Prentice Hall International (UK) Limited, *London*
Prentice Hall of Australia Pty. Limited, *Sydney*
Prentice Hall Canada, Inc., *Toronto*
Prentice Hall Hispanoamericana, S.A., *Mexico*
Prentice Hall of India Private Limited, *New Delhi*
Prentice Hall of Japan, Inc., *Tokyo*
Simon & Schuster Asia Pte. Ltd., *Singapore*
Editora Prentice Hall do Brasil Ltda., *Rio de Janeiro*
Prentice Hall, *Englewood Cliffs*, *New Jersey*

Library of Congress Cataloging-in-Publication Data

Mulvihill, Mary L.
    Human diseases : a systemic approach / Mary Lou Mulvihill. —4th ed.
        p.   cm.
    Includes bibliographical references and index.
    ISBN 0-8385-3928-9
    1. Pathology.   I. Title.
    [DNLM: 1. Medicine.   2. Disease.   WB 100 M961h 1994]
RB111.M83   1994
616—dc20
DNLM/DLC
for Library of Congress   94-8977
                                                           CIP

Acquisitions Editor: Cheryl L. Mehalik
Designer: Janice Barsevich Bielawa

ISBN 0-8385-3928-9
90000

PRINTED IN THE UNITED STATES OF AMERICA

9 780838 539286

To
my husband, Jim, and all my relatives and friends
who have encouraged me in this work.

Contents in Brief

PART I.   MECHANISMS OF DISEASE   1

  1. Introduction to Disease   3
  2. Inflammation, Immunity, and Allergy   11
  3. Neoplasia   31
  4. Hereditary Diseases   45
  5. Dietary Deficiencies and Excesses:
     Malnutrition, Obesity, Alcoholism   63

PART II.   DISEASES OF THE SYSTEMS   83

  6. Diseases of the Blood   85
  7. Diseases of the Heart   103
  8. Diseases of the Blood Vessels   129
  9. Diseases of the Excretory System   147
 10. Diseases of the Digestive System   167
 11. Diseases of the Liver, Gallbladder, and Pancreas   193
 12. Diseases of the Respiratory System   215
 13. Diseases of the Endocrine System   247
 14. Diseases of the Reproductive Systems and
     Sexually Transmitted Diseases   291
 15. Diseases of the Nervous System   323
 16. Diseases of the Bones, Joints, and Muscles   351
 17. Diseases of the Skin   373
 18. Stress and Aging   391
 19. Wellness: Diet and Exercise   407
 Glossary of Terms   417
 References   447
 Answers to Self-Study Questions   449
 Index   451

Contents in Detail

Preface xxiii
Reviewers xxvii
Acknowledgments xxviii

PART I.   MECHANISMS OF DISEASE   1

1. Introduction to Disease   3
   Chapter Outline   3
   Introduction   3
   Abnormal Growth Patterns   5
   Etiology of Disease   5
      Antibiotic Resistant Bacteria   6
   Diagnosis   8
   Chapter Summary   9
   Self-Study   10

2. Inflammation, Immunity, and Allergy   11
   Chapter Outline   11
   Inflammation and Repair   12
   Immunity   15
   Autoimmunity   19
      Lupus Erythematosus   19
   Immune Deficiency   20
      Acquired Immune Deficiency Syndrome (AIDS)   20
      HIV Infection   21
      Precautions for Health-care Professionals   21
      Chronic Fatigue Syndrome   22
   Vaccination   22
   Hypersensitivity—Allergies   23
   Chapter Summary   27
   Self-Study   29

3. Neoplasia 31

Chapter Outline 31
Tumor Formation 31
Malignant Tumors 32

Development of Cancer 32
Causes of Cancer 33
Prevention of Cancer 35
Signs and Symptoms of Cancer 35
Types of Cancer 36
Metastasis 37
Diagnosis of Cancer 37
Treatment of Cancer 39

Benign Tumors 40

Types of Benign Tumors 40

Differences Between Malignant and Benign Tumors 42
Chapter Summary 42
Self-Study 44

4. Hereditary Diseases 45

Chapter Outline 45
Introduction to Heredity 46
Transmission of Hereditary Diseases 47

Autosomal Dominant 47
Autosomal Recessive 48
Sex-linked Inheritance 51

Color Blindness/51 Familial Diseases/53

Abnormal Chromosome Diseases 53

Down's Syndrome 53
Fragile X Syndrome 54

Sex Anomalies 55

Turner's Syndrome 55
Klinefelter's Syndrome 55
Hermaphrodites 56

Congenital Diseases 57
Chapter Summary 59
Self-Study 60

5. Dietary Deficiencies and Excesses:
Malnutrition, Obesity, Alcoholism 63

Chapter Outline 63
Malnutrition 64

Vitamin Deficiencies 65
   Vitamin A Deficiency 65
   Vitamin D Deficiency (Rickets) 66
   Vitamin K Deficiency 66
   Vitamin C (Ascorbic Acid) Deficiency 66
Hypervitaminosis 67
Mineral Deficiencies 67
Anorexia Nervosa 68
Bulimia 70
Obesity 70
   Causes of Obesity 72
   Diseases Aggravated by Obesity 72
   Diagnosis and Treatment of Obesity 73
Alcoholism 75
   Signs and Symptoms of Alcoholism 76
   Effects of Excessive Alcohol on the Central Nervous System/76
   Effects of Alcoholism on the Digestive System/77
   Effects of Alcoholism on the Cardiovascular System/78
   Alcohol and Pregnancy 78
   Treatment of Alcoholism 79
   Chapter Summary 80
   Self-Study 82

PART II.   DISEASES OF THE SYSTEMS 83

6. Diseases of the Blood 85
   Chapter Outline 85
   Composition of Blood 86
   The Anemias 87
      Pernicious Anemia 88
      Hypochromic Anemia 88
      Hemolytic Anemia 88
      Aplastic Anemia 92
      Secondary Anemia 92
   Excessive Red Blood Cells 93
      Primary Polycythemia 93
      Secondary Polycythemia 93
   Bleeding Diseases 93
      Hemophilia 93
      Purpura (Thrombocytopenia) 94

Diseases of White Blood Cells and Blood-forming Tissue   95
    Leukemia   95
    Malignant Lymphomas   97
    Infectious Mononucleosis   98
Diagnostic Procedures for Blood Diseases   99
Chapter Summary   100
Self-Study   101

7. Diseases of the Heart   103
Chapter Outline   103
Structure and Function of the Heart   104
The Relationship Between Heart and Lungs   105
Influence of the Autonomic Nervous System   106
Diseases of the Heart   109
    Coronary Artery Disease   109
    Hypertensive Heart Disease   111
    Cor Pulmonale   112
    Congestive Heart Failure   112
    Congenital Heart Disease   112
    Valvular Diseases   117
    Rheumatic Heart Disease   120
    Infectious Endocarditis   121
Symptoms of Heart Disease   123
Abnormalities of Heart Action   124
Diagnostic Procedures for Heart Action   124
Chapter Summary   126
Self-Study   127

8. Diseases of the Blood Vessels   129
Chapter Outline   129
Blood Vessels and Circulation   129
Structure and Function of the Blood Vessels   131
Diseases of the Arteries   131
    Arteriosclerosis   131
    Atherosclerosis   131
    Thrombosis and Embolism   132
    Aneurysms   135
    Hemorrhages   136
    Raynaud's Diseases   137
Diseases of the Veins   138
    Phlebitis   138
    Varicose Veins   138

Hypertension 140
   Control Mechanisms 140
   Hypertension and Kidney Disease 141
   Primary and Secondary Hypertension 141
   Effects of Hypertension 141
   Treatment of Hypertension 141
Shock 142
Diagnostic Procedures for Vascular Disease 142
Chapter Summary 143
Self-Study 144

9. Diseases of the Excretory System 147
   Chapter Outline 147
   Functions of the Kidneys 148
      The Nephron 148
      Formation of Urine 148
   Diseases of the Kidney 150
      Glomerulonephritis 150
      Acute Glomerulonephritis/150
      Chronic Glomerulonephritis/151
   Renal Failure 152
      Acute Renal Failure 152
      Chronic Renal Failure 153
   Pyelonephritis 153
   Pyelitis 155
   Renal Carcinoma 155
   Kidney Stones 155
   Hydronephrosis 157
   Polycystic Kidney 157
   Diseases of the Urinary Bladder and Urethra 159
      Cystitis 159
      Carcinoma of the Bladder 160
      Urethritis 160
   Diagnostic Tests 161
   Chapter Summary 162
   Self-Study 164

10. Diseases of the Digestive System 167
   Chapter Outline 167
   The Digestive Process 168
   Diseases of the Mouth 170
      Cancer of the Mouth 170

Diseases of the Esophagus 171
    Cancer of the Esophagus 171
    Esophageal Varices 171
    Esophagitis 171
    Hiatal Hernia 171
Diseases of the Stomach 173
    Gastritis 173
    Chronic Atrophic Gastritis 173
    Peptic Ulcers 173
    Gastroenteritis 178
    Cancer of the Stomach 178
Diseases of the Intestines 178
    Appendicitis 178
    Malabsorption Syndrome 179
    Diverticulosis 180
    Diverticulitis 180
    Regional Enteritis (Crohn's Disease) 180
    Chronic Ulcerative Colitis 181
    Salmonella (Food Poisoning) 181
    Carcinoma of the Colon and Rectum 183
    Intestinal Obstructions 184
    Spastic Colon (Irritable Bowel Syndrome) 185
    Dysentery 186
General Disorders of the Digestive Tract 186
    Vomiting 186
    Diarrhea 187
    Constipation 187
    Hemorrhoids 187
Diagnostic Procedures for the Digestive Tract 187
Diseases Indicated by Stool Characteristics 188
Chapter Summary 188
Self-Study 190

11. Diseases of the Liver, Gallbladder, and Pancreas 193
    Chapter Outline 193
    Functions of the Liver 194
    Diseases of the Liver 196
        Jaundice 196
        Causes of Jaundice/197
        Viral Hepatitis 198
        Cirrhosis of the Liver 199
        Carcinoma of the Liver 203

Diseases of the Gallbladder 205
Cholecystitis/205 Gallstones (Cholelithiasis)/206
Structure and Function of the Pancreas 207
Diseases of the Pancreas 208
Pancreatitis 208
Cancer of the Pancreas 210
Diagnostic Tests 211
Chapter Summary 211
Self-Study 212

12. Diseases of the Respiratory System 215
Chapter Outline 215
Structure and Function of the Respiratory System 216
Upper Respiratory Diseases 219
The Common Cold 219
Hay Fever (Seasonal Allergic Rhinitis) 220
Tonsillitis 221
Influenza 222
Lower Respiratory Diseases 222
Chronic Obstructive Pulmonary Disease (COPD) 222
Bronchitis/222 Bronchial Asthma/224
Bronchiectasis 226
Emphysema 227
Pneumothorax 230
Atelectasis 231
Pneumonia 231
Pleurisy 235
Empyema 235
Tuberculosis 236
Tuberculosis of the Kidney/238
Bronchogenic Carcinoma 239
Cystic Fibrosis 240
Sudden Infant Death Syndrome 240
Hiccoughs 241
Diagnostic Procedures for Respiratory Diseases 242
Chapter Summary 243
Self-Study 244

13. Diseases of the Endocrine System 247
Chapter Outline 247
Functions of the Endocrine Glands 248

Structure and Function of the Pituitary Gland 249
  Hormones of the Anterior Pituitary Gland 251
Diseases of the Anterior Pituitary Gland 252
  Hyperpituitarism 252
  Hypopituitarism 253
Function of the Posterior Pituitary Gland 258
  Hyposecretion of the Posterior Pituitary Gland 258
  Diabetes Insipidus 258
Structure and Function of the Thyroid Gland 259
  Structure of the Thyroid Gland 260
  Function of the Thyroid Gland 260
  Effects of Thyroid Hormones 261
  Control of Circulating Thyroxine Level 262
Diseases of the Thyroid Gland 262
  Goiter 262
  Hyperthyroidism 264
  Hypothyroidism 266
  Cretinism 267
Structure and Function of the Adrenal Glands 272
Diseases of the Adrenal Cortex 274
  Hyperadrenalism 274
  Hypoadrenalism 276
Structure and Function of the Parathyroids 278
  Structure of the Parathyroids 278
  Function of the Parathyroids 278
Diseases of the Parathyroid Gland 279
  Hyperparathyroidism 279
  Hypoparathyroidism 280
Endocrine Function of the Pancreas 280
  Hyposecretion of the Pancreas 282
  Diabetes Mellitus (Hyperglycemia) 282
    *Symptoms of Diabetes Mellitus/282 Complications
    of Diabetes Mellitus/283 Treatment of Diabetes Mellitus/283
    Diabetic Coma and Insulin Shock/284 Tests for Diabetes
    Mellitus/285 Education of the Diabetic Patient/286*
Hypoglycemia 286
Abnormalities in Secretion of Sex Hormones 286
  Hypergonadism (Hypersecretion) 286
  Hypogonadism in the Male 287
  Hypogonadism in the Female 287

Diagnostic Procedures for Endocrine Diseases 287
Chapter Summary 288
Self-Study 289

14. **Diseases of the Reproductive Systems and
    Sexually Transmitted Diseases** 291

    Chapter Outline 291
    Function of the Reproductive System 292
    Anatomy of the Female Reproductive System 292
    Physiology of the Female Reproductive System 294
    Diseases of the Female Reproductive System 296

    Pelvic Inflammatory Disease (PID) 296
    Salpingitis 296
    Vaginitis 297
    Inflammation of Bartholin's Glands 297
    Puerperal Sepsis 297
    Neoplasms of the Female Organs 298

    *Carcinoma of the Cervix/298 Carcinoma
    of the Endometrium/298 Fibroid Tumors/298
    Ovarian Neoplasms/299 Hydatidiform Mole/299
    Choriocarcinoma/300 Adenocarcinoma of the Vagina/300
    Neoplasms of the Breast/301 Benign Tumors
    of the Breast/301*

    Menstrual Abnormalities 302
    Premenstrual Syndrome 303
    Toxic Shock Syndrome 303
    Endometriosis 304
    Abnormalities of Pregnancy 305
    Ectopic Pregnancy 305
    Spontaneous Abortion 306
    Toxemia of Pregnancy 306
    Anatomy of the Male Reproductive System 307
    Physiology of the Male Reproductive System 307
    Diseases of the Male Reproductive System 310

    Diseases of the Prostate Gland 310

    *Prostatitis/310 Benign Prostatic Hyperplasia/311
    Carcinoma of the Prostate Gland/311*

    Diseases of the Testes and Epididymis 313

    *Epididymitis/313 Orchitis/313 Testicular Tumors/313
    Impotence/313 Cryptorchidism/314*

    Sexually Transmitted Diseases (STDs) 315

    AIDS (Acquired Immune Deficiency Syndrome) 315
    Gonorrhea 315

Syphilis 316
Genital Herpes 317
Genital Warts 318
Chlamydial Infections 318
Diagnostic Procedures for Reproductive and Sexually
   Transmitted Diseases 319
Chapter Summary 319
Self-Study 320

15. Diseases of the Nervous System 323
   Chapter Outline 323
   A Highly Organized Communication System 324
   Structure of the Nervous System 324
      The Spinal Cord 324
      The Brain 325
      The Autonomic Nervous System 326
   Function of the Nervous System 328
      The Sensory Nervous System 328
      The Motor Nervous System 329
   Diseases of the Nervous System 330
      Infectious Diseases of the Nervous System 330

      *Meningitis/331 Encephalitis/331 Poliomyelitis/332
      Tetanus/332 Rabies/333 Shingles (Herpes Zoster)/334
      Reye's Syndrome/335 Abscess of the Brain/335*

      Degenerative Neural Diseases 335

      *Multiple Sclerosis/335 Amyotrophic Lateral Sclerosis
      (ALS)/337 Parkinson's Disease/337 Huntington's Disease
      (Huntington's Chorea)/338*

   Convulsions 339
      Epilepsy 339
   Developmental Errors 340
      Spina Bifida 340
      Hydrocephalus 341
   Brain Damage 343
      Cerebral Palsy 343
   Cerebrovascular Accident (Stroke) (CVA) 343
      Cerebral Hemorrhage 343
      Thrombosis and Embolism 344
      Transient Ischemic Attack (TIA) 345

Traumatic Disorders 345
   Concussion of the Brain 345
   Contusion 346
   Skull Fractures 346
   Hemorrhages 346
Brain Tumors 346
Diagnostic Procedures for the Nervous System 347
Chapter Summary 348
Self-Study 349

16. Diseases of the Bones, Joints, and Muscles 351
Chapter Outline 351
Interaction of Bones, Muscles, and Joints 352
The Structure and Function of Bones, Joints, and Muscles 352
Diseases of Bone 354
   Infectious Diseases of Bone 354
   Osteomyelitis/354 Tuberculosis of the Bone/355
Bone Diseases of Vitamin and Mineral Deficiencies 355
   Rickets/355 Osteomalacia/356
Secondary Bone Diseases 356
   Osteitis Fibrosa Cystica/356 Osteoporosis/356
   Paget's Disease/357
   Bone Fractures 357
   Neoplasia of Bone 359
   Benign Bone Tumors/359 Malignant Bone Tumors/359
Diseases of the Joints 359
   Dislocations, Sprains, and Strains 360
   Carpal Tunnel Syndrome 360
   Arthritis 361
   Rheumatoid Arthritis/361 Osteoarthritis/363
   Gout 364
   Herniation of Intervertebral Disks (Slipped Disk) 364
   Bursitis 365
Diseases of Muscles 367
   Muscular Dystrophy 367
   Myasthenia Gravis 367
   Tumors of Muscle 368
Diagnostic Tests for Bone, Joint, and Muscle Diseases 368
Chapter Summary 368
Self-Study 370

17. Diseases of the Skin 373

Chapter Outline 373
Functions of the Skin 373
Structure of the Skin 374
Classification of Skin Diseases 376
Infectious Skin Diseases 376

Bacterial Skin Infections 376

Impetigo/376 Erysipelas/377 Abscess/377
Lyme Disease/377

Viral Skin Infections 377
Fungal Skin Infections 379
Parasitic Infestations 379

Hypersensitivity Diseases of the Skin 380

Urticaria (Hives) 380
Eczema 380
Poison Ivy 381
Drug Hypersensitivity 382

Neoplastic Skin Diseases 382

Nevus (Mole) 383
Basal Cell Carcinoma 383
Squamous Cell Carcinoma 383
Malignant Melanoma 385

Metabolic Skin Disorders 386

Acne (Vulgaris) 386
Seborrheic Dermatitis (Chronic Dandruff) 386
Sebaceous Cysts 386
Seborrheic Keratosis 387
Psoriasis 387

Diagnostic Tests for Skin Diseases 388
Chapter Summary 389
Self-Study 390

18. Stress and Aging 391

Chapter Outline 391
Homeostasis and Adaptation to Stress 391
Effects of Stress on the Body 392
Function of the Autonomic Nervous System in Response to Stress 393
Stress and the Adrenal Cortical Hormones 393
Treatment with Cortical Hormones 395
Stress-related Diseases 396

Gastrointestinal Diseases Affected by Stress 396
Migraine Headaches 396

The Cardiovascular System and Stress 397
Sexual Abnormalities Related to Stress 397
The Respiratory System and Stress 398
Skin Diseases Affected by Stress 398
Systemic Changes Produced by Stress 399
Effects of Aging 399
Common Diseases of the Elderly 399

Alzheimer's Disease/401

Care of the Elderly 402
Chapter Summary 403
Self-Study 405

19. Wellness: Diet and Exercise 407
Chapter Outline 407
Wellness 407
Importance of Diet 409
High Fiber–Low Fat Diet 409
Functions of Vitamins 409
Hypervitaminosis 410
Phytochemicals 410
Triglycerides and Cholesterol 410
Cholestrol: Good and Bad 411
Value of Exercise 412
Aerobic Exercise 413
Chapter Summary 413
Self-Study 414

Glossary of Terms 417
References 447
Answers to Self-Study Questions 449
Index 451

Preface

Human Diseases: A Systemic Approach, Fourth Edition, is designed for students pursuing a medical or health-related career. The first three editions of the book have been well received by students and instructors, and have been widely used throughout the country.

The Fourth Edition has been greatly revised with many new topics and features added, while the strengths of the previous editions have been retained. The writing style is clear, concise, and appropriate for students beginning a health science education. Emphasis is placed on the meaning of medical terms as they are introduced and a comprehensive glossary helps students develop a strong medical vocabulary.

The book is divided into two parts. Part I treats the general mechanisms of disease and health problems, and introduces such basic terminology as etiology, prognosis, and signs and symptoms. Concepts such as inflammation, immunity, allergy, and neoplasia are explained. Hereditary diseases and diseases caused by deficiencies or excesses (e.g., malnutrition, obesity, and alcoholism) are described. Part II covers the most commonly occurring diseases of each system (e.g., cardiovascular, excretory, digestive, and respiratory). Normal anatomy and physiology is reviewed at the beginning of each chapter although each chapter's emphasis is primarily the malfunctioning of an organ or organ system. Manifestations of the various diseases and treatment methods are explained. General diagnostic procedures for each system conclude the chapters.

NEW ORGANIZATION

The section on AIDS, although mentioned with sexually transmitted diseases, is now treated in Chapter 2 as failure of the immune system. The coverage has been expanded and updated, and the distinction between HIV infection and full-blown AIDS is clarified.

Cystic fibrosis, formerly treated with diseases of the pancreas, is now covered in Chapter 12 with respiratory diseases; its most devastating manifestation is on the respiratory system.

The descriptions of peptic ulcers and migraine headaches have also been revised.

NEW TOPICS

A new chapter, "Wellness: Diet and Exercise," has been added to reflect the current emphasis on preventive medicine. The value of a high fiber–low fat diet is stressed and replaces the section on rare vitamin deficiency diseases.

Many diseases not previously treated are covered in this edition. They include carpal tunnel syndrome (CTS), sudden infant death syndrome (SIDS), and premenstrual syndrome (PMS). Hereditary diseases, Tay–Sachs disease, and fragile X syndrome are explained. Infectious diseases, salmonella, and Lyme disease are now included. Chronic fatigue syndrome is treated with immune deficiencies.

NEW FEATURES

A chapter opener and brief outline introduce each chapter, providing a sense of direction. "Practical Applications," a new feature, appear throughout the text to add interest and stimulate thought.

At the end of each chapter an in-text Study Guide of true–false, multiple choice, and matching questions is provided to enhance learning. Answers to the self-study questions can be found at the back of the book.

NEW ILLUSTRATIONS

The art work, which is a significant aid to the learning process and a definite attribute of this text, has been redrawn and new illustrations have been added. Line drawings help convey concepts and numerous photographs show disease states. The addition of a second color to the text enhances new design features for increased clarity.

SUPPLEMENTS

■ Instructor's Manual and Test Bank

The Instructor's Manual has been completely rewritten. It now includes a chapter-by-chapter outline, introductory questions stimulating thought and interest, and teaching tips and suggestions. Titles of pertinent films and videos are now listed. Over 700 test questions are also included.

# Reviewers

I wish to thank the following reviewers for their excellent contributions to the fourth edition of *Human Diseases: A Systemic Approach*. They have shared their knowledge and teaching experience and thus helped to make this edition the useful text that it is.

Burt Goldberg
Adjunct Assistant Professor and Research Associate
Pace University
Department of Biology
New York, New York

Neil B. Schanker, MS
Assistant Professor
William Rainey Harper College
Palatine, Illinois

Eric Trunnel, PhD
University of Utah
Department of Health Education
Salt Lake City, Utah

G. Marlene Donavan, RN, BSN, MEd, MSN
Allied Health/School of Nursing
Hocking College
Nelsonville, Ohio

Mary L. Madigan, RT (R)
Bellevue Community College
Bellevue, Washington

Pamela J. Carlton, MS, EMT-P
Professor of Biology and Coordinator of Allied Health Sciences
The College of Staten Island
Staten Island, New York

Acknowledgments

I am sincerely grateful to Robert J. Kapicka, MD, who offered his time to critique the new medical material. His expertise added much to the value of the text. I also am grateful to John Cox, MD, SC, whom I consulted on certain skin diseases. I continue to appreciate the contribution of photographs from David R. Duffell, MD, Chief, Department of Pathology at Northwest Community Hospital in Arlington Heights, Illinois. I am also grateful to Northwest Community Hospital for the use of their medical library.

I wish to thank Ann Sophie, film specialist at William Rainey Harper College, for helping to compile a list of films and videos for the Instructor's Manual. I also appreciate the help of the research librarians at William Rainey Harper College.

I particularly want to express my gratitude to Cheryl L. Mehalik, Senior Editor of Appleton & Lange, who has been so encouraging and helpful during the preparation of this Fourth Edition.

Finally, I am grateful to my readers who, by their enthusiastic response to previous editions, have given me the needed encouragement to write this new one. My hope is that it achieves the purpose for which it was written: that the reader will better appreciate the human body, and understand its workings in health and in disease.

Mary Lou Mulvihill, PhD

In Memoriam

Dr. Mary Lou Mulvihill died during the final stages of completing this book. A dedicated teacher, writer, wife, and friend, it was an honor to know her and to work with her. She will be remembered by many for her generosity of spirit, and enthusiasm for life. This book is dedicated to her memory, a lasting tribute to a life lived fully, and in service to others.

Cheryl L. Mehalik
Senior Editor
Appleton & Lange

HUMAN
DISEASES
A Systemic Approach

Fourth Edition

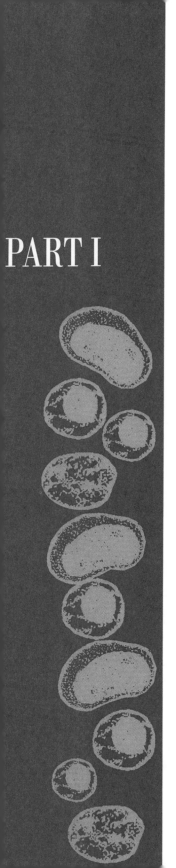

PART I

Mechanisms of Disease

Disease can be the result of many factors: infection, injury, allergy, to name a few. Heredity and malnutrition cause many diseases as does abnormal cell growth or tumor formation. Part I treats these mechanisms of disease.

Chapter
1. Introduction to Disease
2. Inflammation, Immunity, and Allergy
3. Neoplasia
4. Hereditary Diseases
5. Dietary Deficiencies and Excesses

Chapter 1

Introduction to Disease

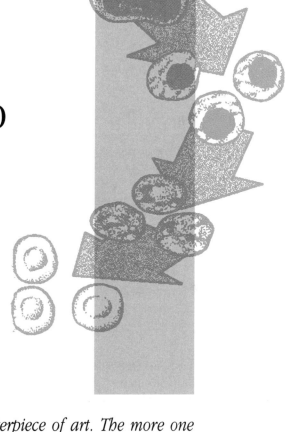

Chapter Outline

- Introduction
- Abnormal Growth Patterns
- Etiology of Disease
- Diagnosis
- Chapter Summary
- Self-Study

*T*he human body is a masterpiece of art. The more one understands the functioning of the body, the greater appreciation one has for it. Even in disease, the body is quite remarkable in attempting to right what is wrong and compensate for it.

INTRODUCTION

Changes constantly occur within the body, and yet a steady state called **homeostasis** is generally maintained. A significant disturbance in the homeostasis of the body triggers a variety of responses that often produce **disease** signs and symptoms. Athletes, for example, develop abnormally high red blood cell counts due to their increased need for oxygen. This is a natural compensatory mechanism to circulate more hemoglobin, but it is a disease symptom in polycythemia, which will be discussed later.

On the Practical Side

MAINTAINING BODY TEMPERATURE— PREVENTING HYPOTHERMIA

A sudden snow storm causes a driver to become temporarily stranded and required to walk for help in the freezing cold. How does the person maintain a normal body temperature in the frigid environment? Superficial blood vessels constrict to prevent heat loss to the environment. Reflex shivering is muscle contraction which produces body heat.

An organ will often enlarge, **hypertrophy,** when it is required to do extra work. The heart enlarges with prolonged high blood pressure as it must continue to pump blood against great resistance. Heart muscle also hypertrophies when the valves are defective because valves that are either too narrow or too wide require extra pumping action. If one kidney fails the other enlarges to meet the needs of the body and compensate for the defective one. When blood flow to the kidneys is inadequate, the kidneys help raise the blood pressure by means of a hormonal secretion. If, however, an organ or body part is not used, it will **atrophy** or, that is, decrease in size or function.

Blood plays several roles in maintaining homeostasis. When tissue is **traumatized,** injured, or becomes infected, blood flow increases to the damaged site. This is vital because the blood carries cells that are specialized to remove harmful substances and cellular debris. Other cells in the blood produce antibodies against invading organisms that cause disease.

Disease is the unhealthy state of a body part, a physiologic system, or the body as a whole; there is a disordered structure or function. Disease often begins at the cellular level. An abnormal gene, acquired through one's heredity or **mutated** (altered), by an environmental factor can start the disease process. Cancer, for example, begins with uncontrolled growth of cells when the genetic information is affected, often by a virus. New research techniques are making it possible to link certain diseases with abnormal gene findings.

ABNORMAL GROWTH PATTERNS

Abnormal growth patterns are the cause of many diseases. An increased number of cells, **hyperplasia** (*plasia*—formation or development), results in tumor formation (Chapter 3). **Hypoplasia,** on the other hand, is the incomplete or underdevelopment of an organ or tissue. Developmental failure, **aplasia,** leads to the absence of a structure or tissue. Aplastic anemia (Chapter 6) is such an example. **Metaplasia** is the conversion of normal tissue cells into an abnormal form following chronic stress or injury. **Dysplasia** (*dys*—painful or disordered) is abnormal development such as a congenital heart defect.

A **functional** condition is one in which there is no organic change such as hypertension, or high blood pressure. Abnormal tissue or function is referred to as a **lesion.** A lesion may be a wound, injury, or pathologic condition. Figure 1–1 summarizes abnormal growth patterns.

ETIOLOGY OF DISEASE

An important aspect of any disease is its **etiology,** or cause. Many familiar diseases are caused by infectious agents, bacteria, viruses, fungi, and parasites. The common cold and flu are viral infections, but abscesses and strep throat are caused by bacteria; fungi and parasites are infectious agents that cause athlete's foot and worm diseases respectively. Some common bacteria are *Streptococci, Staphylococci, Salmonella*, and *E. coli* which will be mentioned throughout the text.

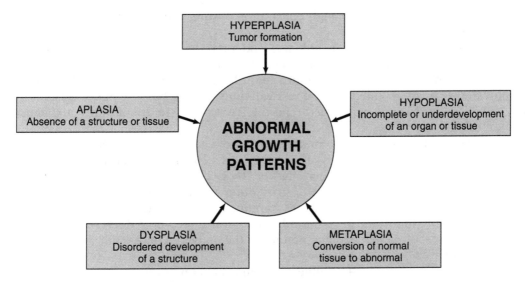

Figure 1–1. Abnormal growth patterns.

On the Practical Side

HANDWASHING—A HEALTHY HABIT

Infection can often be prevented by the simple task of thorough handwashing with soap or detergent, rubbing vigorously for at least 10 seconds. Germs tend to accumulate under fingernails and around cuticles so those areas should get special attention. Disease causing microorganisms are always present on the skin surface but proper handwashing prevents ingesting them or passing them on to others. Hands should always be washed before handling or eating food, when exiting the bathroom, after playing with pets, and handling money.

■ Antibiotic Resistant Bacteria

For 50 years people have been dependent on antibiotics to treat all kinds of bacterial infections. Some diseases such as tuberculosis were thought to be eradicated through the action of antibiotics. Now, however, new and hardier strains of bacteria are developing which can resist the action of antibiotics.

The misuse and overuse of these drugs has caused the problem. Patients have used antibiotics for colds, flu, and other viral infections which are untouched by the drugs. Tons of antibiotics are used by food producers to control infections so the environment has become saturated with them. Bacteria have developed immunity to many antibiotics through constant exposure, a condition known as multidrug resistance.

Bacteria generally live in colonies and reproduce rapidly. When antibiotic treatment is prescribed for a bacterial infection the patient must take the drug for the specified length of time to assure that all the bacteria are destroyed. If not, only the weakest are killed and the rest will multiply and become more resistant to the antibiotic. To counteract this trend the indiscriminate use of antibiotics must be curtailed.

Viruses, minute parasitic organisms, produce disease by invading cells and multiplying within them. They utilize the host cell's raw materials to duplicate their own genetic material, either **DNA** or **RNA.** The virus particles then spill out in great numbers to invade and destroy other healthy cells. Viruses are not affected by antibiotics. The individual's immune system, to be described in Chapter 2 is extremely important in overcoming the viral infection. **Interferon,** a protective substance, is made in small amounts by the body and may act as a broad spectrum anti-viral agent.

The source or cause of an illness or abnormal condition, together with its development, is its **pathogenesis. Pathology** is the branch of medicine that studies the characteristics, causes, and effects of disease. The cellular pathologist studies cellular or microscopic changes; the clinical pathologist utilizes laboratory tests and methods to make a diagnosis. A pathologist may specialize in autopsies or surgical findings.

Many diseases are due to heredity; they are transmitted by a defective gene. Hemophilia, sickle cell anemia, and color blindness are examples of genetic diseases. **Congenital birth defects,** mental or physical, may be due to a developmental error resulting from a maternal infection such as rubella or German measles during pregnancy, the use of certain drugs, or the mother's excessive consumption of alcohol. Some congenital birth defects result from an accident at the time of delivery such as an interference with oxygen supply.

Environmental factors are the cause of many diseases. Skin cancer, for example, can result from excessive exposure to the ultraviolet light rays of the sun, especially in fair-skinned people. The development of leukemia is an occupational hazard for radiologists and the development of cancer is linked to asbestos exposure. Many chemicals found in industrial wastes have been found to cause disease.

Malnutrition causes many diseases that are not always due to the unavailability of food, but rather the inability of the person to use it, which will be explained later. Signs of nutritional deficiency diseases frequently accompany chronic alcoholism.

Stress adversely affects the entire body; it reduces the ability of the immune system to counteract disease. It aggravates some digestive diseases and respiratory ailments—asthma, for example—and other allergic conditions. If the cause of a disease is not known, it is said to be **idiopathic.**

Another important aspect of disease is the way it manifests itself: its signs and symptoms. **Signs** are objective evidence of disease observed on physical examination, such as abnormal pulse or respiratory rate, fever, and **pallor,** or abnormal paleness, whereas **symptoms** are an indication of disease perceived by the patient, such as pain, dizziness, and itching. An attempt will be made throughout this book

On the Practical Side

FINGERNAILS AND HEALTH PROBLEMS

Clubbing or rounding of the fingertips and nails is often caused by a chronic lack of oxygen. The oxygen deficiency may be due to lung or heart disease. Enlargement in the connective tissue is a compensation for the oxygen deficiency. The nail often separates from the nail bed in psoriasis, fungal infection, and in injury. Dark discoloration may accompany cirrhosis, adult-onset diabetes, cancer and aging.

to relate the signs and symptoms of a disease to the specific malfunctioning of the ailment. For example, why does the anemic person feel weak, fatigued, and short of breath? How does a hyperactive thyroid cause weight loss, nervousness, and excessive sweating? Why are the ankles swollen in certain heart conditions?

Certain signs and symptoms occur concurrently in some diseases and the combination of symptoms is referred to as a **syndrome.** Down's syndrome is an example of a disease with concurrent signs; the most prominent are mental retardation, an enlarged, protruding tongue, and a characteristic appearance of the eyes.

DIAGNOSIS

Diagnosis, the determination of the nature of a disease, is based on many factors, including the signs, symptoms, and, often, laboratory results. Laboratory tests include such familiar procedures as urinalysis, blood chemistry, electrocardiography, and radiography. New diagnostic-imaging techniques such as **computerized tomography (CT scan), magnetic resonance imaging (MRI),** radiology, ultrasound, and nuclear medicine provide a visualization never before possible. Diagnostic procedures used in determining various diseases are discussed for each system. A physician also derives information for making a diagnosis from a physical examination, from interviewing the patient or a family member, and from a medical history of the patient and family. The physician, having made a diagnosis, may state the possible **prognosis** of the disease, or the predicted course, and outcome of the disease.

The treatment considered most effective is prescribed and may include medication, surgery, radiation therapy, or possibly psychological counseling. A patient may be advised to change habits of life-style such as overeating, smoking, alcohol abuse, or to avoid a stressful situation if possible.

The course of a disease varies; it may have a sudden onset and short term, in which case it is an **acute** disease. A disease may begin insidiously and be long-lived, or **chronic.** The term *chronic* is derived from the Greek word *chronos* for time. Diseases that will end in death are called *terminal.* The signs and symptoms of a chronic disease at times subside, during a period known as **remission.** They may recur in all their severity in a period of **exacerbation.** Certain diseases, leukemia and ulcerative colitis, for example, are characterized by periods of remission and exacerbation. A relapse at times occurs when a disease returns weeks or months after its apparent cessation.

Complications frequently occur, meaning that a disease develops in a patient already suffering from another disease. Patients confined to bed with a serious fracture frequently develop pneumonia as a complication of the inactivity. Infection of the testes may be a complication of mumps, particularly after puberty. Anemia generally accompanies leukemia, cancer, and chronic kidney disease. Bacterial infection frequently follows certain predisposing factors such as kidney stones, heart defects, and an enlarged prostate gland. The relationships between the diseases that develop secondarily and the original disease will be discussed in later chapters.

The aftermath of a particular disease is called the **sequela,** a sequel. The permanent damage to the heart after rheumatic fever is an example of a sequela, as is the paralysis of polio. The sterility resulting from severe inflammation of the fallopian tubes is also a sequela.

Diseases can be classified in many ways, but in this book they will be considered according to the general mechanisms of disease and in the physiologic systems in which they are a factor. General health problems include allergies, malnutrition, obesity, and alcoholism.

An understanding of disease, its cause, the way it affects the body, effective treatments, and its possible prognosis should enable the health professional to alleviate suffering, anxiety, and fear in those who are ill.

CHAPTER SUMMARY

The body attempts to maintain homeostasis in the midst of ever-changing conditions. It senses a deficiency in the working of an organ and tries to compensate for it. The response to a significant disturbance in the body's homeostasis can resemble the sign of disease.

Disease is an unhealthy state of a body part, a system, or the body as a whole. It may result from a structural anomaly, a functional condition, or trauma. Many factors can cause disease: infectious agents, heredity, environmental conditions, malnutrition, and stress. The cause of a disease is sometimes unknown. Etiology is the cause of a disease. Pathology is the branch of medicine that studies the etiology, characteristics, and effects of disease; in other words, its pathogenesis.

Disease manifests itself by signs and symptoms, objective and subjective indications of its presence. In some diseases a certain combination of signs and symptoms occur as in Down's syndrome.

Diagnoses of disease are based on many factors: signs and symptoms, laboratory tests, physical examination, and patient and family histories. The most suitable treatment is then prescribed. The disease may be acute or chronic; signs of a chronic disease frequently subside or exacerbate.

Diseases may be classified in many ways but in this book they will be considered according to the general mechanisms of disease and the physiologic system in which they occur. Understanding the various aspects of disease enables the health professional to serve those who are ill in a comprehensive manner.

■ Self-Study

True or False

_____ 1. The predicted outcome of a disease is its prognosis.
_____ 2. An increased blood cell count is always a sign of disease.
_____ 3. Exacerbation and remission would characterize a chronic condition.
_____ 4. A body part that is used excessively will atrophy.
_____ 5. When tissue is damaged, blood flow to the site is increased.
_____ 6. A congenital birth defect is caused by a defective gene.
_____ 7. Symptoms are objective evidence of a disease.
_____ 8. Etiology is the cause of the disease.
_____ 9. A sequela is the return of a disease after the symptoms have ended.
_____ 10. Signs may be perceived by the physician.

Match

_____ 11. idiopathic
_____ 12. syndrome
_____ 13. exacerbation
_____ 14. relapse
_____ 15. complication

a) worsening of symptoms
b) cause unknown
c) development of a new disease when another exists
d) return of symptoms after their apparent cessation
e) combination of symptoms

(Answers on page 449)

Chapter 2

Inflammation, Immunity, and Allergy

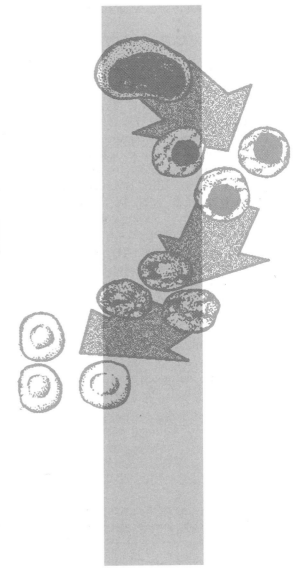

Chapter Outline

- Inflammation and Repair
- Immunity
- Autoimmunity
- Immune Deficiency
- Vaccination
- Hypersensitivity—Allergies
- Chapter Summary
- Self-Study

*T*issues react to local injury, foreign invasion, or irritation by producing an inflammatory response. Although inflammation is painful, it is nature's way of correcting a disorder. Every disease ending in -itis is an inflammatory disease, such as appendicitis, bronchitis, and colitis.

INFLAMMATION AND REPAIR

The cause of the inflammation may be a trauma or injury, such as a sprained ankle or a severe blow. A physical irritant in the tissue—a piece of glass, a wasp sting, or an ingrown toenail—will trigger the response. **Pathogenic organisms** will do the same. Figure 2–1 shows various agents that are capable of stimulating an inflammatory response.

Inflammation should not be confused with infection. Invading pathogenic organisms—bacteria, viruses, fungi, or parasites—are necessary to produce an infection. The invading organisms cause disease by local cellular injury, secretion of a toxin, alteration of DNA by a virus, or by initiating an allergic response. Inflammation, however, is a protective tissue response to injury or invasion by disease-producing organisms.

Vascular changes occur when tissue is traumatized or irritated. Local blood vessels, arterioles, and capillaries dilate, resulting in increased blood flow to the injured area. This increased amount of blood, **hyperemia,** causes the heat and redness associated with inflammation. As the blood flow to the site of the injury or infection increases, more and more **leukocytes,** or white blood cells, reach the area. Certain of these white cells, the neutrophils or **polymorphs,** line up within the capillary walls. The polymorphs are specialized to fight against the invading agent or injury.

The damaged tissue releases a substance called **histamine** that causes the capillary walls to become more permeable. This increased permeability enables

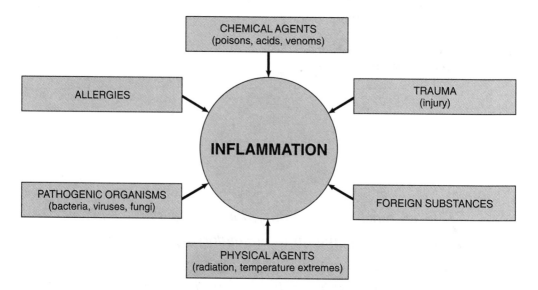

Figure 2–1. Agents capable of stimulating an inflammatory response.

plasma and neutrophils to move out of the blood vessels into the tissue. Neutrophils are **phagocytes** that have the ability to engulf and digest bacteria and cellular debris. The root word, *phag(o),* means to eat. Figure 2–2 shows the vascular changes that occur with inflammation and the movement of the polymorphs to the infected site. The attraction of the white blood cells to the site of inflammation is called **chemotaxis.**

The plasma and white cells that escape from the capillaries comprise the **inflammatory exudate.** This exudate in the tissues causes the swelling associated

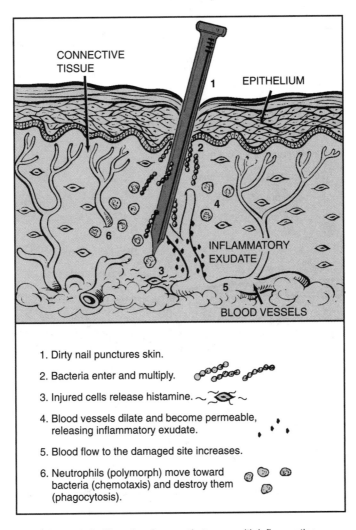

Figure 2–2. Vascular changes that occur with inflammation.

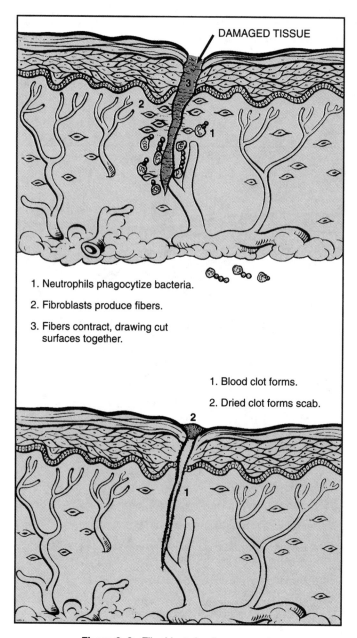

DAMAGED TISSUE

1. Neutrophils phagocytize bacteria.

2. Fibroblasts produce fibers.

3. Fibers contract, drawing cut surfaces together.

1. Blood clot forms.

2. Dried clot forms scab.

Figure 2–3. Fibroblasts healing a wound.

with inflammation. The excess of fluid in the tissues **(edema)** puts pressure on sensitive nerve endings, causing pain. The chief signs and symptoms of inflammation are redness, swelling, heat, and pain. It is the increased blood flow to the damaged or irritated area that causes the redness and heat. The inflammatory exudate is responsible for the swelling and pain.

Bacterial infection may be the cause of an inflammation. Organisms such as **staphylococci** and **streptococci** that produce **toxins** (substances damaging to the tissues) will initiate an inflammatory response. To increase the power of the white cells fighting the infection, the bone marrow and lymph nodes release very large quantities of leukocytes. This increased production of white cells accounts for the elevated white cell count associated with infection. The count may rise to 30,000 or more from the normal range of 7000 to 9000 per cubic **millimeter** of blood (mm³). The excessive production of white cells is called **leukocytosis.**

The polymorphs soon die after ingesting bacteria and toxins. Substances are released from the dead cells, now called pus cells, that liquefy the tissue affected by the toxins. This liquefied tissue—dead polymorphs, inflammatory exudate, and bacteria—make up the thick, yellow fluid known as pus. Other phagocytic white cells, the **monocytes** or macrophages, follow the polymorphs in the process of clearing debris. Inflammatory exudate contains a plasma protein, **fibrin,** essential for the blood-clotting mechanism. Fibrin acts in the damaged tissue by forming a clot, thus walling off the infection and preventing its spread.

Bacteria that cause pus formation are called **pyogenic** bacteria. An inflammation associated with pus formation is a **suppurative** inflammation. Abscesses, boils, and styes are examples of inflammations with suppuration.

Wound healing and repair can occur only when bacteria have been destroyed. Cut edges of tissue will grow together as connective tissue cells **(fibroblasts)** produce fibers that will close the gap. Figure 2–3 shows the fibroblasts and their fibers healing a cut. This is known as scar tissue. Sometimes the connective tissue fibers will anchor adjacent structures together, such as loops of intestine, causing **adhesions.** The problems associated with adhesions will be explained in later chapters.

A scar following surgery or a severe burn is often raised and hard. This is known as **keloid** healing and is really a benign tumor that is harmless. Surgery to remove such a scar is usually ineffective, as the subsequent incision will have a tendency to heal in the same way.

IMMUNITY

The immune reaction of the body provides a strong line of defense against invading organisms. The body recognizes bacteria, viruses, molds, and toxins as something foreign to itself and produces substances to counteract them. The foreign element, generally a protein, that triggers this response is called an **antigen.** The substances produced to fight against the antigen and make it harmless are **antibodies** and **activated lymphocytes,** a type of white blood cell. This type of immunity is *acquired immunity*.

An important part of immunity is the body's **lymphatic system.** It consists of a complex network of thin-walled capillaries carrying lymph fluid, nodes, and organs which help to maintain the internal fluid environment of the body. The lymph nodes are small filtering stations which help fight infection. They produce certain white blood cells, lymphocytes, monocytes, and plasma cells which destroy invading organisms. Organs such as the spleen, tonsils, and adenoids are comprised of lymphoid tissue and function in the body's internal defense (Fig. 2–4).

The body also possesses natural, or *innate immunity*. Examples of innate immunity include destruction of bacteria and other invaders by white blood cells

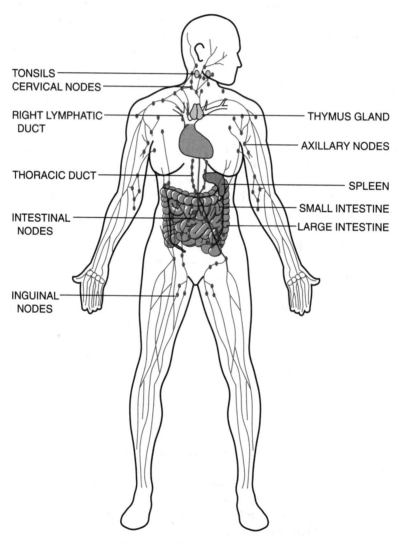

Figure 2–4. The lymphatic system.

(phagocytosis), destruction of swallowed organisms by digestive enzymes and acid secretions of the stomach, and resistance of the skin to invading organisms.

There are two basic types of acquired immunity: circulating antibodies or globulin molecules capable of destroying foreign invaders, and activated lymphocytes. The antibodies provide **humoral immunity** and the activated lymphocytes provide **cell-mediated immunity** (Fig. 2–5). Both types are formed in lymph nodes and lymphoid tissue such as the spleen, bone marrow, tonsils, and adenoids. The lymphoid tissue is placed strategically in the body to intercept invading organisms.

The body recognizes the initial invasion of a foreign substance, a toxin or organism, by a specific chemical compound of its makeup, a protein or large polysaccharide (a complex carbohydrate). These specific substances are called *antigens.*

Two types of lymphocytes provide immunity, the T and B lymphocytes. The lymphocytes responsible for cell-mediated immunity first migrate to and are processed by the thymus gland; hence they are called **T lymphocytes** or activated lymphocytes. The other type of lymphocytes form antibodies and are called **B lymphocytes;** these are responsible for humoral immunity. Processing of the T lymphocytes by the thymus gland takes place shortly before birth and in the early months of infancy. Antibodies and T lymphocytes are each highly specific for one type of antigen.

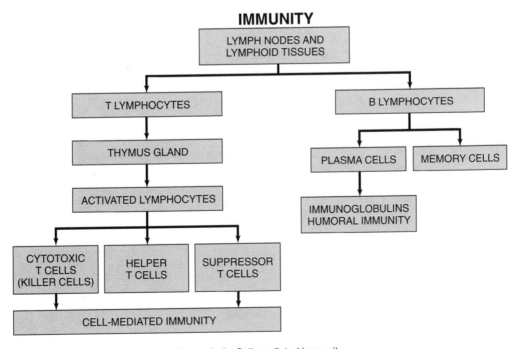

Figure 2–5. Cell-mediated immunity.

A T lymphocyte activated by its antigen reproduces sensitized T cells that enter the lymphatic system and are carried to the blood to circulate through the body. B lymphocytes will produce cells that also secrete antibodies.

Both T lymphocytes and B lymphocytes are activated by antigens. Some T cells are called "helper cells" and further stimulate the B lymphocytes to produce more antibodies. This is done through the helper cell's secretion of chemicals called **lymphokines.** Some activated B lymphocytes are transformed into **plasma cells** and begin to divide at a rapid rate and produce large numbers of antibodies. These are secreted into the lymph and travel to the blood to be circulated through the body.

Some B lymphocytes do not become plasma cells and remain dormant until reactivated by the same antigen. These are called **memory cells** and cause a more potent and rapid antibody response. The secondary response begins more rapidly after exposure to the antigen, produces more antibodies, and lasts for a longer time than the initial response. This is the basis for booster shots following vaccination (Fig. 2–6).

The antibodies are plasma proteins, gamma globulins called **immunoglobulins.** There are several types of immunoglobulins, two of which will be described with hypersensitivity reactions, IgG and IgE. Ig stands for immunoglobulins.

There are several different kinds of T cells, each with different functions: **cytotoxic T cells, helper T cells** and **suppressor T cells.** The virus responsible for AIDS, HIV, causes severe immunodeficiency of T cell functions.

The cytotoxic T cells are often called *killer cells* because they are capable of killing invading organisms. They have on their surfaces receptor proteins that bind

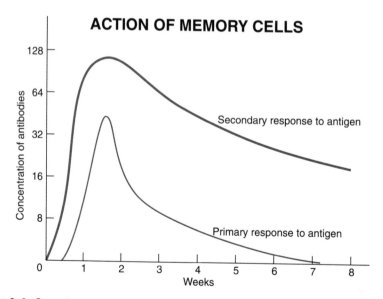

Figure 2–6. Secondary response begins more rapidly after exposure to antigen, produces more antibodies, and lasts for a longer time than initial exposure.

tightly to cells or organisms that contain a specific antigen. Once bound, the cytotoxic T cells release poisonous substances into the attacked cell. Many organisms can be killed by one killer cell. The cytotoxic cells are important in killing cells that have been invaded by viruses. These T cells also can destroy cancer cells.

The helper T cells get their name from the fact that they help the immune system in many ways. They increase the activity of killer cells, B cells, and suppressor T cells. Activated helper T cells secrete lymphokines that increase the response of other types of lymphoid cells to the antigen and activate large cells called macrophages to destroy large numbers of invaders by phagocytosis.

The immune response normally recognizes the difference between the individual's own tissues and those of invaders; this is known as *tolerance.* However, this immune tolerance can fail, and activated T cells and antibodies attack the body's own tissue, causing **autoimmune diseases.** Several of these autoimmune diseases, such as rheumatic fever, glomerulonephritis, myasthenia gravis, and rheumatoid arthritis, are described elsewhere in this book. One very serious autoimmune disease will be considered here, **lupus erythematosus.**

AUTOIMMUNITY

■ Lupus Erythematosus

Lupus erythematosus is a noncontagious inflammatory disease that takes one of two forms, mild or severe. The **discoid** form is only a minor disorder in which red, raised, itchy lesions develop. The lesions characteristically form the pattern of a butterfly over the nose and cheeks. Steroids are administered to relieve the inflammatory symptoms, but there is no treatment to cure the disease.

The serious form is **systemic lupus erythematosus (SLE),** which affects not only the skin but also causes the deterioration of collagenous connective tissue. Systemic lupus can affect the glomeruli of the kidney, causing abnormal excretion of albumin and blood, as well as casts (Chapter 9), in the urine. The red cell, white cell, and platelet counts are low. The lining of the heart and the heart valves may deteriorate. Hypersensitivity to an antigen is thought to be the cause of systemic lupus erythematosus. The antigen may be an allergen outside the body or the patient's own tissue to which the patient has become sensitized, an example of autoimmunity.

Young women are most frequently affected by systemic lupus, which may begin suddenly or insidiously. The patient experiences a rash, and the skin becomes overly sensitive to sunlight. Joint and muscle pains may be accompanied by fever. The lymph nodes and spleen are frequently found to be enlarged. Periods of exacerbation and remission are characteristic of the disease.

There is no specific treatment for systemic lupus erythematosus, but, as with many inflammatory diseases, corticosteroids are administered to control the symptoms. The disease may even be fatal, death frequently being due to kidney or heart failure. The decreased number of leukocytes also reduces resistance to such diseases as pneumonia.

IMMUNE DEFICIENCY

■ Acquired Immune Deficiency Syndrome (AIDS)

One of the most deadly diseases to affect today's population is **acquired immune deficiency syndrome, AIDS.** AIDS destroys the patient's immune system, making the person remarkably susceptible to infection. AIDS originally attacked primarily promiscuous homosexual and bisexual men and drug users who shared hypodermic needles. Now, however, the spread of AIDS is rapidly increasing among young women.

In some cases, recipients of blood transfusions given before blood screening was done developed AIDS. Reliable tests for the presence of the virus now minimize the risk of contracting it through contaminated blood transfusion. Children born to infected mothers have also contracted AIDS, either in utero or during the passage through the birth canal. The virus has also been detected in breast milk.

The causative agent of AIDS is the **human immunodeficiency virus (HIV),** a retrovirus, i.e., it carries its genetic information as RNA rather than DNA. The virus infects certain white blood cells of the body's immune system, namely the helper T-4 lymphocytes, and destroys their ability to fight infection. The virus replicates itself within the lymphocyte, killing it, and spreading to others. These lymphocytes normally activate antibody producing B-cell lymphocytes, thus the body's immune response is blocked. The affected person becomes especially susceptible to a rare type of pneumonia caused by *Pneumocystis carinii.* Kaposi's sarcoma, a rare slow-growing cancer is also noted more frequently, as are other opportunistic infections.

Symptoms include unexplained weight loss, generalized **lymphadenopathy** (enlarged lymph nodes), diarrhea, fever, and night sweats in the early stages. **Encephalopathy** (chronic, destructive, or degenerative condition of the brain) and **dementia** (organic loss of intellectual function) occurs in a high percentage of AIDS patients with advanced disease.

HIV has been isolated from the blood and semen of AIDS patients, and is transmitted principally by direct intimate contact involving mucous membrane surfaces. The virus cannot penetrate skin but enters through natural body openings and open wounds. It is transmitted through all forms of unprotected intercourse where there may be tiny tears in the mucous membrane lining; transmission rate is very high with anal intercourse.

There is a long and variable latent period of 2 to 8 years between HIV infection and the development of full-blown AIDS. An individual who tests positive for HIV may manifest some of the signs of AIDS such as flulike symptoms when first infected, but may recover and be symptom-free for some period of time. The long, latent period increases the risk of spreading the infection as the patient is not aware he has the disease. Once infected, the person is infected for life, and the mortality rate is 100%. There have been no reported recoveries to date. Once diagnosed with full-blown AIDS, the chance of surviving more than three years is around one in ten.

■ HIV Infection

Even before full-blown AIDS develops, the virus is destroying the immune system of the HIV positive individual. Studies have shown that large amounts of virus are present during the asymptomatic stage of the disease. The virus resides in high concentration in lymph nodes where it continues to increase. Eventually a threshold is crossed and the infected person develops one of the distinctive infections or other manifestations that characterize AIDS.

The CDC (Centers for Disease Control) has revised the HIV classification system for more accurate surveillance of AIDS cases. It provides a recommended standard for monitoring the number of infected cells, CD4+ T-lymphocytes. CDC has also added pulmonary TB, recurrent pneumonia, and invasive cervical cancer to the list of AIDS-indicator diseases.

■ Precautions for Health-care Professionals

Health-care professionals must exercise great precautions when handling blood or bodily secretions of AIDS patients. Several workers have contracted the virus by accidental sticks. The best protection against HIV exposure is consistent adherence to the universal recommendations of the CDC and the guidelines required by the Occupational Safety and Health Administration (OSHA), which are as follows.

OSHA requires employers to train employees who are at risk of exposure to blood-borne pathogens; training must be held during work hours and at no cost to employees. Appropriate instruction on handwashing, the use of gloves, gowns, and protective eye covering, and the proper disposal of sharps must be provided. Information must be given on the facility's Exposure Control Plan, blood-borne disease symptoms and modes of transmission, and use and limitations of risk-reduction methods. Employees must be informed of hepatitis B vaccination availability (Chapter 11), actions to take in case of emergencies, and procedures to follow if exposure incidents occur.

Warning labels bearing the biohazard symbol (Fig. 2–7) in fluorescent orange or orange-red must be part of, or securely affixed to, containers used to store,

BIOHAZARD

Figure 2–7. Required warning on potentially hazardous material.

transport, or dispose of potentially infectious material. Refrigerators and freezers used for such material must also be labeled. Red bags or red containers may be substituted for labels on containers of infectious wastes.

Development of a vaccine to prevent the spread of AIDS has not yet been possible. The genetic makeup of the AIDS virus varies greatly from strain to strain which complicates the attempt to develop an AIDS vaccine. HIV tends to mutate frequently or change which adds to the difficulty of producing a vaccine.

Researchers around the world are working toward designing drugs to effect a cure for AIDS. They are utilizing their knowledge of the manner in which HIV infects the immune system's T cells. Prior to this knowledge of the virus's attachment to T4 lymphocytes and their destruction, a variety of drugs used for other purposes were tested. AZT, originally formulated as an anticancer drug, was the only one which had any effect. AZT does not cure AIDS but reduces the symptoms and prolongs life. It extends the symptom-free period between HIV infection and the onset of AIDS. However, AZT loses its effectiveness with time. Newer, less toxic drugs are now being formulated.

■ Chronic Fatigue Syndrome

Chronic fatigue syndrome is a peculiar disease which affects primarily young professionals in the prime of life. It has been dubbed "yuppie flu" because of the class of individuals affected. The flulike symptoms include severe and persistent fatigue, muscle and joint pain, and fever. The victim experiences difficulty in concentrating and trouble in remembering.

The cause and cure are unknown although much research has been done on the disease. It was thought at first to be psychosomatic or the result of depression, but changes have been found in the patient's immune system. No particular virus has been proven to be the cause but blood tests have shown an immune response consistent with a viral infection.

VACCINATION

Two types of artificial immunity can be administered, active and passive immunity. In **active immunity** the person is given a vaccine or a toxoid as the antigen, and he or she forms antibodies to counteract it. A **vaccine** consists of a low dose of dead or deactivated bacteria or viruses. Because the organisms have been specially treated to deactivate them, they cannot cause disease. As protein foreign to the body, these antigens do trigger antibody production against them. A **toxoid** works similarly. It consists of a chemically altered toxin, the poisonous material produced by a pathogenic organism. Having been treated chemically, the toxin will not cause disease. It will, however, stimulate the immune response.

This type of immunity, in which cells are exposed to an antigen and begin to form the corresponding antibodies, is long-lived. This kind of protection is given to prevent smallpox, polio, and diphtheria. Time is required to build up immunity, and a booster shot is frequently given for a stronger effect. Once cells have been

ACTIVE IMMUNITY	PASSIVE IMMUNITY
PERSON FORMS ANTIBODIES	PREFORMED ANTIBODIES RECEIVED (usually in immune horse serum)
VACCINE (deactivated bacteria or virus) OR TOXOID (chemically altered toxin)	
LONG-LIVED IMMUNITY (requires time)	SHORT-LIVED IMMUNITY (acts immediately)

Figure 2–8. Differences between active and passive immunity.

sensitized to these viruses, bacteria, or toxins, they will continue to produce antibodies against them.

What if a person is exposed to a serious disease such as hepatitis, tetanus, or rabies and has no immunity against it? It takes time to build antibodies and time is limited. In this case, the person is given **passive immunity,** doses of preformed antibodies from immune serum of an animal, usually a horse. This type of immunity is short-lived but acts immediately. Figure 2–8 contrasts active and passive immunity.

HYPERSENSITIVITY—ALLERGIES

Closely related to the concept of immunity is **allergy,** or **hypersensitivity.** Some diseases are actually the result of an individual's immune response, which causes tissue damage and disordered function rather than immunity. The immune phenomena is destructive rather than defensive in the individual who is supersensitive or allergic (atopic) to an antigen. Hypersensitivity diseases or allergic diseases may manifest themselves locally or systemically.

The abnormal sensitivity to pollens, dust, dog hair, certain foods or chemicals, is the result of abnormally formed antibodies or immunoglobulins. The genetic makeup of the hypersensitive individual causes the formation of IgE rather than IgG immunoglobulins. The abnormal immunoglobulins have an affinity for certain cells, basophils and **mast cells,** and attach to them. Mast cells are in connective tissue and contain **heparin, serotonin, bradykinin,** and **histamine.** As the antigen attaches to the antibody, the mast cells break down and release the above-named chemicals. Histamine causes the dilation of the blood vessels and makes them susceptible to plasma leakage. The leakage of plasma into the tissues causes **edema,** or swelling, which when localized in the nasal passages results in the familiar congestion and irritation of hay fever. If the tissue damage and edema are near the skin, the welts and itching of hives may appear. Antihistamines are quite effective in the treatment of hives but less so for hay fever. A typical allergic reaction is illustrated in Figure 2–9.

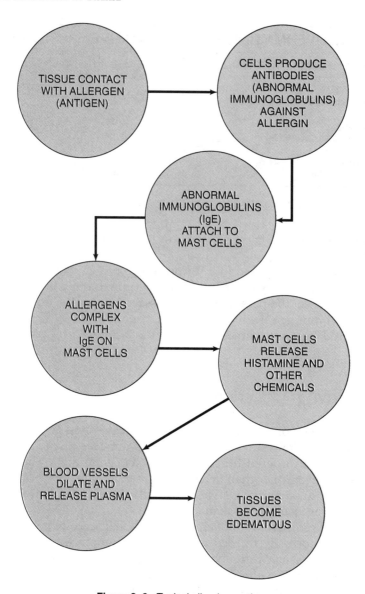

Figure 2–9. Typical allergic reaction.

Allergy shots can desensitize the hypersensitive person. Small amounts of the offending antigen are administered and concentrations gradually increased. This gives the allergic person time to build proper antibodies, subsequently reducing the amount of tissue damage.

The hypersensitivity reaction **(anaphylaxis)** can also be systemic and life-threatening and require immediate treatment. It can result from a penicillin injection, bee, wasp, or hornet sting, or certain foods such as peanuts in the allergic individual. Another cause of anaphylaxis can be an intravenous injection of iodine-containing dyes used in certain exams such as the intravenous pyelogram, IVP (Chapter 9).

Less severe signs may include skin flush, hives, swelling of lips or tongue, wheezing, and abdominal cramps. Life-threatening signs include weakness and collapse due to low blood pressure, inability to breathe, and seizures.

The most vital therapy is prompt intramuscular injection of **epinephrine (adrenalin).** Certain allergic individuals have to carry epinephrine with them, which can be self-injected in an emergency.

The mechanisms of the systemic anaphylactic reaction are the same as in the local response, that is, abnormal antibodies attach to mast cells and basophils with the release of histamine and other powerful chemicals. There is a generalized change in capillary permeability leading to hypotension, low blood pressure, and shock. Smooth muscle contraction in the respiratory tract causes respiratory distress resembling asthma. Fluid in the larynx may threaten to obstruct the airways and necessitate a **tracheotomy,** creation of an opening into the trachea to facilitate passage of air or evacuation of secretions.

On the Practical Side

MEDICAL ALERT BRACELETS

A life may be saved in an emergency by providing medical personnel with vital information. Bracelets, necklaces, and/or wallet cards can alert caregivers to severe allergies such as penicillin, bee or wasp stings, or certain foods. Insulin-dependent diabetics can be identified if encountered while in a coma or insulin shock and unable to speak for themselves.

Anaphylactic shock can occur in anyone if large quantities of antigen are introduced intravenously when large numbers of antibodies are already present. The best example of this reaction is an incompatible blood transfusion. A person with type A blood has A antigens on the red cells, and antibodies against type B blood in the serum. If the person receives a type B transfusion, the antigens and antibodies will interact. The red blood cells will **agglutinate,** or clump together, and **hemolyze** (rupture) (see Fig. 2–10). The cellular damage triggers the release of histamine from mast cells, causing blood vessels to dilate and thus drastically reducing blood pressure. In addition, the capillaries become very permeable and plasma

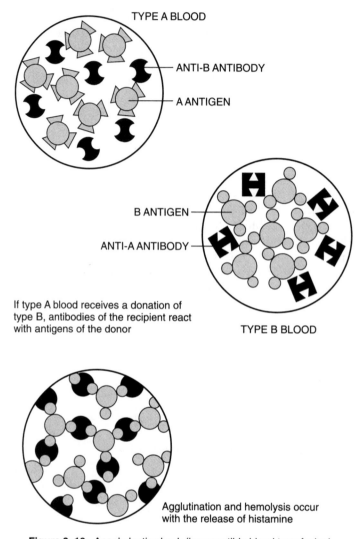

TYPE A BLOOD

ANTI-B ANTIBODY

A ANTIGEN

B ANTIGEN

ANTI-A ANTIBODY

If type A blood receives a donation of
type B, antibodies of the recipient react
with antigens of the donor

TYPE B BLOOD

Agglutination and hemolysis occur
with the release of histamine

Figure 2–10. Anaphylactic shock (incompatible blood transfusion).

leaks out, reducing blood volume, which further reduces blood pressure. Low
blood pressure causes a poor return of venous blood to the heart, and cardiac output is drastically reduced. Blood pools rather than circulates, and death can follow. This serious type of reaction is known as **anaphylactic shock.** Figure 2–11
shows this sequence of vascular events.

Another type of allergic reaction can occur in anyone but is a delayed reaction. Initial exposure to an antigen is required before any antibodies are formed.
For example, the first time one contacts poison ivy there will be no reaction. However, the cells may become sensitized to it and will begin making antibodies

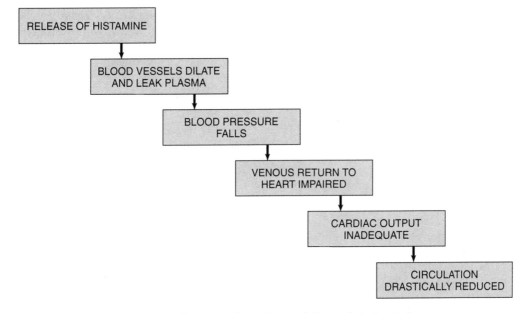

Figure 2–11. Sequence of vascular events in anaphylactic shock.

against the poison ivy antigen. On the next exposure the typical rash and irritation associated with poison ivy will develop. This is the type of reaction in contact dermatitis (Chapter 17) and the tuberculin test. Tissue and organ rejections are also examples of delayed hypersensitivity reactions.

Another example of the delayed allergic reaction would be an Rh positive (Rh$^+$) blood transfusion to an Rh negative (Rh$^-$) recipient. Rh$^-$ blood means that the Rh antigen or factor is not present. This transfusion would cause no trouble, but in the transfusion the Rh$^-$ recipient is exposed or sensitized to the **Rh factor** and begins to form antibodies against this foreign protein. Subsequent Rh$^+$ transfusions would cause clumping and rupture of red blood cells. Rh incompatibility during pregnancy is also a delayed allergic reaction. An Rh$^-$ mother can become sensitized by the fetus' Rh$^+$ blood and make antibodies that destroy the fetal red blood cells. This does not generally occur during the first pregnancy, as the mother has not yet become sensitized. Rh incompatibility is examined more closely in Chapter 6.

CHAPTER SUMMARY

Tissues react to injury, foreign invasion, or irritation by producing an inflammatory response. Although painful, inflammation is a protective tissue function. Inflammation should not be confused with infection, which requires the invasion of pathogenic organisms. Vascular changes produce the characteristic signs of inflammation, namely redness, swelling, heat, and pain.

The immune reaction provides the body with a strong defense against invading organisms. The body recognizes substances foreign to itself, antigens, and produces substances to counteract them—antibodies and activated lymphocytes. Antibodies produce humoral immunity; activated lymphocytes produce cell-mediated immunity.

The two types of lymphocytes are T cells processed by the thymus gland and B lymphocytes that are responsible for humoral immunity. Different kinds of T lymphocytes include killer cells, helper cells, and suppressor cells.

The lymphatic system plays an important part in the immune system. The lymph nodes are small filtering stations which help fight infection. They also are the site of lymphocyte production and of other white blood cells which destroy invading organisms.

An abnormality in the immune system can cause disease when the body becomes hypersensitive to its own tissue and destroys it. This is known as autoimmunity. Systemic lupus erythematosus is such a disease. The most serious failure in the immune system is acquired immune deficiency syndrome, or **AIDS**.

Artificial immunity can be provided by vaccination. In active immunity the individual is given a vaccine or a toxoid and actively makes antibodies to counteract it. Preformed antibodies are given in passive immunity.

Allergies can be considered a side effect of immunity. Allergic diseases are the result of an immune response that causes tissue damage and disordered function rather than immunity. Hypersensitivity to harmless substances is the result of abnormally formed immunoglobulins in the allergic person. Allergies range in severity from local tissue damage, as in hay fever and hives, to a systemic anaphylactic reaction that can be life-threatening.

■ Self-Study

True or False

_____ 1. Bacteria, viruses, or fungi are always present in an inflammation.

_____ 2. Leukocytes are present in inflammatory exudate.

_____ 3. Blood vessels in an inflamed area constrict.

_____ 4. The fluid that oozes out of capillary walls during inflammation is pus.

_____ 5. Leukocytosis occurs in bacterial infections.

_____ 6. Substances produced to fight infection are called antigens.

_____ 7. A vaccine or a toxoid produces active immunity.

_____ 8. A severe allergic reaction elevates blood pressure.

_____ 9. Preformed antibodies are administered in passive immunity.

_____ 10. Epinephrine (adrenalin) is administered in severe allergic reactions.

_____ 11. Edema results from excessive fluid in the tissues.

_____ 12. Histamine constricts small blood vessels.

_____ 13. Anaphylactic shock causes an elevation in blood pressure.

_____ 14. Antihistamines may be helpful in treating hives.

_____ 15. An individual's immune response can be destructive in nature.

Match

_____ 16. hyperemia

_____ 17. fibrin

_____ 18. pyogenic bacteria

_____ 19. anaphylactic shock

_____ 20. abnormal immunoglobulins (IgE)

a) drastically reduced circulation

b) helps wall off infection

c) suppurative inflammation

d) increased blood flow to damaged area

e) allergic individual

Multiple Choice

_____ 21. Activated lymphocytes provide _____ immunity.
   a. humoral
   b. cell-mediated

_____ 22. _____ produce cells that secrete antibodies.
   a. B lymphocytes
   b. T lymphocytes

_____ 23. Some activated _____ are transformed into plasma cells.
   a. T cells
   b. B lymphocytes

_____ 24. The virus responsible for AIDS causes severe immunodeficiency of
   _____.
   a. B lymphocytes
   b. T-cell function

_____ 25. Lymphokines are secreted by _____.
   a. activated helper T cells
   b. B cells

(Answers on page 449)

Chapter 3

Neoplasia

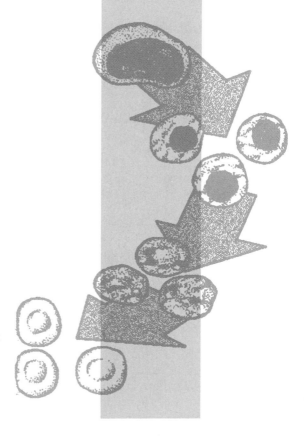

Chapter Outline

- Tumor Formation
- Malignant Tumors
- Benign Tumors
- Differences Between Malignant
  and Benign Tumors
- Chapter Summary
- Self-Study

*T*he discovery of a lump or a mass can be a frightening experience as one's first thought is often the possibility of cancer. The swelling or tumor may indicate a serious condition or it may be relatively harmless.

TUMOR FORMATION

Formation of such tumors is called **neoplasia.** Swelling caused by new and abnormal growth is called a **neoplasm.** A neoplasm is a mass of new cells that grows in a haphazard fashion with no control and serves no useful function. Neoplasms are divided into two classes: **malignant** and **benign.** A malignant neoplasm tends to worsen and possibly cause death whereas a benign neoplasm is noncancerous. There is a great difference in the growth rate of various tumors. At times there may be a period of remission when the progress of the growth seems to be temporarily halted. Remission can occur spontaneously or may follow a type of therapy.

MALIGNANT TUMORS

Cancer is a malignant tumor, a growth that can affect any organ. It is often fatal and is the second leading cause of death in the United States. The exact cause of cancer is not known, but one of many different factors triggers the initial cellular change that leads to the tumor formation. Cancer is an invasive type of tumor, and many forms send fingerlike projections into underlying tissue. This manner of penetration resembles the claws of a crab, hence the name cancer from the Latin word for crab, *cancri.* As the tumor continues to grow, normal cells are destroyed.

The malignancy can grow into a normally open space and then block the lumen of an organ. This pattern of growth can obstruct the esophagus, the intestines, or the respiratory tract. As the tumor grows it can exert pressure and cause pain.

The surface of the mass often ulcerates, which can lead to hemorrhage and infection. The ulceration allows bacteria to enter the open lesion. The debilitated patient often has impaired immunity due to improperly functioning bone marrow, if that is a site of the malignancy, or the result of chemotherapy that suppresses the production of leukocytes. The key features of malignant tumors are their uncontrolled growth and tendency to **metastasize,** to spread to other sites.

The rapid growth of the malignant tumor uses up the body's nutrients, its supply of glucose, and amino acids, which, coupled with the patient's inability to eat, causes severe weight loss. The patient becomes weak and emaciated in appearance; this condition is referred to as **cachexia.**

■ Development of Cancer

Extensive research has transformed cancer into a highly curable chronic disease and one that is potentially preventable. Development of cancer **(carcinogenesis)** requires a long period of time, often decades, from the initial exposure to the carcinogen, the cause of the cancer, to the malignancy. In other words, there is a latent period.

Cancer development includes three stages, **initiation, promotion,** and **progression.** Initiation is the stage in which there is a genetic change in a cell, an altering of the DNA by some agent, chemical, radiation, or an oncogenic virus, a virus capable of causing cancer. During the promotion stage these altered cells proliferate and resemble benign neoplasms, which can either regress to normal-appearing tissue or evolve into cancer. Sometimes the individual's own immune system can reverse carcinogenesis. Removing or avoiding the causative agent at this stage can prevent the development of cancer. The third stage, progression, includes a change from a precancerous to a malignant lesion at which time growth rate increases and the malignancy can invade and metastasize. These devastating aspects of cancer occur late in the process of carcinogenesis. Figure 3–1 illustrates the steps in carcinogenesis.

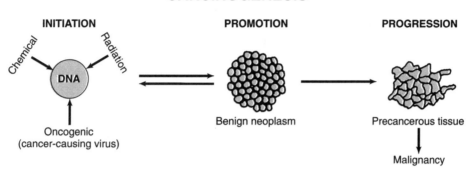

Figure 3–1. Development of cancer.

■ Causes of Cancer

What are some of the possible causes of cancer? Environmental agents may be a factor; in various geographic areas there is a higher frequency of certain types of cancer than in others. Air, soil, or water pollutants may be carcinogenic (cancer-causing). There is a genetic predisposition for some particular cancers, as certain family histories of the disease indicate. Radiation is known to cause skin cancer in certain people who are overexposed to the ultraviolet light of the sun and/or artificial tanning. Individuals affected may have an inherited sensitivity to solar radia-

On the Practical Side

SUN SCREENS AND TANNING SPAS

A deeply tanned body is considered by many to be beautiful, but the sunlight that produced the tan has already done its damage. Prolonged exposure to the ultraviolet (UV) light rays of the sun causes premature aging of the skin, wrinkles, liver spots, and a leathery texture. Most importantly, it causes premalignant lesions, warty growths called keratoses, and skin cancer. Fair-skinned individuals are the most susceptible but no one is exempt from the danger. Sun screens, lotions with an SPF (sun protection factor) of at least 15, should be used when exposure to the sun is necessary.

Popular tanning spas which provide a year-round tan also provide a great risk for developing skin cancer.

tion, and a combination of genetic makeup and radiation may cause the cancer. Fair-skinned people have the highest risk of developing skin cancer.

Workers in the field of radiation and radiology must take great precautions to prevent exposure to the harmful rays. This includes x-ray technicians and people using radioactive material in laboratories. Survivors of atom bomb explosions have shown a high incidence of leukemia and thyroid cancers as a result of the radiation they received. Certain chemicals used in industry have caused cancer in many workers. A large number of persons working with a particular dye developed cancer of the bladder. Inhalation of asbestos, benzedrine, and arsenic is known to have caused lung cancer. These cancer-causing substances are called *chemical carcinogens*. Intensive research is being done today to study relationships between food preservatives, elements of cosmetics, and plastics such as vinyl chloride in the development of cancer.

Hormones are related to certain forms of cancer, at times stimulating the growth of the cancer and in other cancers used for treatment. A benign mole never becomes malignant before puberty, the time when the sex hormone level increases. Cancer of the prostate gland is stimulated by the male hormone testosterone, but its growth is inhibited by estrogen therapy. The ovaries are sometimes removed after breast cancer surgery to prevent estrogen stimulation of other tu-

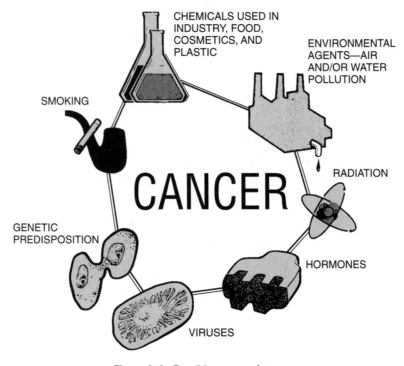

Figure 3–2. Possible causes of cancer.

mors. Many forms of cancers are more common in either men or women, which seems to indicate a hormonal relationship. A virus has been shown to cause some kinds of cancer in humans.

Viruses invade cells and may alter the genetic material of the cell. This could account for the abnormal cell divisions and rapid growth observed in malignant tumors. Possible causes of cancer are summarized in Figure 3–2.

■ Prevention of Cancer

The sites most responsible for cancer deaths are lungs, breast, and colon and many of these cancers can be prevented by changes in life-style. Cigarette smoking and use of tobacco products cause about 30 percent of all cancers. Cigarette smoking is considered the single most preventable cause not only of cancer but of diseases such as heart disease, chronic bronchitis, and emphysema. Diet and nutrition also play a significant role in reducing the risk of cancer. Reduction of fat intake and the inclusion in the diet of fruits, vegetables, and fiber have been found to reduce the risk of breast and colon cancer. Vitamin A in the diet, specifically carotene-containing foods, has a protective effect against lung cancer.

Early detection of a potential malignancy is extremely significant in preventing carcinogenesis. Widespread use of the Papanicolaou **(Pap)** smear has greatly decreased the incidence and mortality from invasive cervical cancer. The use of mammography has led to early detection of breast cancer, which can be cured.

The association between sex and cervical cancer has been known for many years. Studies show that early sexual activity and multiple partners increase the incidence of cervical cancer. A high rate of sexually transmitted diseases, multiple pregnancies, and early age at first pregnancy are often linked to this cancer. The **human papillomavirus** (HPV) responsible for genital warts (Chapter 14) seems to be the causative agent in uterine cervical carcinoma.

■ Signs and Symptoms of Cancer

Signs and symptoms of cancer vary with the site of the malignancy. Pain is usually not an early sign of cancer. It is only when the mass has grown, causing an obstruction or putting pressure on nerve endings, that pain is experienced. Infection frequently accompanies cancer and may cause pain.

There are certain warning signs that a cancerous tumor might be present. Abnormal bleeding or discharge from a natural body opening such as the rectum or vagina may be an indication of a malignancy. Blood in the urine, sputum, or vomitus should be investigated. This bleeding may not be due to cancer at all, but it is a precautionary measure to have it checked.

A thickening or lump, particularly in the breast, indicates a tumor or a cyst. A **cyst** is a sac or capsule containing fluid and is usually harmless. The tumor might well be benign, but the possibility of a malignancy exists, and it should be examined by a physician. The American Cancer Society urges women to perform monthly self-examinations of each breast and to have mammography on a regular basis.

Another sign of a possible cancer is a persistent cough or hoarseness. A growth in the respiratory tract, or one pressing on it, acts as an irritant in stimulating the cough reflex.

A change in bowel activity, intermittent constipation and diarrhea, may indicate an obstruction in the colon. Difficulties in urination such as urgency, burning sensations, and the inability to start the stream of urine may signal a tumor in the urinary system. In men, it may signal a tumor of the prostate gland.

Normally the body has excellent healing ability. If a sore or an ulceration fails to heal after a period of time there is some reason for it, and the lesion should be examined. A mole may change color, darken, enlarge, or become itchy. This can signal a transition from a benign growth to one that is malignant.

A person experiencing difficulty in swallowing **(dysphagia)** or loss of appetite **(anorexia)** may have some kind of obstruction in the upper gastrointestinal tract. These symptoms, particularly if accompanied by rapid weight loss, are significant.

A severe anemia may indicate internal bleeding from a malignant lesion or malfunctioning of the bone marrow due to replacement of normal tissue by cancerous cells. Chemotherapy and/or radiation also affect the blood-clotting mechanism. Excessive production of a hormone can signal a tumor, benign or malignant, of an endocrine gland. Figure 3–3 lists warning signs that may indicate a malignancy. The first letter of each word spells the acronym, CAUTION.

■ Types of Cancer

There are two major types of cancer, carcinoma and sarcoma; the suffix *oma* means a tumor. **Carcinoma** is the more common form, affecting epithelial tissues, skin, and mucous membranes lining body cavities. Tumors of the skin are called **epidermoid carcinomas.** Carcinoma is also the malignancy of glandular tissue such as the breast, liver, and pancreas. Cancerous glandular tumors are known as **adenocarcinomas;** the prefix *adeno* always refers to a gland. Although these tumors develop in either epithelial or glandular tissue, they invade deeper and surrounding tissues. Cancer of the mouth, lung, and stomach are examples of carcinoma. Figure 3–4 shows an adenocarcinoma of the stomach.

Sarcoma is the less common cancer, but it spreads more rapidly and is highly malignant. Connective tissue tumors, such as tumors of bone, muscle, and cartilage, are sarcomas. Rapidly growing tumors show little differentiation, and this lack of form is referred to as **anaplasia,** the prefix *an* meaning without and *plasia*,

The American Cancer Society lists several signs of cancer, the first letter of each word spelling the acronym, **CAUTION**.

Change in bowel or bladder habits
A sore that does not heal
Unusual bleeding or discharge
Thickening or lump in breast or elsewhere
Indigestion or difficulty in swallowing
Obvious change in wart or mole
Nagging cough or hoarseness

Figure 3–3. Warning signs of cancer.

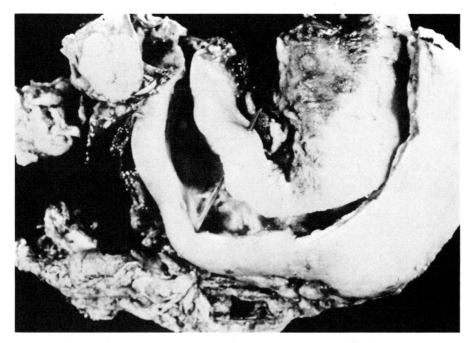

Figure 3–4. Adenocarcinoma of the stomach. White area is the greatly thickened stomach wall. (*Courtesy of Dr. David R. Duffell.*)

form. These rapidly growing, undifferentiated tumors are the most responsive to radiation treatment. Figure 3–5 contrasts carcinoma and sarcoma.

■ Metastasis

Unfortunately, when a malignant tumor develops in an organ such as the breast or prostate gland, it tends to spread to other parts of the body. This spread of the cancer to distant sites is known as **metastasis.**

Carcinoma spreads principally through the lymph vessels, affecting the lymph nodes. This is the reason for removal of the axillary lymph nodes in a radical mastectomy (removal of the breast). Regional lymph nodes are removed in surgical operations for malignant tumors of the colon. Carcinoma can also spread through the bloodstream. Malignant tumors of the liver that have developed through metastases are seen in Figure 3–6.

The metastasis of sarcoma is generally through the blood vessels. Clusters of cancer cells can break off from the primary sites and travel as emboli to the liver, lungs, brain, or other organs. Frequently, it is a secondary site of cancer that is discovered first.

■ Diagnosis of Cancer

X-ray techniques, particularly those using contrast dyes, can show the site of a mass or tumor. The tumor can only be diagnosed as malignant through micro-

	CARCINOMA	SARCOMA
AFFECTS	EPITHELIAL AND GLANDULAR TISSUE	CONNECTIVE TISSUE
EXAMPLES	SKIN, BREAST, AND LIVER CANCER	CANCER OF BONE, MUSCLE, AND CARTLAGE
INCIDENCE	MORE COMMON	LESS COMMON
GROWTH RATE	SLOWER	FASTER
METASTASIS	PRINCIPALLY THROUGH LYMPH VESSELS	PRINCIPALLY THROUGH THE BLOOD

Figure 3–5. Distinctions between carcinoma and sarcoma.

scopic examination of the cells and tissue. All tumors removed surgically must be sent to a pathology department for this study. When a suspected tumor is **biopsied,** a small sample is removed and examined microscopically for abnormalities. A technique known as the *frozen section* enables the pathologist to determine immediately whether the sample is malignant. This is extremely helpful during

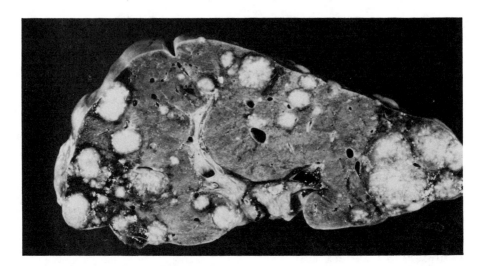

Figure 3–6. Malignant tumors of the liver that have metastasized from other sites. (*Courtesy of Dr. David R. Duffell.*)

surgery. A sample of the tissue is sent to the laboratory, the surgeon waits for the result, and then determines the extent of the surgery required based on the report. Further examination of the tissue generally follows.

Another means of obtaining cells for microscopic examination is through scrapings, washings, and secretions from suspected areas. This is called **exfoliative cytology.** It takes advantage of the fact that cancer cells in the early stages tend to be cast off or shed. This technique is helpful in diagnosing early cancer of the bronchus and uterus. It is the principle of the Pap smear, which was named for its originator, Dr. George N. Papanicolaou. Fine needle aspiration is also used to suction cells from a tumor for microscopic examination.

There are different stages of cancer development. The pre-invasive stage means that the tumor has not yet penetrated into underlying tissues. If cancer of the cervix can be determined at this stage through the Pap smear, surgical removal offers good prognosis.

Once the cancer has become invasive its total removal is very difficult. The edges of the malignant tumor are poorly defined and if it is not entirely removed the cancer will recur. If the tumor has metastasized, surgery is of little benefit.

Pathologists grade tumors by the microscopic appearance of the suspected cells. Grading is helpful in determining proper treatment. The following table shows how tumors are graded.

Grade	Appearance	Survival Rate
1	Tumor cells differentiated and closely resemble parent tissue	High
2 & 3	Tumor cells moderately or poorly differentiated	Moderate
4	Tumor cells so undifferentiated that tissue origin cannot be readily recognized	Low

Staging neoplasms is a means of estimating how much the tumor has spread. A system has been developed by which tumors are staged according to their size and extent, number of lymph nodes involved, and metastases of the primary tumor.

■ Treatment of Cancer

Surgery and radiation therapy are very effective in the early stages of breast and uterine cancer and other cancers that are readily accessible. Fast-growing, undifferentiated tumors respond best to radiation therapy; radiation has a greater destructive action on fast-growing cells than on normal cells. Leukemia and Hodgkin's disease, a malignancy of the lymph nodes and lymphoid tissue, respond well to radiation and chemotherapy. Hormonal therapy, a type of chemotherapy, is used to treat cancer of the prostate, either by removal of the androgen sources, which stimulate the tumor growth, or by administration of estrogens, which inhibit it. Chemotherapy, the use of antineoplastic agents that are metabolic inhibitors and cell-killing chemicals, is effective in treating leukemia and many other cancers. Side effects from the potent chemicals include gastrointestinal disturbances, loss of hair, and reduced immunity. The latter is due to an abnormal decrease in the number of circulating white blood cells, **leukopenia.**

On the Practical Side
HAIR LOSS WITH CHEMOTHERAPY

The chemicals used in treating cancer destroy rapidly dividing cells of the tumor. The chemicals, however, affect not only malignant cells, but all rapidly dividing cells. This includes the epidermal cells of the hair follicle that give rise to hair. As these cells are killed by the chemotherapy, hair is lost. Hair growth usually resumes following treatment as previously dormant epidermal cells become active.

BENIGN TUMORS

Benign tumors are different from malignant tumors. Benign growths are generally encapsulated with clearly defined edges, which makes their removal from surrounding tissue relatively easy. **Benign** tumors do not metastasize nor do they recur after surgical removal. Only rarely do these tumors ulcerate and bleed. A benign tumor differentiates somewhat in its development and resembles the structure from which it grew.

This does not mean that benign tumors pose no threat. A tumor on the brain or in the spinal cord, even if it is benign, puts pressure on nerves and seriously affects the functioning of the nervous system. Any tumor can obstruct a passageway such as the trachea, shutting off the air supply, or the esophagus, making it impossible to swallow. A benign tumor of a gland can cause oversecretion of its hormone with very serious effects. If a tumor of the anterior pituitary gland develops before puberty, the increased secretion of growth hormone leads to the development of a giant. An adrenal gland tumor produces an oversecretion of androgens (male sex hormones) and causes masculinization of females.

■ Types of Benign Tumors

Tumors are classified according to the tissue in which they develop. A common benign tumor is the **lipoma,** a soft, fatty tumor that develops in adipose (fat) tissue. As it grows it pushes normal tissue aside. Lipomas are commonly found on the neck, back, and buttocks—anyplace where there is fat.

A **myoma** is a tumor of the muscle; the prefix *myo* refers to muscle. These tumors are rare in voluntary muscle but do develop in smooth or involuntary muscle. Myomas are the tumors of the uterus referred to as *fibroids*. Fibroid tumors are also called **leiomyomas,** specifying a tumor of smooth muscle. Leiomyomas are the tumors most commonly found in women. If the tumors are small they may cause no symptoms, but if they become large they can cause menstrual problems or difficulties during a pregnancy, even spontaneous abortion.

The typical red birthmark, or "port-wine" stain, is another type of benign tumor. It is an **angioma,** a tumor composed of blood vessels. Lymph vessels can also comprise an angioma, but since lymph is colorless a tumor of this type is colorless. An angioma is one type of benign tumor that is not encapsulated. Advanced laser technology is now being used effectively to gradually erase port-wine stains.

The common mole is a benign tumor called a **nevus** and like the angioma it is not encapsulated. This tumor of the skin contains a black pigment called *melanin* and is sometimes called a *melanoma*. There is also a cancerous condition known as **malignant melanoma,** so the name nevus is better used when the tumor is benign. The nevus is congenital but may not be apparent until later in life; it usually enlarges at puberty. This benign tumor can change to a malignant melanoma. An increase in size and pigmentation, bleeding, or itchiness may indicate this transformation to the malignant type. Figure 3–7 shows an enlarging mole on a woman's back.

An epithelial tumor that grows as a projecting mass on the skin, or from an inner mucous membrane, is a **papilloma** or polyp. The common wart is an example of a papilloma. This tumor has a fixed base with a stalk growing from it. A growth of this type in the intestinal tract or uterus can be moved back and forth on the stalk and become irritated.

A benign tumor of glandular tissue is an **adenoma.** It often develops in the breast, thyroid gland, or in mucous glands of the intestinal tract. The adenoma is an example of a benign tumor that resembles the structure from which it develops.

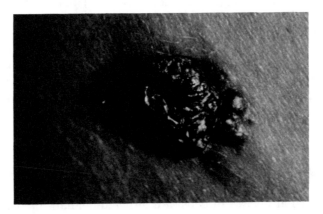

Figure 3–7. Enlarging mole on back, increasing in size over 2 or 3 months. Patient died in 10 months despite radical surgery. (*Courtesy of Dr. Barry A. Goldsmith.*)

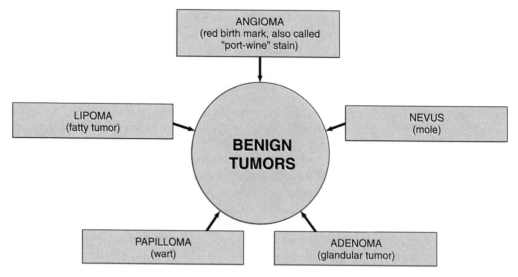

Figure 3–8. Examples of benign tumors.

Glands and ducts are found within the tumor, and it may be secretory. Various benign tumors are summarized in Figure 3–8.

A unique benign tumor of the ovary is the **teratoma,** or dermoid cyst. Lining the cyst is epidermis, skin with its usual appendages: hair, oil and sweat glands, even teeth. The cyst contains oily material from the sebaceous (oil) glands. The teratoma probably stems from some primitive cell that has the potential of developing in several directions. When these cysts develop on a long pedicle, or stalk, twisting may occur and cause acute abdominal pain; surgical removal is then necessary.

DIFFERENCES BETWEEN MALIGNANT AND BENIGN TUMORS

Malignant tumors are usually larger and more irregular in shape than benign tumors. Benign tumors are generally encapsulated, whereas malignant ones are not. A malignancy is invasive and penetrating, destroying underlying tissue; this is not characteristic of benign tumors. Malignant tumors grow at a faster rate than benign tumors and metastasize, setting up new colonies of cells at distant sites. Benign tumors resemble the tissue in which they developed, but malignant tumors lack form.

CHAPTER SUMMARY

Neoplasms, abnormal masses of cells, are either malignant or benign. Malignant tumors are invasive and spread by metastasis. Infection, hemorrhage, and anemia are often complications of cancer.

The development of cancer is a slow process that includes three stages: initiation, promotion, and progression. The process can be interrupted or reversed by removing or avoiding the cause of the cancer.

Many cancers are preventable by avoiding such causes as smoking, overexposure to ultraviolet light, and chemical pollutants. Early detection and treatment of cancer can often bring about a cure. Pathologists grade tumors by the microscopic appearance of the suspected cells which is helpful in determining treatment.

Carcinoma is the more common major type of cancer. It affects epithelial tissues and glands and spreads principally through the lymph system. Sarcoma affects bone, muscle, and cartilage and spreads rapidly through the blood.

Cancer is treated by surgery, radiation, and chemotherapy, depending on the type and the location.

Benign tumors are generally encapsulated, and they neither metastasize nor recur after surgical removal. They tend to resemble the tissue from which they developed.

■ Self-Study

True or False

_____ 1. Carcinogenesis is a rapid process.

_____ 2. Hodgkin's disease responds well to radiation and chemotherapy.

_____ 3. Sarcoma generally spreads faster than carcinoma.

_____ 4. A benign tumor of the thyroid is an adenoma.

_____ 5. A genetic change in a cell occurs during the initiation stage of cancer development.

_____ 6. Pain is an early symptom of cancer.

_____ 7. Carcinogenesis can be reversed.

_____ 8. Malignant epithelial tumors are carcinomas.

_____ 9. Anaplastic tumors are most sensitive to radiation.

_____ 10. Cancer of the uterus is sarcoma.

_____ 11. Benign tumors can metastasize.

_____ 12. Surgery is the recommended procedure for treating fast-growing, undifferentiated tumors.

_____ 13. Hormonal therapy is effective for benign tumors.

_____ 14. Hormones can both cause cancer growth and be used in therapy.

_____ 15. Cancer of a mucous gland is an adenocarcinoma.

_____ 16. A leiomyoma is a tumor of skeletal muscle.

_____ 17. A papilloma may become malignant.

_____ 18. Carcinoma spreads principally through lymph vessels.

_____ 19. Chemotherapy can impair immunity.

_____ 20. Cancers of bone and cartilage are carcinomas.

Match

_____ 21. nevus

_____ 22. "port-wine" stain

_____ 23. myoma

_____ 24. thyroid tumor

_____ 25. stalked projection

a) angioma

b) fibroids

c) filled with melanin pigment

d) adenoma

e) papilloma

(Answers on page 449)

Chapter 4

Hereditary Diseases

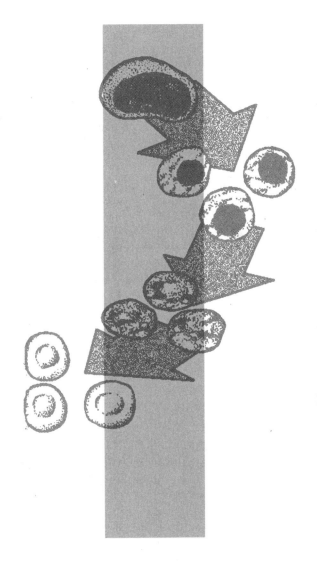

Chapter Outline

- Introduction to Heredity
- Transmission of Hereditary Diseases
- Abnormal Chromosome Diseases
- Sex Anomalies
- Congenital Diseases
- Chapter Summary
- Self-Study

*H*ave you ever been startled by observing a particularly strong family resemblance? How is this similarity between brothers and sisters, children and parents, and even between cousins explained? You can say, "It's because of their genes," which is true, but what about two brothers of the same parents who do not resemble each other at all? How does this phenomenon called inheritance work?

INTRODUCTION TO HEREDITY

All genetic information is contained in the nucleus of each cell, and each time the cell divides, in growth and repair, the information is passed on to the daughter cells. The vehicle of transmission is the DNA molecule, which duplicates itself when a cell is about to divide, providing an exact copy for each daughter cell.

On the Practical Side
IDENTIFICATION BY FINGERPRINTS

The value of fingerprints and footprints has increased greatly not only at crime scenes, but in the identification of abducted infants and children. No two sets of fingerprints are identical. The dermis, or true skin, projects upward into the epidermis in curving parallel ridges forming the pattern of fingerprints and footprints.

DNA, which stands for **deoxyribonucleic acid,** is the blueprint for protein synthesis within the cell. Proteins form a structural part of the cell and comprise the enzymes, the biological catalysts, that control cellular activity. Some of the genetic disorders that will be discussed result from the lack of a particular enzyme and are referred to as *inborn errors of metabolism.*

At the time of cell division, the DNA is assembled into units called **chromosomes.** Each human cell contains 46 chromosomes divided into 23 pairs. Half of the chromosomes were inherited from each parent. The chromosomes contain thousands of **genes,** each of which is responsible for the synthesis of one protein. Forty-four of the chromosomes are called **autosomes,** and two are called the X and Y, or the sex, chromosomes, the ones that determine the sex of the person. A combination of XY chromosomes results in a male, and XX chromosomes in a female. This chromosomal composition of the nucleus is called the **karyotype** of the cell. The karyotype can be visualized microscopically and photographed to determine chromosomal abnormalities.

The genes inherited from each parent for a particular trait such as eye color, hair color, and hair type occupy a particular site on a chromosome and are called **alleles.** If the pair of genes are similar, the person is **homozygous** for that trait. If the genes are different, one for dark and one for light hair, for example, the person is **heterozygous.** Some genes always produce an effect and are said to be **dominant.** The result of the dominant gene is the same whether a person is homozygous or heterozygous. The gene for brown eyes, for example, is dominant to that for blue eyes. Other genes are **recessive** and only manifest themselves when the person is homozygous for the trait. This is significant in many hereditary diseases.

Certain factors may cause a deviation from the basic principles of inheritance that have been described. Some genes are codominant, so that both are expressed. An example of codominant genes is found in blood type AB. The gene for the A factor is inherited from one parent and that for the B factor from the other, but both genes are expressed. At times a dominant gene is not fully expressed, a condition known as reduced penetrance.

Spontaneous **mutations** or changes in the DNA structure occur at times, and they become permanent hereditary alterations if the gonads are affected. Mutations can result from viral activity, chemical action, and radiation. The effect of the mutation may be slight and go unnoticed or it may be lethal. Serious mutations are generally incompatible with life and cause the death of a fetus and spontaneous abortion.

The environment interacts with heredity, as seen in certain diseases. A predisposition to develop allergies is inherited, but contact with an offending antigen is required for sensitization to it. As an example, a person is not born allergic to ragweed but develops the hypersensitivity on exposure, and a fair-skinned person can develop cancer when overexposed to the ultraviolet light of the sun. Obesity develops through a combination of heredity and dietary habits.

TRANSMISSION OF HEREDITARY DISEASES

Many of the diseases described throughout this book are called *hereditary* or *familial diseases*. In this chapter, the mechanism of transmission will be explained. Some diseases are inherited from a single autosomal dominant gene. One such defective gene causes Huntington's chorea, a disease described in Chapter 15, and another causes polydactyly, explained next. Other diseases are inherited as autosomal recessives, with one defective gene being inherited from each parent, making the person homozygous for that trait. Cystic fibrosis is such a disease. A third type of inheritance is sex-linked, with the defective gene on the X chromosome. Color blindness and hemophilia are examples of sex-linked inherited diseases.

■ Autosomal Dominant

A defective dominant gene is usually transmitted from a parent who is heterozygous for the trait. If the other parent is normal for the particular condition, 50 percent of their children have the chance of being affected and manifesting the genetic defect. The remaining children will be homozygous for the recessive gene and be normal. This is illustrated in Figure 4–1. The disease appears in every generation, with males and females being equally affected. Exceptions to the rule are minimal.

Polydactyly, extra fingers or toes, is an example of an autosomal dominant disorder. A boy or girl inheriting the defective gene from either parent will have

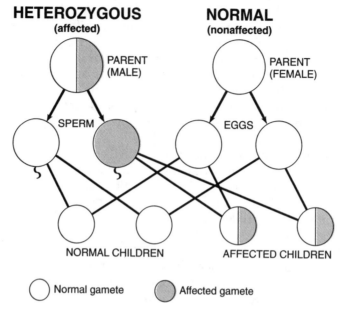

HETEROZYGOUS
(affected)

NORMAL
(nonaffected)

PARENT
(MALE)

PARENT
(FEMALE)

SPERM

EGGS

NORMAL CHILDREN

AFFECTED CHILDREN

Normal gamete   Affected gamete

Figure 4–1. Transmission of autosomal dominant disorders (50 percent chance for an affected child).

the abnormality. **Achondroplasia** is another disorder resulting from one defective dominant gene (Fig. 4–2). The word element *chondro* refers to cartilage, *plasia* to formation, and the prefix *a* means a lack. In this disease, cartilage formation in the fetus is defective. Normally, the fetal skeleton develops as cartilage that is gradually replaced by bone. In achondroplasia the defective cartilage formation results in improper bone development and **achondroplastic dwarfism.** The long bones of the arms and legs are short, the trunk of the body is normal in size, the head is large, and the forehead very prominent. The person develops sexually, has normal intelligence, and is muscular and agile.

■ Autosomal Recessive

These diseases manifest themselves only when a person is homozygous for the defective gene. Two parents who are both carriers of the recessive gene are themselves heterozygous for the trait and do not have the disease. There is a 25 percent chance that their children will be affected. Two out of four will be carriers and one will be normal. This is shown in Figure 4–3. The recessive gene appears more frequently in a family, and close intermarriage, as between first cousins, increases the risk of the particular disease.

Phenylketonuria, also called PKU, is an example of autosomal recessive gene inheritance. The PKU patient lacks a specific enzyme that converts one amino acid, phenylalanine, to another, tyrosine. This mechanism is illustrated in Figure 4–4. As a result, high levels of phenylalanine and its derivatives build up in the

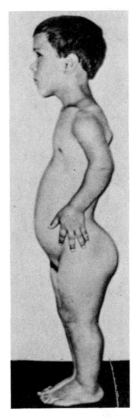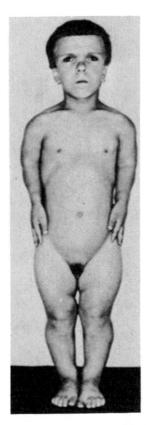

Figure 4–2. A 12-year-old achondroplastic dwarf. Note the disproportion of the limbs to the trunk, the curvature of the spine, and the prominent buttocks.

blood and are toxic to the brain, interfering with normal brain development. If the condition is not diagnosed and treated early, severe mental retardation results. Physical development proceeds normally, but the child is very light in color. Production of the pigment melanin is impeded because of inadequate tyrosine, a result of the missing enzyme. The child may manifest disorders of the nervous system, such as a lack of balance, and may possibly suffer convulsions.

To prevent the serious mental retardation that accompanies PKU, newborn babies are routinely screened for the disease. If it is found, a synthetic diet is prescribed that eliminates phenylalanine. Good results have been achieved with this treatment. The diet is unpleasant, and controversy exists as to the length of time the diet must be maintained. To begin treatment immediately, by excluding phenylalanine during the earliest years of life, seems to be the most critical factor in preventing mental retardation.

Galactosemia is another example of an inborn error of metabolism resulting from autosomal recessive inheritance. The person with this disease lacks the en-

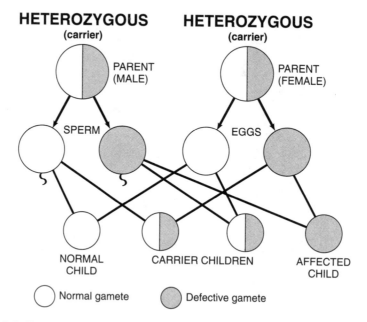

Figure 4–3. Transmission of recessive disorders (25 percent chance for an affected child).

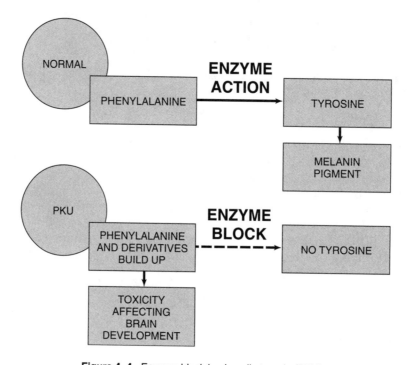

Figure 4–4. Enzyme block in phenylketonuria (PKU).

zyme necessary to convert galactose, a sugar derived from lactose in milk, to glucose. Galactose accumulates in the blood and interferes with development of the brain, liver, and eyes. If untreated, mental retardation develops. The liver becomes enlarged and cirrhotic, and ascites fluid (see Chapter 11) accumulates in the abdominal cavity. Intestinal distress results in vomiting and diarrhea. Early diagnosis and treatment of galactosemia can prevent these signs, and development will then proceed normally. The treatment consists of eliminating lactose from the diet.

Sickle cell anemia, a severe anemia generally confined to blacks, will be described in Chapter 6. The manner of inheritance is best explained in the context of genetic diseases. Sickle cell anemia is an autosomal recessive disorder, in which the hemoglobin is abnormal, resulting in deformed red blood cells. The improperly formed cells become lodged in capillaries and block circulation, causing necrosis and **infarcts,** death of tissues. The sickle-shaped red blood cells rupture easily, and they are removed from the circulation by the spleen. The depletion of red blood cells results in severe anemia.

The person with sickle cell anemia is homozygous for the trait by inheriting one defective gene from each parent. A person who is heterozygous for sickle cell anemia has both normal and abnormal hemoglobin and possesses the sickle cell trait. The person is mildly anemic, but the one defective gene provides an advantage. The person with sickle cell trait has an immunity against malaria that is significant in tropical climates where malaria abounds.

Tay–Sachs is an autosomal recessive condition which affects primarily families of Eastern Jewish origin. An enzyme deficiency causes abnormal lipid metabolism in the brain which results in progressive mental and physical retardation. Symptoms appear by 6 months of age when no new skills are learned, convulsions occur, and blindness may develop. A cherry-red spot may be seen on each retina. Children usually die between 2 and 4 years of age. There is no specific therapy for the condition so care treats the symptoms.

■ Sex-linked Inheritance

Diseases of sex-linked inheritance generally result from defective genes on the X chromosome, as the Y chromosome is small and carries very few genes. A recessive gene on the single X chromosome of a male is unmasked, and the trait is expressed. A female may be heterozygous for the gene, having a recessive gene on the one X chromosome but a normal gene on the other X. That female is then a carrier of the disease, and she has a 50% chance of transmitting the gene to half of her sons and daughters. An affected male transmits the disease only to his daughters, as they receive his X chromosome. His sons are unaffected, as the Y chromosome is normal. This is illustrated in Figure 4–5. The abnormalities of **sex-linked inheritance** are generally confined to the male and are transmitted by the female. In a rare case, the female may have the sex-linked disease if she is homozygous for the recessive gene.

Color Blindness. Color blindness, the inability to distinguish between certain colors, is a disorder of sex-linked inheritance. It is generally confined to males, al-

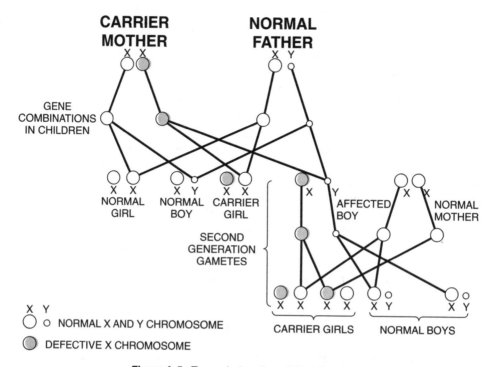

Figure 4–5. Transmission of sex-linked disorders.

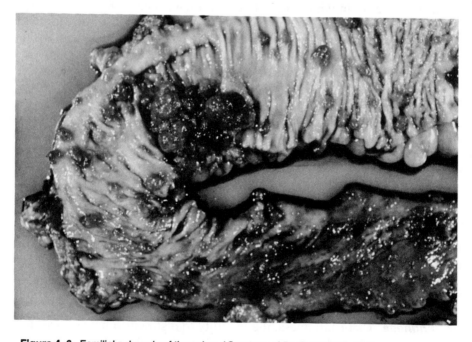

Figure 4–6. Familial polyposis of the colon. (*Courtesy of Dr. David R. Duffell.*)

though it is possible for a female to be color-blind if she receives the recessive gene from each parent, which is rare.

The gene for color blindness is on the X chromosome, but the gene for normal vision is dominant to it. A male with the recessive gene on his one X chromosome will express the trait and be color-blind.

The defect that causes color blindness is apparently in certain specialized receptors of the retina called cones. There are three types of receptors that are stimulated by wavelengths of the primary colors: red, green, and blue. Impulses are then sent to the brain and interpreted. The color-blind person is most frequently unable to distinguish reds and greens. There is no correction for color blindness.

Familial Diseases. Some diseases appear in families, but the means of inheritance are not understood. Examples of diseases with a higher incidence in certain families are epilepsy, diabetes, cardiovascular problems, allergies, and familial polyposis (Fig. 4–6). The cause of these diseases does not seem to be a single gene but the effect of several genes working together.

ABNORMAL CHROMOSOME DISEASES

The hereditary diseases that have been described so far result from a defective gene. Abnormalities in the chromosomes, either in their number or structure, cause other disorders. At times, chromosomes fail to separate properly during cell division, causing one daughter cell to be deficient and one to have an extra chromosome. The loss of an autosomal chromosome is usually incompatible with life because each autosome contains a large number of essential genes. A fetus affected by this condition is generally spontaneously aborted. The loss of a sex chromosome or the presence of an extra one is less serious, but many abnormalities accompany the condition.

■ Down's Syndrome

Down's syndrome is an example of a disorder caused by the presence of an extra autosomal chromosome. Chromosome 21 is in triplicate, which is called **trisomy 21.** The extra chromosome results from **nondisjunction,** the failure of two chromosomes to separate as the gametes—the egg and sperm—are being formed.

The Down's syndrome child is always mentally retarded. The excessive enzyme production from the extra genes may have a toxic effect on the brain. The child can be taught simple tasks and is generally very affectionate.

The life expectancy of a child with Down's syndrome is relatively short due to complications that accompany the condition. Congenital heart diseases are common, and there is a greater susceptibility to respiratory tract infections, including pneumonia. There is also a higher incidence of leukemia than in a normal child.

The Down's syndrome child has a very characteristic appearance. The eyes appear slanted due to an extra fold of skin at the upper, medial corner of the eye; the tongue is coarse and often protrudes; and the nose is short and flat. The child is usually of short stature, and the sex organs are under-developed. A straight crease extends across the palm of the hand, and the little finger is often shorter than normal (Fig. 4–7).

The incidence of Down's syndrome is higher in mothers over 35 than in younger women, and the risk increases with age.

■ Fragile X Syndrome

A condition of mental and physical disability that results from an abnormality on the X chromosome is known as **fragile X syndrome.** It affects principally males although females may also be affected. Females are the carriers of the defective gene. The combination of sex chromosomes, X and Y, determines the sex of an individual, XX being female and XY male. The female carrier having the defective gene on one X chromosome, has a good gene on the other as a compensator. She may have some degree of mental retardation or learning disabilities and exhibit some of the signs of the syndrome. However, the male has the defective gene on his only X chromosome and therefore it usually manifests itself. The fragile X chromosome appears to have a broken end and the genetic abnormality somehow affects the connections in the brain cells. Scientists have very recently identified this gene and are presuming that it incorrectly makes a protein required by the brain.

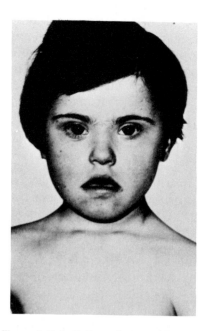 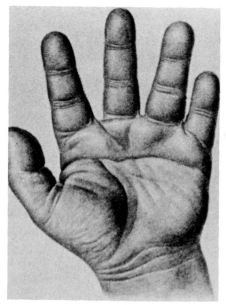

Figure 4–7. Left. Face of a 5-year-old girl with Down's syndrome. Note widely set eyes, underdeveloped bridge of the nose, partially open mouth, and protruding tongue. **Right.** Short, broad hand of a 9-year-old Down's syndrome patient, showing shortened fifth finger and transverse crease across palm.

The child may appear normal at first, but be slow in his development. His behavior may be abnormal, avoiding eye contact, exhibiting tantrums unexplainably, flapping his hands and even biting them. Certain physical characteristics may be noted as the child grows; a large head, long face, pronounced ears, and possibly double jointedness. His movements may be clumsy and poorly coordinated. Large testicles become especially noticeable at puberty.

Many of the children are hyperactive, easily distractible, and act impulsively. They are overly stimulated by all types of stimuli, sound, sight, touch, and smell and often respond by tantrums and disruptive behavior. Language characteristics, repetitive speech, unusual rhythm, inability to pronounce multisyllable words or complete a sentence, help to distinguish a fragile X child.

The degree of mental disability of a fragile X child is difficult to assess because of his hyperactivity, poor attention span, and impulsive behavior. These children usually function higher than their IQs would indicate.

Many physical problems are associated with fragile X syndrome, some of which are the result of connective tissue abnormality. Eye problems are common and are often caused by muscle weakness; muscle tone in general is poor.

The principal mental defect is sensory integration dysfunction, the inability to screen out or inhibit sensations. As a result the child is overwhelmed by them and responds with tantrums and uncontrolled behavior.

There is no cure for fragile X syndrome, but great strides have been made in enabling these children to sort out sensations so that they can react to some and disregard others. Intensive sensory integration therapy (S.I.), the process by which sensory input is organized to be used appropriately, is especially effective when administered at an early age.

SEX ANOMALIES

■ Turner's Syndrome

One of the sex chromosomes is missing in **Turner's syndrome,** resulting in a karyotype of 45,XO. The patient appears to be female, but the ovaries do not develop; thus, there is no ovulation or menstruation, and the person is sterile. The nipples are widely spaced, the breasts do not develop, and the person is short of stature and has a stocky build. Congenital heart disease, particularly coarctation of the aorta (described in Chapter 7), frequently accompanies Turner's syndrome. Facial deformities are often present. Figure 4–8 shows a patient with Turner's syndrome.

■ Klinefelter's Syndrome

An extra sex chromosome is present in **Klinefelter's syndrome,** and the patient's karyotype is 47,XXY. This person appears to be a male but has small testes that fail to mature and produce no sperm. At puberty, with the development of secondary sex characteristics, the breasts enlarge and a female distribution of hair de-

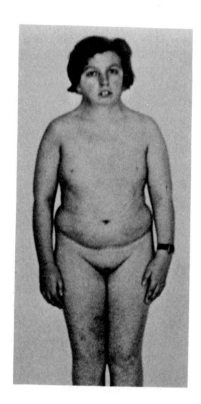

Figure 4–8. A 21-year-old patient with Turner's syndrome. The chest is broad and the nipples are small and pale. Pubic hair is totally lacking.

velops. There is little facial hair, and the general appearance is that of a eunuch. The person is tall (with abnormally long legs), is mentally deficient, and is sterile (Fig. 4–9).

■ Hermaphrodites

The number of true **hermaphrodites** who have both testes and ovaries is small. Pseudohermaphrodites do develop, and they have either testes or ovaries, usually nonfunctional, but the remainder of the anatomy is mixed. This condition is referred to as sex reversal, in which the chromosomal sex is different from the anatomic sex. Sex reversal occurs during fetal life. The sex glands are neutral during the first few weeks after conception, but the male gonads differentiate at about the sixth week under the influence of masculinizing hormone. In the absence of an adequate amount of this hormone, ovaries develop, and the individual is anatomically female but chromosomally male (XY).

Some cases of pseudohermaphroditism result from excessive production of sex hormones from the adrenal cortex. An affected female develops male secondary sexual characteristics at a very early age. The external genitalia of pseudohermaphrodites resembles that of both males and females. A pseudohermaphrodite is shown in Figure 4–10.

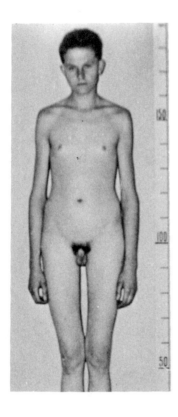

Figure 4–9. A 19-year-old patient with Klinefelter's syndrome. Extremities are excessively long, pubic hair is scanty, and genitals are underdeveloped. Body proportions resemble those of a eunuch.

CONGENITAL DISEASES

Congenital diseases are those appearing at birth or shortly after, but they are not caused by genetic or chromosomal abnormalities. Congenital defects usually result from some failure in development during the embryonic stage, or first 2 months of pregnancy. Congenital diseases cannot be transmitted to offspring.

Various factors—inadequate oxygen, maternal infection, drugs, malnutrition, and radiation—can interfere with normal development. Rubella, or German measles, contracted by the mother during the first trimester of pregnancy, can produce serious birth defects. The rubella virus is able to cross the placental barrier and affect the central nervous system of the embryo, causing mental retardation, blindness, and deafness. Cerebral palsy and hydrocephalus can develop as a result of the viral infection.

Syphilis can be transmitted to a developing fetus and cause multiple anomalies—structural deformities, blindness, deafness, and paralysis; children with congenital syphilis may become insane. Syphilitic infection of a fetus frequently results in spontaneous abortion or a stillbirth. A mother with syphilis should be treated for it before the fifth month of pregnancy to prevent fetal infection. A child

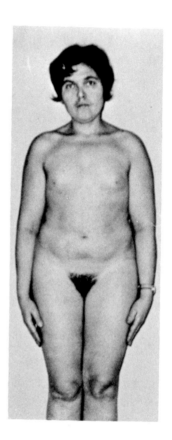

Figure 4–10. A 22-year-old patient with pseudohermaphroditism, reared as a girl because of ambiguous genitalia. Surgery and tissue studies showed the gonads to be testes.

born with syphilis should be treated immediately with penicillin, but considerable irreversible damage may have already occurred.

The tragic effect of the drug thalidomide, used during pregnancy many years ago, alerted the public to the danger of drugs to the developing embryo. Babies who had been exposed to thalidomide before birth were born without limbs or had flipperlike appendages.

Many congenital defects result from improper closure of a structure or failure of parts to unite. Congenital heart diseases are discussed in Chapter 7. Spina bifida, an improper union of parts of the vertebral column, is explained in Chapter 15. Congenital defects of the alimentary tract include various types of obstructions. The absence or closure of a normal body opening or tubular structure is called **atresia.** Atresia occurs in various parts of the gastrointestinal tract. The lack of an opening from the esophagus to the stomach is esophageal atresia; it is frequently accompanied by an abnormal opening between the esophagus and the trachea.

Intestinal atresia is a complete obstruction of the intestine, resulting in vomiting, dehydration, scanty stool production, and distention of the abdomen. The bile ducts are blocked in biliary atresia, and the inability to secrete bile into the duodenum causes severe jaundice to develop. The liver and spleen become greatly enlarged. Another congenital obstruction of the intestinal tract is **pyloric stenosis,** in which the circular sphincter muscle is hypertrophied, closing the opening between the stomach and the duodenum. Symptoms include projectile vomiting, dehydration, constipation, and weight loss. Corrective surgery has been very effective in removing these congenital obstructions of the intestinal tract, just as it has been for congenital heart disease.

CHAPTER SUMMARY

Genetic information is conveyed from parents to their children through the complex activity of the DNA molecule, which duplicates itself when a cell is about to divide. DNA provides a blueprint for protein synthesis in the daughter cells and comprises the genes that are arranged on the chromosomes, with half being received from each parent. Some genes are dominant and are always expressed, whereas others are recessive and require two similar genes for the expression of a trait. One pair of chromosomes, the X and Y chromosomes, determines the sex of the fetus.

Certain diseases are inherited by children just as physical traits are. Some diseases develop if only a single dominant autosomal gene is received. An example of this is Huntington's chorea, a devastating disease of the central nervous system. Other diseases develop only if a recessive gene is received from each parent, as is the case in phenylketonuria. Other diseases are sex-linked, affecting primarily males but being transmitted through females. This is the inheritance pattern in color blindness, hemophilia, and fragile X syndrome. Some diseases are found within families but are not attributable to a particular gene. The action of several genes seems to be responsible. Epilepsy, diabetes, and allergies are thought to be caused in this way.

In addition to diseases inherited by specific genes, gross chromosomal abnormalities result in other disorders. Down's syndrome is caused by chromosome 21 being in triplicate (trisomy 21). A missing or extra sex chromosome produces sex anomalies and usually mental retardation.

Certain conditions are apparent at birth or soon after, but they are not the result of genetic or chromosomal abnormalities. These are congenital diseases caused by various factors during early development. Certain heart malformations, absence of a natural body opening, or failure of a structure to close are examples of congenital diseases. These diseases are not passed on to offspring.

■ Self-Study

Mark the Answer

If a disease is caused by an autosomal dominant disorder, MARK A.
If a disease is caused by sex-linked inheritance, MARK B.
If a disease is caused by recessive inheritance, MARK C.
If a disease is caused by an autosomal chromosome abnormality, MARK D.
If a disease is caused by an abnormal number of sex chromosomes, MARK E.

_____ 1. Turner's syndrome

_____ 2. Phenylketonuria

_____ 3. Achondroplasia

_____ 4. Color blindness

_____ 5. Down's syndrome

_____ 6. Polydactyly

_____ 7. Hemophilia

_____ 8. Sickle cell anemia

_____ 9. Klinefelter's syndrome

_____ 10. Huntington's chorea

True or False

_____ 11. Klinefelter's syndrome results from lack of a sex chromosome.

_____ 12. A Turner's syndrome patient appears to be female.

_____ 13. A Down's syndrome patient has an extra autosomal chromosome.

_____ 14. Cerebral palsy is genetically transmitted.

_____ 15. If one parent is normal and the other has one defective gene for an autosomal dominant disorder, 50% of their children may be affected.

_____ 16. If one parent is normal and the other is a carrier for cystic fibrosis, all of their children will be normal.

_____ 17. The gene for color blindness is on the Y chromosome.

_____ 18. A defective dominant gene is usually transmitted from a parent who is heterozygous for the trait.

_____ 19. Phenylketonuria (PKU) is caused by autosomal recessive gene inheritance.

_____ 20. A person with sickle cell anemia is heterozygous for the trait.

(Answers on page 449)

Chapter 5

Dietary Deficiencies and Excesses: Malnutrition, Obesity, and Alcoholism

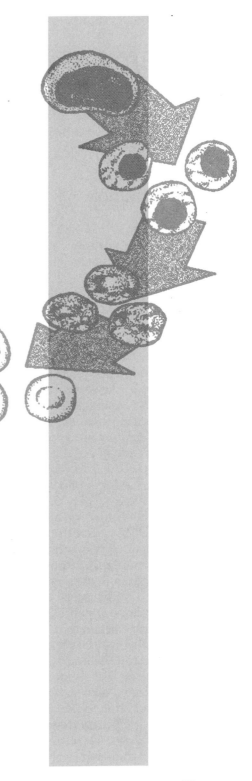

Chapter Outline

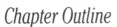

- Malnutrition
- Vitamin Deficiencies
- Hypervitaminosis
- Mineral Deficiencies
- Anorexia Nervosa
- Bulimia
- Obesity
- Alcoholism
- Chapter Summary
- Self-Study

D *isease can result from a dietary deficiency such as malnutrition or from excess as in obesity and alcoholism. Psychoneurotic diseases, anorexia, and bulimia, are examples of diseases involving dietary deficiency or excess.*

MALNUTRITION

Diseases that may be classified as nutritional diseases stem from a wide range of causes. Malnutrition caused by poverty, ignorance, or the unavailability of proper foods comprises one end of the spectrum, whereas excessive intake due to obesity, hypervitaminosis, or alcoholism is at the other extreme.

The concept of malnutrition is generally associated with an inadequate availability of food, but one can suffer nutritional deficiencies in the midst of plenty. Several diseases that will be discussed in this book are actually nutritional diseases in that they deprive the body of essential dietary elements.

Various malfunctionings of the gastrointestinal system (Chapter 10) prevent the use of nutrients in the diet. The absence of gastric, intestinal, and pancreatic enzymes to digest proteins, carbohydrates, and lipids deprives the body of these nutrients. Pancreatitis (Chapter 11), for example, interferes with digestion when the diseased pancreas is unable to function. Digestive disturbances that cause persistent vomiting or diarrhea also result in malnutrition.

Not only is the digestion of foodstuffs essential for proper nourishment, but the end products of digestion must be absorbed through the intestinal wall. Bile secretion, essential for the absorption of lipids, including the fat-soluble vitamins A, D, E, and K, may be inadequate for such reasons as liver dysfunction, a diseased gallbladder, or obstruction of the bile ducts. The malabsorption syndrome (Chapter 10) causes the loss of essential nutrients in the stools. Pernicious anemia (Chapter 6) develops in the absence of gastric intrinsic factor needed for absorption of vitamin B_{12} from the digestive tract. This condition occurs even if vitamin B_{12} is present in the diet.

Impaired blood circulation through the liver due to cirrhosis or severe hepatitis (Chapter 11) deprives the body of proteins normally synthesized by the liver. The storage of nutrients in the liver is also diminished when the organ is severely damaged. The liver normally stores glucose (as **glycogen**), vitamins, and iron.

Diabetes mellitus (Chapter 13) is a nutritional disease in which glucose cannot enter the cells to be used in the absence of insulin. Glucose is lost in the urine, and the untreated diabetic metabolizes fat reserves and even tissue protein.

In addition to the diseases already described that cause malnutrition, the failure to eat properly is associated with other problems that will be discussed in this chapter. A disease of psychoneurotic origin in which willful starvation leads to total emaciation and even death, will be explained.

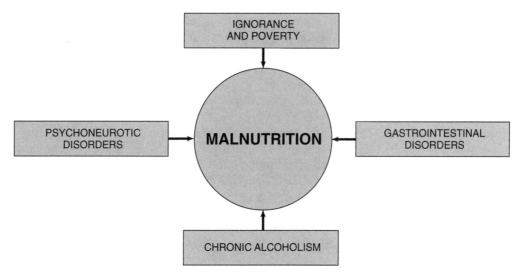

Figure 5–1. Possible causes of malnutrition.

The effect on the body of excessive food intake that leads to obesity, and of toxicity that results from hypervitaminosis, will be discussed. The medical aspects of alcoholism, many of which are related to malnutrition, will also be explained. Figure 5–1 summarizes causes of malnutrition.

VITAMIN DEFICIENCIES

The importance of vitamins included in a healthful diet will be discussed in Chapter 19 on Wellness. The following vitamin deficiencies result in various disorders.

■ Vitamin A Deficiency

Vitamin A is essential for vision because it is an essential component of **rhodopsin,** the pigment that absorbs light in the rods of the retina. A lack of vitamin A results in an inability to see in dim light, a condition known as **night blindness.**

It is thought that vitamin A contributes to the integrity of mucous membranes—those membranes that line the respiratory, gastrointestinal, and urogenital tracts. In the absence of vitamin A, the membranes become dry and susceptible to cracking, permitting the entrance of infectious organisms. The **conjunctiva,** the membrane that lines the eyelids and covers the eyeball, also becomes dry and cracked, making it a target for infection.

Vitamin A deficiencies are most commonly seen in parts of India and China where the diet is limited. The condition also exists when vitamin A is present in the diet but cannot be used because of malabsorption (Chapter 10).

Vitamin A is derived from a plant pigment, **carotene,** which is converted into vitamin A by the liver. Dairy products, egg yolks, and vegetables are good sources of vitamin A.

■ Vitamin D Deficiency (Rickets)

Rickets is a bone disease in children in which calcification is impaired, resulting in weak, deformed bones (Chapter 16). Vitamin D is essential for the absorption of calcium from the gastrointestinal tract. Rickets develops when vitamin D is deficient in the diet. The lack of vitamin D in adults results in a softening of the bones, a disease known as **osteomalacia** (Chapter 16).

Rickets and osteomalacia can be prevented by a diet that includes vitamin D fortified milk. Exposure to sunlight also provides a source of vitamin D, as ultraviolet light converts a substance in the skin (sterol) to vitamin D. Rickets and osteomalacia can be treated by administering vitamin D concentrate and improving the diet, and by exposure to sunlight. Vitamin deficiency diseases are summarized in Figure 5–2.

■ Vitamin K Deficiency

Vitamin K is essential to the blood-clotting mechanism and is made in the intestine by bacterial action. The liver synthesizes an enzyme, **prothrombin,** with the aid of vitamin K. This enzyme initiates the chain reaction in the blood coagulation process. In the absence of prothrombin, hemorrhaging occurs. Excessive use of antibiotics can destroy the normal flora (naturally occurring bacteria) of the intestine and thus prevent the production of vitamin K.

■ Vitamin C (Ascorbic Acid) Deficiency

A lack of vitamin C prevents proper formation of the cementing substance that holds epithelial cells together. This causes capillary walls to be weak and to rup-

DEFICIENT VITAMIN	DISEASE	MANIFESTATIONS	TREATMENT AND/OR PREVENTION
VITAMIN C		BLEEDING GUMS AND HEMORRHAGES INTO TISSUES	CITRUS FRUITS AND GREENS
VITAMIN A	NIGHT BLINDNESS	POOR VISION IN DIM LIGHT; DRY, CRACKED MUCOUS MEMBRANES	DIET INCLUDING DAIRY PRODUCTS, AND VEGETABLES
VITAMIN D	RICKETS, OSTEOMALACIA	WEAK, DEFORMED BONES	VITAMIN D SUPPLEMENTS, VITAMIN D FORTIFIED MILK, AND EXPOSURE TO SUNLIGHT
VITAMIN K		TENDENCY TO HEMORRHAGE	NORMAL DIET

Figure 5–2. Effects of vitamin deficiencies.

ture easily, resulting in hemorrhage into surrounding tissues. Small black-and-blue spots appear all over the body as a result of the rupture of blood vessels. Anemia may develop over a period of time and manifest itself by weakness, palpitation, and breathing difficulties.

The gums are particularly affected and they bleed easily. The open lesions provide an entry for bacteria, and, as the gum tissue becomes necrotic, the teeth loosen and fall out. Synthesis of **collagen,** a fibrous protein in connective tissue, is impaired, causing wounds to heal poorly.

A vitamin C deficiency can be prevented by a diet that includes fresh fruits and vegetables, particularly tomatoes, citrus fruits, and greens. The activity of the vitamin is lost by heating and drying.

HYPERVITAMINOSIS

An excess of vitamins, particularly of vitamins A and D, can be harmful because the excess produces a toxicity **(hypervitaminosis).** Children can become very ill after swallowing a large number of vitamin pills, and they can experience gastrointestinal disturbances and drowsiness. A generalized edema develops that even increases intracranial pressure. The affected child is irritable and fails to gain weight. The symptoms are reversible once the toxicity has subsided.

Excessive vitamin D causes too much calcium to be absorbed from the gastrointestinal tract. **Hypercalcemia** results in deposits of calcium in organs such as the kidney, heart, lungs, and the walls of the stomach. The digestive system is affected, and excessive thirst and polyuria develop. Some of the damage to the tissues may be irreversible.

MINERAL DEFICIENCIES

Minerals are only required in minute amounts, but a lack of them has serious consequences. An inadequate level of **calcium** prevents proper bone formation and maintenance, as described in Chapter 16. A calcium deficiency also interferes with the blood-clotting mechanism. One type of anemia develops in the absence of the **iron** needed to form hemoglobin. One type of goiter results from insufficient **iodine.**

Potassium may be adequate in the diet but missing from the body under certain conditions. An excessive secretion of aldosterone causes a loss of potassium through the kidneys. A prolonged loss of fluid through vomiting or diarrhea removes potassium, as will the action of certain diuretics. The muscles are weak in a potassium deficiency and the heart muscle is particularly affected.

Sodium is usually adequate in the diet but may be lacking in Addison's disease (Chapter 13), in which aldosterone is not secreted by the adrenal cortex. Sodium is essential for the transmission of nerve impulses and muscle contraction. The principal functions of minerals are summarized in Figure 5–3.

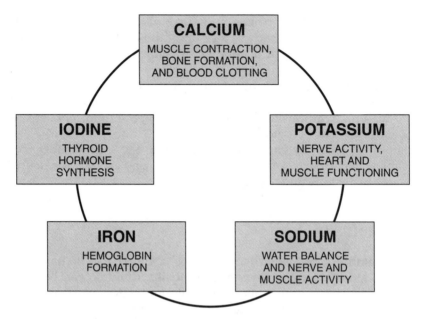

Figure 5–3. Minerals and their principal functions.

ANOREXIA NERVOSA

Anorexia nervosa is a disease of psychoneurotic origin in which the aversion to food leads to emaciation and malnutrition. Anorexia nervosa is most common in teenage girls, and the incidence of the disease has greatly increased in recent years. The nation's obsession with thinness is now even affecting preteens. The disease is rare in males and older age groups. The desire to be thin and the patient's misconception of her own body size underlie the onset of the disease. The girl may have been socially normal before the initial dieting or may have shown some social maladjustments.

The anorexia nervosa patient actually starves herself, yet denies that she is not eating adequately. Personality changes are noticeable as she becomes irritable, full of anxiety, and depressed. She may become hostile toward her parents who encourage her to eat and to see a doctor, and family relationships become strained.

Anorexia nervosa is not an accurate name for this disease. *Anorexia* means loss of appetite, but the patient with this disease experiences hunger and may be obsessed with food. She may elaborately prepare food for others but not for herself. Counting calories and weighing food becomes ritualistic. She often prepares her food—consisting primarily of fruits, vegetables, and cheese—when she is alone and sure that no one is giving her extra calories. At least she does not suffer from a vitamin deficiency, but she avoids all carbohydrates.

Hunger may cause occasional orgies of overeating, and the patient then induces vomiting and uses laxatives excessively. She exercises strenuously, increasing the weight loss. The girl becomes absolutely emaciated in appearance. Her face is gaunt with protruding bones, yet she denies that she is thin and even perceives herself as fat. An anorexia nervosa patient is seen in Figure 5–4.

Amenorrhea, the absence of menstruation, always accompanies anorexia nervosa. The ovaries stop producing estrogen and gonadotropins are not secreted by

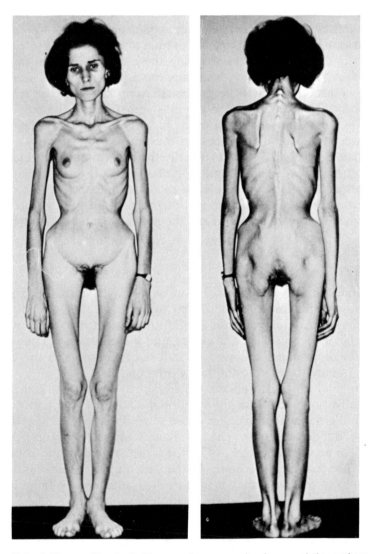

Figure 5–4. A 19-year-old patient with anorexia nervosa showing emaciation and premature aging. Note protruding bones, muscle atrophy, and sunken abdomen. Patient is about 5′ 6″ tall and weighs 66 pounds.

the anterior pituitary. Amenorrhea occurs early in the disease, so it is not considered a result of malnutrition. A possible hypothalamic disturbance is indicated in which releasing factors for the gonadotropins are not being secreted. In rare cases of males with anorexia nervosa, the levels of gonadotropic hormones and testosterone are also decreased.

The patient with anorexia nervosa rejects the suggestion to see a physician. If the person can be persuaded to be examined, the findings include low blood pressure, decreased heart rate, and anemia. Dehydration caused by the induced vomiting and excessive use of laxatives results in a depletion of potassium. This deficiency causes muscular weakness and heart abnormalities. A lowered resistance due to malnutrition makes the patient susceptible to infections.

Treatment is directed toward correcting the malnutrition and the abnormal psychological state. Hospitalization is usually required to assure close observation of eating and bathroom habits. The patient may resist eating the required diet, fearing that she will become fat. The therapist must assure the patient that the weight she gains will help to make her more attractive and improve her health. Cooperation between the patient and therapist is essential to recovery.

The psychological problems that underlie the disease must be uncovered and proper psychotherapy given as the condition of anorexia nervosa is extremely serious. The patient can actually starve herself to death, and her depressed state may make her suicidal. Even after an apparent recovery, close supervision is required as relapses of the disease are common and the mortality rate is quite high.

BULIMIA

Bulimia, a gorge–purge syndrome, is the opposite of, yet similar to, anorexia nervosa. Teenage girls and women in their early twenties are the usual victims of this condition. As in anorexia nervosa, the goal of the patient is to avoid weight gain. Bulimics may be of average weight or obese, and therefore the disease may not be detected. Food-eating binges followed by induced vomiting and the use of laxatives and diuretics are the manifestations of this condition.

The detrimental long-term effects include tooth decay, constant sore throat, and swollen salivary glands from the abnormal acidity of the induced vomiting. Dehydration and electrolyte imbalance cause serious disturbances, and liver damage is common. Sudden death from heart failure or stomach rupture is possible.

Bulimia, like anorexia nervosa, is linked to a psychoneurotic condition such as depression. The patient is therefore treated with antidepressants and psychological counseling. The condition may persist through much of the bulimic's life, and management, rather than cure, is often the ultimate goal.

OBESITY

The problem of obesity affects many people in our mechanized, modern society. Machines, appliances, and modes of transportation reduce the need for expending energy to obtain food. High-calorie foods attractively packaged are readily available and easy to prepare. Life styles that include TV snacks, eating late at night, and a diet of "fast foods" contribute to the high incidence of obesity in the country.

Obesity is a nutritional disorder in which an abnormal amount of fat accumulates in adipose tissue. Adipose tissue is found under the skin, around organs such as the kidney, and in the omentum and mesentery of the peritoneal cavity. Adipose tissue acts as a reserve energy supply and as an insulating material against body heat loss. An excess of fat tissue is harmful, putting an undue strain on the heart and interfering with the contraction of muscles.

The distribution of fat varies in males and females and may be genetically determined. Men accumulate fat in the upper trunk and not in the arms and legs, but women store fat in the lower trunk and in the arms and legs. Women also have more subcutaneous fat than men, which is probably an effect of the female sex hormones. Estrogen given in high dosage in birth control pills, for example, often causes a weight gain.

Obesity develops when an excess of calories is consumed for the energy expended by a person. Too much food or too little exercise causes the deposition of fat. The rate of fat synthesis is faster than the mobilization of fat to active muscles for the production of energy.

On the Practical Side

ARTIFICIAL SWEETENERS

The popular artificial sweetener, Nutra Sweet (aspartame) is used in many soft drinks, foods, and for table use. Very small quantities of Nutra Sweet are required compared to table sugar (sucrose) because of its intense sweetness. This greatly reduces caloric intake. Nutra Sweet does not have the bitter aftertaste of saccharine, a long-time substitute for sugar.

A person is considered obese if his or her weight is 15 to 20 percent more than the ideal weight given in standard life insurance height–weight tables. These tables give the proper weight ranges for men and women of light, medium, and heavy frames. A person is overweight if the upper limit of the appropriate range is exceeded.

■ Causes of Obesity

Obesity generally results from overeating high-calorie foods—refined sugar and fats—and from insufficient exercise. Genetic factors are probably involved, as obese children tend to have parents who are overweight. Obesity that develops in children is due to the formation of an increased number of adipose cells, the number of which may be genetically determined.

Culture and environment also play a part in the obesity of children. Excessive intake of food may be encouraged, and, too often, good behavior is rewarded with foods such as cookies and candy. This overfeeding of children sets a regulatory system of the hypothalamus at a level that will maintain the habit of overeating.

The central nervous system regulates food intake. An area of the hypothalamus contains the "satiety center," which has an inhibiting effect on the "feeding center." The satiety center senses when enough food has been eaten and it inhibits the feeding center from stimulating further food intake. Eating should be directed toward relieving genuine hunger. The obese person tends to eat because food is available, tastes good, or looks attractive.

Adult-onset obesity results from an enlargement of already existing adipose cells rather than from an increase in their number. The number of adipose cells formed in childhood is irreversible, and for this reason a child's diet should be carefully controlled to prevent excessive weight gain throughout life. Rarely is obesity due to a hypoactive thyroid, a popular misconception. Excessive water retention is not a cause of obesity. Adipose cells, which are filled with fat, contain very little water.

Psychological factors can cause obesity if a person's reaction to stress often precipitates a desire for food as a means of satisfaction.

■ Diseases Aggravated by Obesity

Excessive weight poses many problems, both psychologic and physical. The obese person feels unattractive and may become withdrawn. Children who are obese have difficulty participating in sports, are often teased about their weight, and are hurt by their peers.

Cardiovascular problems accompany obesity, and the death rate due to these ailments is significantly higher among the obese than among those who are not. Atherosclerosis develops as a result of the high level of serum lipids. Excessive fat deposits in heart muscle interfere with its contractions, the heart is overworked as it pumps blood through the extensive vascularity of the adipose tissue, and the left ventricle enlarges. Hypertension is often a complication of obesity.

Respiratory difficulties of hypoventilation with carbon dioxide retention occur when the chest wall cannot be moved adequately. Fat deposits interfere with contraction of the diaphragm and the other respiratory muscles. Inadequate oxygenation of the brain results in lethargy or somnolence.

Osteoarthritis, a degenerative joint disease, is aggravated by excessive weight. As will be explained in Chapter 16, osteoarthritis affects primarily weight-bearing joints: the knees, hips, and lower spine. Flat feet also worsen due to obesity.

Varicose veins frequently develop in the obese, as the excessive adipose tissue interferes with the return of blood from the legs. Diaphragmatic hernias and gall-bladder disease are also more common in overweight people.

Maturity-onset diabetes occurs far more often in those who are obese than in those who are not. A habit of excessive carbohydrate intake overtaxes the **beta cells,** the insulin-producing cells of the pancreas, and they cease functioning. One of the most serious complications of diabetes is atherosclerosis, to which obese people are already prone.

The liver is an important organ for the metabolism of fat, but when fat is in excess, metabolic disturbances occur, and fat accumulates in the liver. The fatty infiltration severely injures the liver cells, so they are no longer able to function. This condition is known as "fatty liver" and occurs in chronic alcoholism as well as in obesity. The complications of obesity are summarized in Figure 5–5.

■ Diagnosis and Treatment of Obesity

Comparison of a person's weight with the standard height–weight tables mentioned previously, is the best way to diagnose obesity. Another mechanism to measure the thickness of subcutaneous fat is with an instrument called a skin-fold caliper. The percentage of body fat can then be determined using a special chart.

Obesity is treated with diet, exercise programs, and drugs, but the most effi-

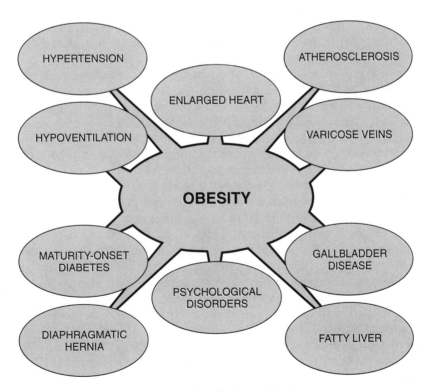

Figure 5–5. Complications of obesity.

cient method is diet. Weight loss is a slow, painful process and requires great effort. The loss of one to three pounds per week is considered ideal. An obese patient may lose weight successfully at the beginning of a diet and then reach a plateau, at which time no weight is lost and even a slight gain may occur. Although this is normal, it is very discouraging to the patient, who then may stop dieting.

Appetite depressants, **amphetamines** and related compounds, may be prescribed at the beginning of a diet regimen while the patient is establishing new eating habits. The use of amphetamines must be carefully controlled to prevent side effects. These drugs can cause excessive nervousness, restlessness, insomnia, dry mouth, and constipation.

A good diet should be balanced nutritionally and include protein, some unsaturated fat, and enough carbohydrate to provide glucose to the cells and to minimize the feeling of hunger. Vitamins and minerals should be provided through a balanced diet. Mild reduction in the use of table salt will prevent excessive retention of water. The patient must learn to change eating habits and to train the appetite so that weight will not be regained once the strict diet is completed.

Reduction diets that take into account the patient's size, sex, physical activity, and desired speed of weight loss are the most satisfactory. Women usually lose weight on a diet of 500 to 1000 calories per day and men lose on a diet of 1500 to 2000 calories.

Fad diets or crash diets are rarely successful and may even be harmful by causing malnutrition or metabolic disturbances. These diets do not help the obese person to change eating habits or train the appetite; weight lost on fad diets is generally regained. The adipose cells are not destroyed with weight loss, but only shrink in size and refill easily with fat when the diet is stopped. An exercise program should accompany the reducing diet; the strenuousness of the exercise depends on the physical condition of the person. Great exertion is required to burn up calories, but even a regular program of walking can increase muscle tone.

Obesity is easier to prevent than to overcome. By establishing proper eating habits in childhood, an excessive number of adipose cells will not be formed if the diet is nutritionally high but calorically low. Control of diet is particularly important if a child has a genetic tendency toward obesity.

Excessive weight gain occurs often during certain periods of childhood, infancy, early school age, and puberty. In women, pregnancy and the menopause are times when weight is easily gained, and special care should be taken to avoid excessive caloric intake. The avoidance of sugar in the form of pastries and soft drinks, and fat in cream, fried foods, gravy, and salad dressing will limit caloric intake and subsequent adipose tissue development. Alcohol is also very high in calories—100 calories per ounce—and has no nutritional value.

Weight reduction in the overweight person dramatically improves the physical ailments associated with obesity. Blood pressure is reduced, the level of circulating lipids that cause atherosclerosis is lowered, and the distress of osteoarthritis is lessened. Diabetes is more easily controlled when excessive weight is lost. The self-image of the obese person who successfully loses weight is greatly improved, and the psychological change makes the effort worthwhile.

On the Practical Side

YO YO DIETING

Yo Yo dieting may be dangerous. Weight lost on commercial diets or with commercial products is usually regained as soon as normal eating is resumed. Severe dieting lowers the rate at which calories are burned; when food intake increases after dieting the body uses fewer calories and stores more fat. A long-term study showed that great fluctuations in weight increased the risk of coronary heart disease.

ALCOHOLISM

Alcoholism is a serious disease with far-reaching consequences. It disrupts marriages, adversely affects children, and threatens job security. Physical damage to the alcoholic is extensive, affecting the nervous system, the cardiovascular system, and the gastrointestinal tract particularly. The American Medical Association supports the following definition of alcoholism: "Alcoholism is an illness characterized by significant impairment that is directly associated with persistent and excessive use of alcohol. Impairment may involve physiological, psychological, or social dysfunction."

The alcoholic is totally dependent on the drug, alcohol, and centers life around it, making sure of an adequate supply and opportunity to drink. The use of other drugs with alcohol frequently compounds the problem. Most authorities agree that there is no single cause of alcoholism but that a combination of factors contribute to its onset and progression. There is no conclusive evidence that it is caused by a genetic factor.

Many psychological problems have been proposed as the cause of alcoholism: emotional disturbances during childhood, a feeling of insecurity, hostility, depression, and countless others. While any of these factors may play a part in the complex etiology of alcoholism, none is considered the sole cause.

Sociological setting may be a factor in the development of the disease. In some circles, heavy drinking is considered a socially sanctioned behavior. Parties are not considered complete without alcohol, and often the host or hostess will encourage the guests to have "one more drink" when they have already had too much. The effects of alcohol on the nervous system include a feeling of relaxation and a release from anxieties, tension, and fears. As this experience is repeated through heavy drinking, alcohol becomes the habitual response to the problems of life.

■ Signs and Symptoms of Alcoholism

Alcoholism can have an insidious and gradual onset. The alcoholic generally experiences feelings of guilt and denies that drinking has become a problem. He or she begins to drink surreptitiously, drinks early in the day, and gulps down drinks when the opportunity arises. Periods of intoxication become regular and more serious, and blackouts are common, with periods of complete amnesia. Behavior becomes irresponsible, resulting in arrest for drunken driving, frequent absenteeism from work, and family problems. The alcoholic resents any discussion about drinking and generally resists treatment.

A physician may suspect alcoholism in a patient whose face is flushed and who shows a tremor about the mouth and tongue. Coarse tremors of the hands are observed, the patient may appear nervous and complain of digestive or motor disturbances. Further examination of the patient reveals other complications of alcohol abuse. Long-term abuse of alcohol takes its toll on the digestive system, the cardiovascular system, and the brain. Malnutrition often accompanies alcoholism depriving the patient of essential nutrients such as vitamins for cellular activity.

Effects of Excessive Alcohol on the Central Nervous System. Alcohol is a depressant on the central nervous system. Large quantities of alcohol interfere with the transmission of nerve impulses in the brain and affect coordination, speech, and judgment. A very high concentration of alcohol in the blood can even suppress the respiratory, cardiac, and vasomotor centers of the brain, causing shock and death.

The effect of alcohol on the central nervous system depends on the amount and the time span in which it was consumed. Alcohol is rapidly absorbed from the gastrointestinal tract into the blood. Some is absorbed from the stomach, but most alcohol absorption is from the duodenum. Drinking "on an empty stomach" is not only irritating to the gastric mucosa, but the alcohol is more rapidly absorbed by the blood when there is nothing in the duodenum to delay gastric emptying.

Alcohol is carried to the liver through the portal vein and is then circulated through the body. Most metabolism and detoxification of alcohol actually occurs in the liver, but the rate of the reaction is limited. Enzymes convert alcohol to acetaldehyde and other fragments that are burned to produce energy.

The effect of excessive alcohol ingestion wears off when it has been metabolized. This causes a period of nerve excitability, a release from the depressive effect, that accounts for the "morning-after" tremors. The effectiveness of another drink in overcoming the shakiness leads to a physical dependence on alcohol that becomes stronger as alcoholism progresses.

Long-term excessive consumption of alcohol can cause a condition known as the **organic brain syndrome.** Its manifestations include impaired judgment, poor powers of concentration, and memory lapses. The symptoms progress with continued drinking, but they may be reversed with abstinence.

Wernicke's encephalopathy is a brain disease often associated with chronic alcoholism, although it may have other causes such as thiamine deficiency. Wernicke's disease is a medical emergency in which the patient becomes mentally confused and disoriented and may suffer delirium tremens. Eye movements are abnormal and double vision may be experienced. **Nystagmus**—involuntary, rapid movement of the eyeball—is characteristic of the disease. The muscular coordination necessary for standing and walking is impaired. Treatment includes a highly nutritious diet and vitamin B supplements, particularly thiamine. If prompt treatment is administered, the symptoms can be reversed.

Thiamine, a B vitamin, is a coenzyme necessary for carbohydrate metabolism, and the lack of this vitamin particularly affects the cardiovascular and nervous systems. Nerve fibers become demyelinated, interfering with the transmission of nerve impulses. "Pins and needles" sensations are experienced, and the limbs become weak and numb. This can develop in chronic alcoholics who do not eat adequately. The effect on the nervous system causes mental confusion, an unsteady walk, and a paralysis of the muscles that move the eyes.

The effect of a niacin deficiency on the nervous system is variable, ranging from chronic depression to violent, irrational behavior. Degeneration of neurons in the brain results from the lack of this vitamin. Chronic alcoholics and drug addicts may develop the disease in the absence of adequate nutrition. The symptoms may be reversed through an improved diet and large doses of vitamin supplements.

Effects of Alcoholism on the Digestive System. Alcohol in excess is an irritant to the gastric mucosa, causing erosion and ulceration of the tissue. Gastritis is often a complication of alcoholism, as will be explained in Chapter 10. Ulceration that occurs due to the irritating effect of alcohol, particularly on an empty stomach, can lead to serious hemorrhaging. Some alcoholics experience nausea and vomiting in the morning after heavy drinking and are able to suppress the symptoms with another drink. This enables them to continue drinking during that day, and the cycle repeats itself.

Liver ailments caused by alcoholism are discussed in Chapter 11. Excessive alcohol has a toxic effect on the liver cells, causing tissue destruction and fibrosis. Alcoholic hepatitis and cirrhosis interfere with essential functions of the liver. Blood-clotting disturbances result from the inability of the liver to synthesize plasma proteins essential to coagulation, and hemorrhages in the gastrointestinal and urogenital tracts are common. Severe **ecchymoses**—hemorrhagic spots—develop in the skin and mucous membranes. **Epistaxis,** or bleeding from the nose, also results from the deficiency of proteins essential to clotting. **Esophageal varices,** described in Chapter 8, are a complication of cirrhosis and may lead to a fatal hemorrhage.

Feminization of the male cirrhosis patient results from a hormonal imbalance. The nonfunctioning liver is unable to inactivate estrogen secreted by the adrenal cortex, and the **hyperestrogenism** that develops causes enlargement of the breasts **(gynecomastia)** and testicular atrophy. Pubic and axillary hair becomes sparse.

Pancreatitis, although it has other causes, is often related to chronic alcoholism (Chapter 11). The disease destroys the pancreas through enzymes that are abnormally released into the tissue. The patient generally experiences nausea, vomiting, and severe pain. As the pancreas becomes more and more necrotic, the likelihood of hemorrhaging increases. Treatment includes a nonirritating diet with no fat or alcohol.

Delirium tremens, DTs, is a medical emergency caused by heavy drinking over a long period of time and may occur after withdrawal from heavy alcohol intake. The symptoms include delirium with illusions and vivid hallucinations that are terrifying to the patient. The patient is extremely restless and shakes uncontrollably. The metabolic rate is increased, causing excessive sweating.

The patient with delirium tremens requires hospitalization in a quiet restful atmosphere. Attendants should show a calm, reassuring manner and observe the patient carefully to prevent self-injury. A comprehensive medical examination is essential to determine if there are any other complications such as signs of heart failure or pneumonia. The patient is very susceptible to respiratory tract infections because of lowered resistance.

Fluid, electrolyte, and nutritional balance must be maintained, and this may require intravenous feeding. Sedation may be required, but it must be administered with caution to prevent overdosage. When the patient is able to take food, the diet should be high in protein and carbohydrates but low in fat and include vitamin B supplements. The complications of chronic alcoholism are summarized in Figure 5–6.

Hepatic coma develops in the final stages of advanced liver disease. This is caused by an accumulation of ammonia in the blood, which has a toxic effect on the brain. The ammonia accumulates when the liver is unable to detoxify it and form urea, the normal breakdown product of protein metabolism. The hepatic coma patient has periods of stupor or coma and manifests neurologic abnormalities. The flapping of outstretched arms is characteristic of the uncontrolled muscular contractions.

Oxygen or a combination of oxygen and carbon dioxide, the stimulus for the respiratory center of the brain, must be administered. Airways must be cleared using mechanical aids. If the patient is in shock, intravenous fluids or blood transfusions are required.

Effects of Alcoholism on the Cardiovascular System. Chronic alcoholism leads to progressive cardiac failure. Alcohol reduces the force of heart muscle contractions and an **arrhythmia,** a deviation from the normal rhythm of the heart beat, develops. The heart enlarges, and thrombi frequently form in the coronary arteries. Fatty infiltration of the heart muscle generally occurs. If cirrhosis accompanies the alcoholism, circulation is impaired further as congestion develops in the veins. A severely damaged liver interferes with blood flow through the portal vein, causing a back pressure in the vessels emptying into it.

■ Alcohol and Pregnancy

There is an increasing awareness of how a mother's excessive consumption of alcohol during pregnancy affects the developing fetus. Alcohol diffuses into the bloodstream of the fetus through the placenta, just as nutrients and oxygen do. Be-

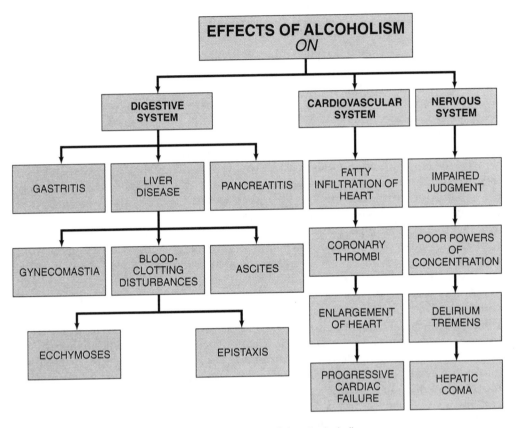

Figure 5–6. Complications of chronic alcoholism.

cause of its small size, the fetus is significantly affected by the alcohol and is likely to be born with physical and mental defects. The earliest weeks of pregnancy are the most critical for development and the most dangerous time for the mother to drink excessively.

Babies of alcoholic mothers are frequently born with **fetal alcohol syndrome.** Mental retardation is the most serious component of the syndrome, but physical growth before and after birth is also retarded. Heads tend to be smaller than those of normal babies, and limb and joint abnormalities are common. A characteristic facial appearance, particularly of the mouth and eyes, develops. The eye slits are small, the nose is short and pugged, and the jaws are underdeveloped. The babies are often born suffering withdrawal symptoms, manifested by stiffness and irritability. Fetal alcohol syndrome is most likely to occur if the mother has had a drinking problem for 5 to 10 years.

■ Treatment of Alcoholism

Alcoholism is a treatable chronic disorder that is best controlled by early intervention and continuing attention. The treatment is directed toward enabling the alcohol-dependent patient to deal with problems and environment without using alcohol.

The best treatment for a particular alcoholic patient depends on the person. The patient may deny having a drinking problem and resist treatment for a time, but with the help of a physician, family member, employer, or friends, he or she may come to realize the need for assistance. Once the drinking problem has been recognized and the patient is willing to be treated, numerous facilities and resources are available.

Alcoholics Anonymous has been extremely effective for countless people and is very widespread geographically in its operation. Alcoholism Information Centers are listed in telephone books and offer valuable suggestions. Many programs are offered for alcoholics by church organizations, the Veterans Administration, employers, and local community organizations.

The mental and physical health of the alcoholic patient determines the most appropriate type of treatment. A personal physician, a psychotherapist, group therapy, or behavior-modification programs are among the options. The emphasis is always directed toward rehabilitation.

Admission to a general or psychiatric hospital is often required for serious alcoholism problems. Comprehensive alcohol treatment centers are also available where the physical and mental problems of the alcoholic can be treated. Delirium tremens and hepatic coma are medical emergencies requiring hospitalization.

Other facilities include detoxification centers for the acutely intoxicated, who once would have been put in jail. Half-way houses or recovery houses are helpful for the alcoholic who is adjusting to coping with life without alcohol. Relapses occur, but as with any chronic illness, they should not indicate that the treatment has failed. The alcoholic who achieves control of the disease sees life in a new light and believes that the struggle was worth it.

CHAPTER SUMMARY

Malnutrition develops from a wide variety of causes: the unavailability of required nutrients, diseases that prevent use of ingested food, chronic alcoholism, eating unbalanced meals, and psychoneurotic disorders.

Vitamins are essential parts of cellular enzyme systems and must be obtained from fruits and vegetables because the body cannot synthesize them. Various diseases develop as a result of specific vitamin deficiencies.

A nutritional disease that is becoming quite common among young girls in this country is anorexia nervosa, in which the patient starves herself to the point of emaciation and even death. Psychoneurotic problems underlie the disease, and the girl has a misconception about her own body size, envisioning herself as fat when, in fact, she is extremely thin.

Another problem related to food intake is obesity. Excessive eating and inadequate exercise are generally the cause of the problem. Obesity is a serious condition that adversely affects the cardiovascular and respiratory systems and may lead to maturity-onset diabetes mellitus. Gallbladder disease and osteoarthritis are also aggravated by obesity.

The excessive consumption of alcohol over a prolonged period of time seriously impairs body functioning. Chronic alcoholism can lead to many diseases of the digestive system—gastritis, pancreatitis, cirrhosis of the liver—and is frequently accompanied by malnutrition. The cardiovascular system is affected together with the central nervous system. Manifestations of the effect of alcohol on the brain are impaired judgment, poor powers of concentration, and memory lapses. The medical emergencies, hepatic coma and delirium tremens, result from long-term alcohol abuse.

Treatment for the nutritional diseases discussed in this chapter is a balanced diet with adequate vitamin supplementation. Treatment for obesity includes diet, exercise, and, often, psychological counseling or group therapy. Alcoholism is treated medically and psychologically in a variety of ways, all of which are directed toward rehabilitation of the patient physically, mentally, and socially.

■ Self-Study

True or False

_____ 1. The activity of vitamin C is lost by heating and drying.
_____ 2. Bleeding gums may be associated with vitamin C deficiency.
_____ 3. Vitamin D deficiency causes osteomalacia in adults.
_____ 4. Vitamin D deficiency is essential for the blood-clotting mechanism.
_____ 5. Vitamin A contributes to the integrity of mucous membranes.
_____ 6. An anorexia nervosa patient suffers from a severe vitamin deficiency.
_____ 7. High acidity causes tooth decay in bulimia.
_____ 8. Lack of calcium causes goiter.
_____ 9. Obesity in adults results from formation of new adipose cells.
_____ 10. Amenorrhea is associated with anorexia nervosa.

Match

_____ 11. epistaxis
_____ 12. hyperestrogenism
_____ 13. delirium tremens
_____ 14. echymoses
_____ 15. nystagmus

a) uncontrolled rapid eye move ments
b) bruises
c) medical emergency
d) severe nose bleed
e) gynecomastia

Match

_____ 16. calcium
_____ 17. sodium
_____ 18. iodine
_____ 19. iron
_____ 20. potassium

a) thyroid hormone production
b) water balance and nerve activity
c) bone formation
d) heart and muscle function
e) hemoglobin production

(Answers on page 449)

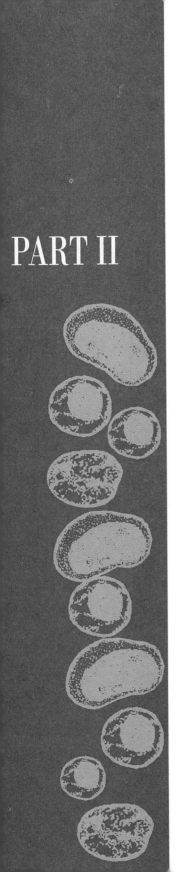

PART II

Diseases of the Systems

Each system can malfunction in its own unique way. Part II describes the normal structure and function of each system, and relates the diseases of the system to an organ or system failure.

Chapter

6. Diseases of the Blood
7. Diseases of the Heart
8. Diseases of the Blood Vessels
9. Diseases of the Excretory System
10. Diseases of the Digestive System
11. Diseases of the Liver, Gallbladder, and Pancreas
12. Diseases of the Respiratory System
13. Diseases of the Endocrine System
14. Diseases of the Reproductive System and Sexually Transmitted Diseases
15. Diseases of the Nervous System
16. Diseases of the Bones, Joints, and Muscles
17. Diseases of the Skin
18. Stress and Aging
19. Wellness: Diet and Exercise

Chapter 6

Diseases of the Blood

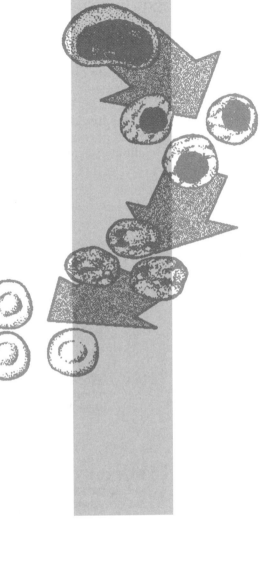

Chapter Outline

- Composition of Blood
- The Anemias
- Excessive Red Blood Cells
- Bleeding Diseases
- Diseases of White Blood Cells and Blood-Forming Tissue
- Diagnostic Procedures for Blood Diseases
- Chapter Summary
- Self-Study

*O*ur life depends on an adequate blood supply to all body tissues. Blood distributes oxygen, nutrients, salts, and hormones to the cells, and carries away the waste products of cellular metabolism. Blood also provides a line of defense against infection, toxic substances, and foreign antigens.

COMPOSITION OF BLOOD

Red bone marrow and lymph nodes are the blood-forming tissues of the body. **Erythrocytes,** or red blood cells, and **platelets** are made in red bone marrow; **leukocytes,** or white blood cells, are made in both red marrow and lymph tissue. These formed elements comprise about 45 percent of the blood, and plasma, the remaining 55 percent. The ratio of formed elements, mostly red cells, to whole blood is called the **hematocrit.**

Erythrocytes normally number about 5 million/mm^3 of blood in males, and about 4.5 million/mm^3 of blood in females. Red blood cells are biconcave in shape

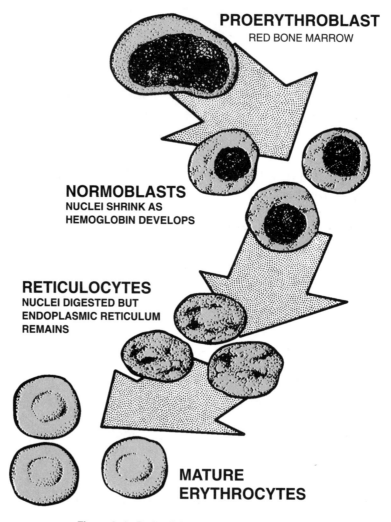

Figure 6–1. Red cell development—erythropoiesis.

and when mature possess no nucleus. The **hemoglobin** contained within the red cells is responsible for carrying oxygen throughout the body. The amount of hemoglobin is normally about **16 grams per 100 milliliters** (16g/dl) of blood in males, about 14 g/dl of blood in females.

The process of red cell formation is called **erythropoiesis.** This takes place in the red marrow of flat bones such as the sternum, hip bones, ribs, and skull bones. A hormone, **erythropoietin,** synthesized principally by the kidney, stimulates this cell development. As erythrocytes mature, they go through several stages before entering the circulation. They begin as large, nucleated, primitive cells called **proerythroblasts** and at this stage possess no hemoglobin. The proerythroblasts multiply, but daughter cells, called **normoblasts,** are small. The normoblasts contain a nucleus, but it begins to shrink as the cytoplasm fills with hemoglobin synthesized by the endoplasmic reticulum. The nucleus is eventually digested and absorbed, and the cell is then called a **reticulocyte.** When the reticulum is lost, the cells become mature erythrocytes ready to circulate. Figure 6–1 illustrates red cell formation. Maturation of erythrocytes is more a degenerative process than one of differentiation, which makes these cells unique. Understanding this developmental pattern is important because certain serious blood conditions are evident when immature red cells, normoblasts, or reticulocytes, are found in the circulation. Examples of these conditions will be discussed.

THE ANEMIAS

One of the most common blood diseases is anemia. Although there are many kinds of anemia and as many causes, there is one common denominator: a reduction in the amount of oxygen-carrying hemoglobin. **Anemia** can result from a loss of red blood cells due to prolonged bleeding or rupture of the cells, **hemolysis.** Anemia can also be caused by the improper formation of new red blood cells, which can be the result of poorly functioning bone marrow or an iron or vitamin deficiency. Erythrocytes are unusual because they do not possess a nucleus and therefore cannot divide to form new cells. The life span of red blood cells is about 120 days, and new cells must constantly replace those that die.

Certain symptoms are common to all anemias. The anemic person is generally pale (a condition called *pallor*) and the mucous membrane of the mouth is light in color, as is the nail bed. This lack of normal color is due to hemoglobin deficiency. Fatigue and muscular weakness accompany the disease because of the inadequate oxygen supply to the cells and tissues. The anemic person experiences **dyspnea,** or shortness of breath. To meet the need for more oxygen, the respiration rate is quickened and the patient experiences palpitations of the heart as it attempts to pump more blood to the tissues.

The anemias may be classified in several ways; they will be considered here on the basis of their causes. It is important for the physician to diagnose the cause of a patient's anemia, for this is what must be treated. The iron prescribed appropriately for one type of anemia is ineffective, even harmful, for another type.

■ Pernicious Anemia

Pernicious anemia is a blood disease in which the red blood cells are few in number, although each cell contains the normal amount of hemoglobin. In this disease the body is unable to use certain elements in the diet that are essential for proper blood cell formation. Two factors are necessary for erythrocytes to mature: an **intrinsic factor** found in normal gastric juice and an **extrinsic factor,** vitamin B_{12}. The intrinsic factor acts as a carrier for vitamin B_{12}, enabling the vitamin to be absorbed from the small intestine and into the blood. The intrinsic factor is not secreted in pernicious anemia, so in its absence, vitamin B_{12} cannot be absorbed even if it is present in the diet. Red cells cannot develop properly, which causes the anemia. The red cell count falls significantly and many immature forms of erythrocytes—normoblasts and reticulocytes—are found.

The signs of pernicious anemia are a low red cell count, low hematocrit, and absence of the intrinsic factor. Hydrochloric acid normally found in the stomach is also absent. Digestive disturbances occur, and the tongue appears sore with a smooth, glazed look. The lack of vitamin B_{12} also causes disturbances in the nervous system such as numbness and tingling sensations in the hands and feet. Pernicious anemia responds well to vitamin B_{12} given by injection.

■ Hypochromic Anemia

In hypochromic anemia the number of red cells is adequate but the amount of hemoglobin per cell is reduced. The word **hypochromic** means lighter than normal color. Since it is hemoglobin united with oxygen that gives red cells their color, this deficiency causes the cells to appear pale and washed-out. Hypochromic anemia is an iron-deficiency anemia that can result from chronic blood loss from an ulcer, a malignant lesion, or **menorrhagia** (excessive bleeding during menstruation). A diet deficient in iron can also cause this type of anemia. Hypochromic anemia frequently develops after a pregnancy during which the mother's iron supply has been depleted through red blood cell development in the fetus. This anemia responds well to treatment with large doses of iron.

■ Hemolytic Anemia

Certain anemias are due to the rupturing of red blood cells and are classed as hemolytic anemias. With the hemolysis of the cells, hemoglobin is released into the plasma. The hemoglobin itself breaks down, yielding another colored pigment, **bilirubin,** which is normally detoxified by the liver and converted into bile. This pigment is orange, and as it accumulates in the plasma, it causes a **jaundiced**—yellow or orange—appearance in the tissues. Some hemolytic anemias are acquired through an environmental factor, whereas others are hereditary; a gene for imperfect red cell formation is transmitted.

Sickle cell anemia is an example of an inherited red cell deficiency and is generally confined to blacks (see Chapter 4). Neither the hemoglobin molecule nor the cell itself can form properly. The cells are crescent- or sickle-shaped (see Fig. 6–2) and tend to rupture. The rapid destruction of erythrocytes stimulates produc-

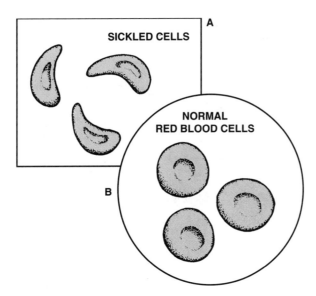

Figure 6–2. Sickled red blood cells **(A)** compared with normal red blood cells **(B)**.

tion of new red cells, but at a rate faster than they can mature. As a result, many reticulocytes and nucleated red cells enter the circulation.

The symptoms of sickle cell anemia include jaundice of the sclera (the white of the eye); pain in the arms, legs, abdomen; and recurrent fever. In a crisis period, headache, paralysis, and convulsions can develop from a cerebral blood clot that forms as a result of the abnormally viscous blood. There is no effective treatment for sickle cell anemia; only the symptoms can be treated.

Spheroidal or spherocytic anemia results from cell formation that is spherical rather than biconcave. The abnormal shape of the cell makes it fragile and susceptible to rupture. A characteristic symptom of this disease is jaundice caused by the release of hemoglobin. The spleen becomes enlarged, **splenomegaly,** due to an accumulation of red cells, many of which are immature. The immature cells result from hyperactivity of the bone marrow as it attempts to compensate for the red cell destruction. The spleen is often removed **(splenectomy)** to prevent the misshapen cells from becoming trapped in the spleen and rupturing. The splenectomy renders the patient very susceptible to infection since the defense provided by the spleen has been lost.

Hemolytic anemias can be acquired. An allergic reaction to drugs such as the sulfonamides may cause this condition. The malarial parasite also causes hemolysis of red cells and severe anemia.

Erythroblastosis fetalis, hemolytic anemia of the newborn, can result when the mother is Rh⁻ and the fetus has Rh⁺ blood inherited from the father. Although the fetal and maternal circulations are separate, fetal blood can reach the mother's blood through ruptures in the placenta occurring at delivery. The mother then becomes sensitized to the Rh factor of the fetus and makes antibodies against it. If

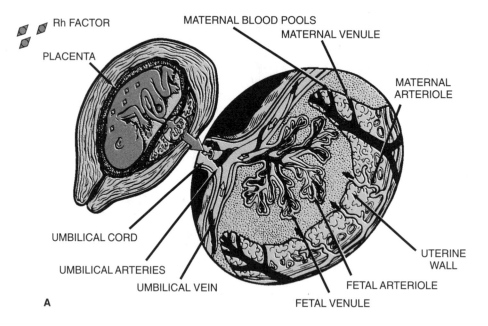

A

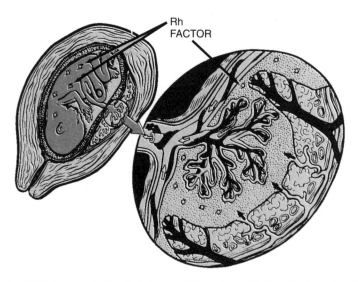

B

Figure 6–3. (A) Rh incompatibility: Rh⁺ fetus of Rh⁻ mother. **(B)** Sensitization of mother: Rh factor enters mother's blood through ruptures in placenta at time of delivery. (*Continued*)

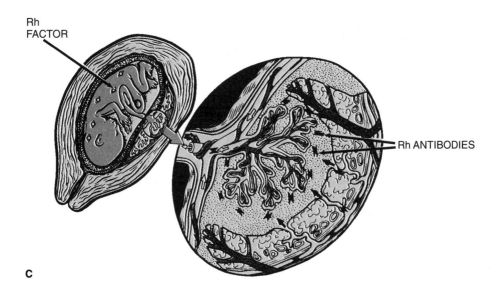

C

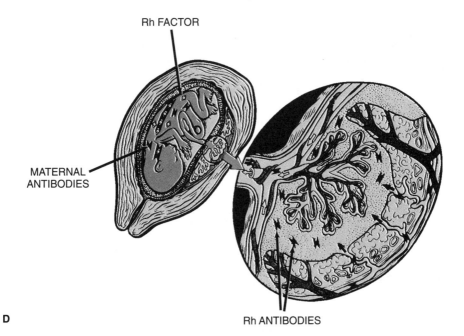

D

Figure 6–3. (C) Subsequent pregnancy: mother sensitized to Rh factor makes antibodies against it. **(D)** Maternal antibodies enter fetal circulation: antibodies destroy fetal Rh⁺ red cells causing severe anemia.

these antibodies reach the fetal blood through the placenta in subsequent pregnancies, the red cells of the fetus will be hemolyzed. The destruction of the cells stimulates rapid production and release of new cells before they mature. Therefore, many erythroblasts appear in the fetal blood. The name **erythroblastosis** means an abnormal increase, *osis,* of erythroblasts, immature cells. The severity of this disease ranges from mild anemia with jaundice to death of the fetus. The first child is usually not affected, but in subsequent pregnancies the possibility of erythroblastosis increases. Rh incompatibility is illustrated in Figure 6–3.

Medical science has developed a technique to prevent this condition. The Rh⁻ mother is given a vaccine of Rh immune globulin within 24 hours of delivery or aborting an Rh⁺ infant. The vaccine prevents antibody production against the Rh factor. This treatment is effective only if the mother is not already immune to the Rh factor; that is, she has had no previous Rh⁺ pregnancies. Blood testing to determine if Rh incompatibility exists is an essential part of prenatal care.

■ Aplastic Anemia

If the bone marrow fails to function, another type of anemia, **aplastic anemia,** results. The bone marrow stops producing erythrocytes, leukocytes, and platelets. The patient then is not only anemic but cannot fight infection, a leukocytic function, and has a bleeding tendency due to platelet depletion. Exposure to excessive radiation, certain drugs, and industrial poisons can cause the bone marrow to stop functioning. This is a very serious condition, and regular blood transfusions are generally necessary. Aplastic anemia is now being treated quite successfully with bone marrow transplants.

■ Secondary Anemia

If anemia is the result of another disease, it is referred to as **secondary anemia.** It generally accompanies chronic kidney disease, leukemia, and cancer. In this ane-

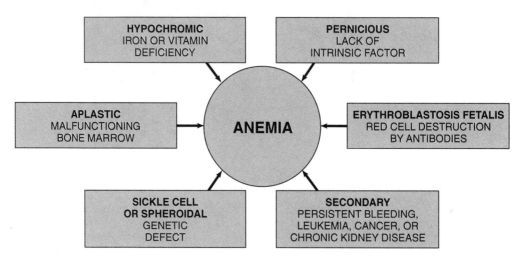

Figure 6–4. Types of anemia and their causes.

mia the number of cells is near normal but the amount of hemoglobin is low. The best treatment is the administration of iron. The types of anemia and their causes are summarized in Figure 6–4.

EXCESSIVE RED BLOOD CELLS

■ Primary Polycythemia
The effects of a red blood cell (RBC) deficiency have been considered. What about an excessive RBC count? This condition, polycythemia, has detrimental effects and is caused by hyperactivity of red bone marrow. In polycythemia the erythrocytes can number 7 to 11 million/mm³ of blood. The hematocrit of a person with polycythemia may be as high as 70 to 80 percent compared to the normal of 45 percent. The elevated cell count increases blood volume; this raises the blood pressure, placing an increased workload on the heart. Blood flow is reduced due to increased viscosity and a tendency to clot. The hyperactivity of the bone marrow is sometimes due to a tumorous condition. The excessive number of red cells gives the skin a purplish appearance. Mucous membranes are extremely red, and the eyes appear bloodshot. The spleen, a reservoir for erythrocytes, is always enlarged. Leukocytes and platelets, also produced in the bone marrow, show elevated counts which is important for diagnostic purposes. Treatment is aimed at reducing the red cell count and the blood volume. Periodic bloodletting **(phlebotomy)** is used to reduce the volume and radiation therapy to decrease red cell production.

■ Secondary Polycythemia
The body often compensates for an inadequate oxygen supply by producing an excessive number of erythrocytes. This can occur when no disease condition exists. Natives of very high altitudes have elevated red cell counts because of the low oxygen content in the air. Trained athletes often have high red cell counts because their muscles have an increased need for oxygen. This compensatory mechanism is called **erythrocytosis** or secondary polycythemia.

In certain diseases of the circulatory and respiratory systems, secondary polycythemia can also occur. It frequently accompanies congenital heart diseases, congestive heart failure, and emphysema. These diseases will be discussed later.

One factor distinguishes secondary polycythemia, or erythrocytosis, from primary polycythemia. In erythrocytosis only the red cell count is elevated, but in polycythemia all blood cell types produced in the bone marrow are affected.

BLEEDING DISEASES

■ Hemophilia
The mechanism for control of bleeding is defective in some people. Hemophilia is a blood disease that results from this inability to clot normally. It is strictly a

hereditary disease, generally affects only males, and is transmitted by females (see Chapter 4). The hemophiliac can experience prolonged and severe bleeding from even a minor cut or injury. Internal bleeding occurs, often into the joints, causing intense pain and injury. This inability to clot blood is due to the lack of a plasma protein required in the chain reaction of coagulation. Blood platelets, essential in the clotting mechanism, are normal in the hemophiliac. Treatment includes transfusions of whole blood or plasma and the administration of clotting protein concentrates.

■ Purpura (Thrombocytopenia)

A deficiency in the number of platelets, which initiate the blood-clotting process, causes spontaneous hemorrhages in the skin (Fig. 6–5), mucous membranes of the mouth, and internal organs. Small, flat, red spots called **petechiae,** appear, or larger hemorrhagic areas **(ecchymoses),** may develop. Gastrointestinal and urogenital hemorrhages, as well as severe nosebleeds, may also occur. The disease is known as **purpura,** or **thrombocytopenia.** Thrombocyte is another name for platelet, and the suffix, *penia*, means a scarcity.

The disease may result from impaired platelet production, antibodies to platelets, or from an allergic response to drugs. Thrombocytopenia may also be idiopathic, that is, of unknown origin. In the latter case, the patient may have a history of bleeding after injury or minor surgery such as a tooth extraction. The condition is referred to as **ITP,** for **idiopathic thrombocytopenia purpura.**

Corticosteroids are generally administered, but if the hemorrhagic condition is chronic, the spleen is often removed (a splenectomy), as it is a major site of platelet destruction.

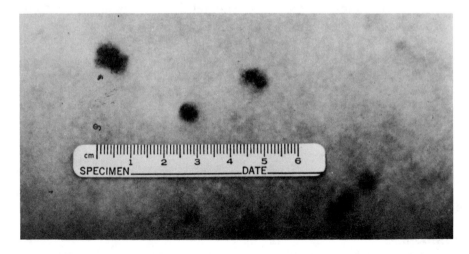

Figure 6–5. Photograph of ecchymotic hemorrhages in the skin. (*Courtesy of Dr. David R. Duffell.*)

DISEASES OF WHITE BLOOD CELLS AND BLOOD-FORMING TISSUE

■ Leukemia

Leukemia is cancer of the tissues that form white blood cells, the bone marrow, or lymph tissue as well as the white blood cells. The leukocyte count is extremely elevated from the normal range of 7000 to 9000/mm^3 of blood to 200,000 to 1 million/mm^3 of blood.

The signs and symptoms of leukemia include fever, swollen lymph nodes, **lymphadenopathy,** joint pain, and abnormal bleeding (Fig. 6–6). Anemia, with its

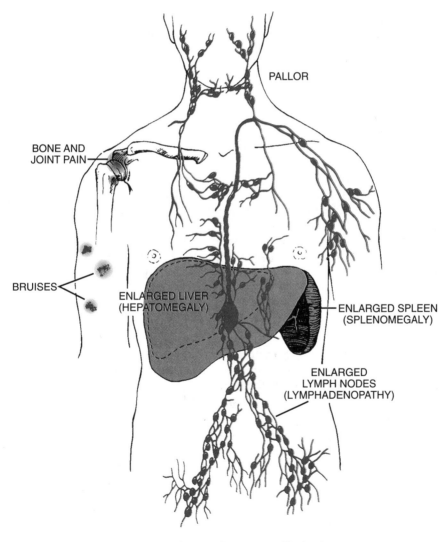

Figure 6–6. Signs and symptoms of leukemia.

manifestation of weakness, shortness of breath, and heart palpitation, accompanies the leukemia. Red blood cells are overwhelmed by the malignant white cell proliferation and cannot develop properly in the malignant bone marrow. Organs where blood is stored, the spleen and liver, become greatly enlarged with the infiltration of white cells. Figure 6–6 summarizes signs and symptoms of leukemia.

The cancerous tissues grow at a rapid rate, using up the body's nutrients, thus causing weight loss. White blood cells, the principal cells in fighting infection, are produced faster than they mature, so they are unable to fight infection normally. The patient becomes highly susceptible to infection and must be protected against exposure to bacteria. As the number of leukocytes increases, the number of platelets decreases; this interferes with the blood-clotting mechanism, causing a tendency to hemorrhage and to bruise.

The two kinds of leukemia are named on the basis of the site of the malignancy. If the cancer is in the bone marrow it is called **myelogenous** leukemia; the primitive white cells in this tissue are called *myelocytes*. In myelogenous leukemia it is granulocytes that are greatly increased, whereas both red blood cell and platelet production are decreased.

The other type of leukemia is **lymphocytic,** or cancer of the lymph nodes. The lymphocytes in this case are the only white cells that are increased, but they become disproportionately high in number and are immature and ineffective. Figure 6–7 gives a comparison of leukemia types.

The cause of leukemia is unknown, but it may be due to a virus, or exposure to radiation may be a factor. A high incidence of leukemia has been found in people exposed to fallout from nuclear weapons. Heredity may also play a part in its etiology.

Both kinds of leukemia can be chronic or acute. Acute lymphocytic leukemia is the more common form in children; it affects immature cells. Acute lymphocytic leukemia has an abrupt onset and progresses rapidly. Acute myelogenous leukemia is more common in adults. Chronic leukemias have a prolonged course and may be either type. More mature cells are affected.

Progress is being made in controlling leukemia and even curing it. Treatment goals include eliminating leukemic cells through chemotherapy and the use of antineoplastic agents to inhibit growth of cancerous tissue. The patient's ability to tolerate adverse affects of treatment is enhanced and psychosocial support is given. There are three stages of chemotherapy treatment—induction, consolidation, and maintenance. The induction stage utilizes intensive chemotherapy to induce complete remission. The largest number of leukemic cells are destroyed at this time. Intermittent cycles of chemotherapy are given during the consolidation stage to eliminate any remaining leukemic cells. If complete remission is achieved, the patient enters the maintenance stage, which is designed to continue the remission. Low doses of chemotherapeutic agents given in combination every 3 to 4 weeks prevent leukemic cells from returning to the bone marrow.

Depending on the type of leukemia, 50 to 90 percent complete remission is possible, which means that there is no evidence of the leukemia in serum studies and the bone marrow returns to normal.

TYPE	INCIDENCE	SIGNS AND SYMPTOMS	PROGNOSIS
Acute myelogenous leukemia (AML)	Most common non-lymphocytic leukemia Usually develops in persons between ages 30 and 60 Slightly more common in men	Usual: anemia, pallor, fatigue, weakness, fever Possible: bleeding, bruising, bone and joint pain, headache, enlarged lymph nodes, liver and spleen, recurrent infections	Generally poor Death usually results from infection or hemorrhage
Acute lymphocytic leukemia (ALL)	Most common cancer in children Usually diagnosed before age 14 (peak incidence between ages 2 and 9) Males slightly more affected than females	Usual: anemia, pallor, fatigue, weakness, swollen lymph nodes, recurrent infections Possible: bleeding, bruising and headache	Generally good (inital treatment usually induces remission in 95% of patients) Overall cure rate is 50%
Chronic myelogenous leukemia (CML)	About 20% of blood cancers Usually affects adults between ages 40 and 60	Usual: loss of appetite, weight loss, fatigue, weakness, enlarged spleen and liver Possible: bleeding, bruising, bone and joint pain, fever, enlarged lymph nodes	Generally poor Average survival time of 3 years No treatment produces satisfactory results
Chronic lymphocytic leukemia (CLL)	Most common form of blood cancer in industrial countries Affects primarily older adults, males more frequently than women	Usual: loss of weight loss, enlarged lymph nodes and spleen Possible: fever	Depends on patient's age, signs, and symptoms Median survival time is 4 to 6 years

Figure 6–7. Comparison of leukemia types.

■ Malignant Lymphomas

Lymphomas include several types of malignancies of lymphoid and reticuloen-dothelial tissue. The origin of the disease is thought to be a virus that interferes with normal lymphocyte production. Patients have a significantly impaired immune system.

Lymphomas have been classified based on the cell type involved and include lymphocytic lymphoma, histiocytic lymphoma, and Hodgkin's disease. Lympho-cytic lymphoma is very similar to chronic lymphocytic leukemia. It affects the elderly and runs a prolonged course. In histiocytic lymphoma the cells are poorly differentiated. The disease has a low cure rate. Lymphomas usually do not spill malignant cells into the bloodstream as occurs in leukemia.

Hodgkin's disease, of which there are several forms, is the most common type of lymphoma. Diagnosis is made on the presence of a characteristic cell

On the Practical Side

BONE MARROW TRANSPLANTATION

Bone marrow transplantation is now being used effectively to treat aplastic anemia, certain types of leukemia, sickle cell anemia and other diseases of the blood and blood-forming tissue. Recent advances in technology reduce the need for a match between donor and recipient. Certain cells of the immune system, T lymphocytes, which would cause rejection are removed from the donor's bone marrow. The remaining suspension of normal bone marrow cells is given like a blood transfusion. The cells enter the general circulation of the recipient and grow in the bone marrow cavities.

found in lymphoid tissue. Hodgkin's disease is thought to be of viral or infectious origin. It manifests itself as a painless swelling in one lymph node, fever, and weight loss. The disease may progress and affect other lymph tissue and organs. The malignancy responds well to radiation and chemotherapy if it is localized in one or two areas. The disease is characterized by long periods of remission, and the cure rate is good if treated early. One form of Hodgkin's disease affects primarily young adults and more often men than women.

■ Infectious Mononucleosis

Many children and young adults experience **infectious mononucleosis.** The symptoms are rather vague—mild fever, marked fatigue, sore throat, and swollen lymph nodes. The patient also has a peculiar putrefactive bad breath. Blood tests show an elevated white cell count with an abnormally high percentage of atypical lymphocytes that resemble monocytes. Mononucleosis results from the **Epstein–Barr herpes virus,** which infects the upper respiratory tract. Diagnosis is based on the presence of antibodies to the virus. The swollen cervical lymph nodes are the response to the virus. Patients with "mono" usually test positive within 5 to 7 days of onset but it may not show up for 10 to 14 days.

Viral diseases do not respond to antibiotics; therefore, antibiotics are not effective in treating infectious mononucleosis. Bed rest is required if the patient has a fever, and adequate sleep is necessary. There are generally no restrictions on normal activity except avoidance of contact sports. The tender, enlarged spleen is susceptible to injury.

Mononucleosis is not a particularly contagious disease. It may be transmitted by kissing and is sometimes called the "kissing disease." Because it often affects young college students who may be under stress it is also referred to as the "college disease."

DIAGNOSTIC PROCEDURES FOR BLOOD DISEASES

Blood tests are extremely significant diagnostically for systemic diseases as well as specific blood conditions. Blood tests reveal cholesterol levels, important enzyme levels, electrolyte (salt) balances, as well as blood components.

A bone marrow smear may be done when certain blood disorders are suspected. The smear is obtained by introducing a sharp needle into the bone marrow cavity (usually of the iliac crest) and withdrawing a sample of the marrow. The test shows if the bone marrow is adequately manufacturing normal red and white blood cells and platelets. The smear is particularly helpful in diagnosing aplastic and pernicious anemias, leukemia, and purpura when used in conjunction with other tests.

A **total white blood cell count (WBC)** can suggest infection or inflammation as well as a serious blood disease. Additional testing is required if warranted by the clinical condition of the patient.

A **differential white blood cell count** can reveal abnormalities in the ratio of leukocyte types. Figure 6–8 lists conditions indicated by an increased number of specific leukocyte types.

Important tests in the determination of anemia and polycythemia are the red blood cell count (RBC) and hematocrit or packed cell volume (PCV). The word *hematocrit* means to separate blood, which is done when a blood sample is centrifuged to separate cells from plasma. The ratio of cells, mostly red blood cells, to the total sample measures roughly the concentration of erythrocytes. Hemoglobin content of a venous blood sample can be determined in several ways and is expressed in grams of Hb/100 ml blood.

A variety of laboratory tests are used to determine the nature and extent of coagulation disorders. **Bleeding time** is a screening test in which a small stab wound is made in the earlobe or forearm. The time required to stop the bleeding and form a platelet clot is recorded. Bleeding time is prolonged in thrombocytopenia, severe liver disease, leukemia, and aplastic anemia. Blood platelets are normal in hemophilia; missing factors in the coagulation chain are determined by other tests.

Type of Leukocyte Increased	Cause
Neutrophils	Bacterial infections, inflammatory disorders, certain drugs, stress
Eosinophils	Allergies, parasitic infestations
Lymphocytes	Viral infections
Monocytes	Severe infections when controlled

Figure 6–8. Conditions indicated by an increased number of specific leukocyte types.

CHAPTER SUMMARY

The principal diseases of the blood considered have been those involving erythro-cytes, leukocytes, and platelets. Each of these formed elements of the blood has a specific function. If any is insufficient in number, improperly formed, or imma-ture, that function cannot be adequately performed. In distinguishing the various anemias, the symptoms were related to their cause, and the best treatment for each was explained. The inability to clot blood and prevent hemorrhaging was seen in hemophilia and purpura. In one a protein factor in plasma was lacking, and in the other platelets were too few in number. A malignancy of blood-forming tissues and blood cells causes leukemia. Its complications of anemia, susceptibility to infection, and a tendency to hemorrhage were considered. The incidence, signs, and symptoms and the prognosis of the various leukemias were compared. Malig-nant lymphomas were classified, the most common of which is Hodgkin's disease. Infectious mononucleosis caused by the Epstein–Barr herpes virus was described. Finally, the significance of the various blood tests was explained.

■ Self-Study

True or False

_____ 1. Hemolytic anemia can be acquired.

_____ 2. A differential white blood cell count shows increased lymphocytes in bacterial infections.

_____ 3. The main function of red blood cells is to fight infection.

_____ 4. Aplastic anemia is best treated by administration of iron.

_____ 5. The number of platelets is normal in hemophilia.

_____ 6. Erythroblastosis fetalis is a hereditary disease.

_____ 7. In erythrocytosis only the RBC's are increased.

_____ 8. In myelogenous leukemia red blood cell and platelet production are decreased.

_____ 9. ITP (idiopathic thrombocytopenia purpura), is a hereditary disease.

_____ 10. The hematocrit of a person with polycythemia is elevated.

Match

_____ 11. pernicious anemia   a) round RBC's

_____ 12. hypochromic anemia   b) failure of bone marrow

_____ 13. sickle cell anemia   c) iron deficiency

_____ 14. aplastic anemia   d) lack of intrinsic factor

_____ 15. congenital spheroidal anemia   e) affects mostly blacks

Multiple Choice

_____ 16. Erythroblastosis fetalis can only occur when _____.
   a. the father is Rh⁻ and the mother is Rh⁺
   b. both parents are Rh⁻
   c. the mother is Rh⁻ and the father is Rh⁺

_____ 17. Jaundice would occur in _____.
   a. aplastic
   b. sickle cell
   c. pernicious anemia

_____ 18. Which of the following anemias are hemolytic?
1. aplastic
2. congenital spheroidal
3. sickle cell
4. pernicious
5. hypochromic
   a. 2 and 4
   b. 1 and 3
   c. 2 and 3
   d. 3 and 5

_____ 19. Cells contain normal amounts of hemoglobin, but are few in number
in _____.
a. hypochromic anemia
b. sickle cell anemia
c. pernicious anemia

_____ 20. The Epstein–Barr herpes virus causes _____.
a. pernicious anemia
b. thrombocytopenia
c. infectious mononucleosis

(Answers on page 449)

Chapter 7

Diseases of the Heart

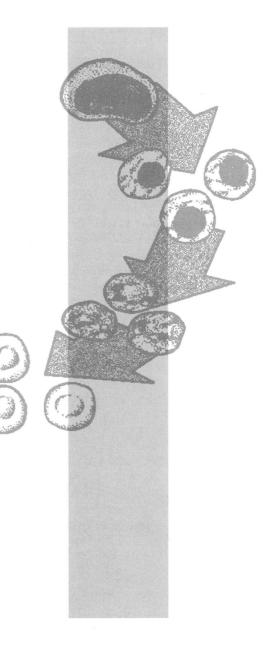

Chapter Outline

- Structure and Function of the Heart
- Relationship Between Heart and Lungs
- Influence of the Autonomic Nervous System
- Diseases of the Heart
- Symptoms of Heart Disease
- Abnormalities of Heart Action
- Diagnostic Procedures for Heart Diseases
- Chapter Summary
- Self-Study

*N*o one questions the importance of a well-functioning heart. It is the pump that keeps blood flowing to all the cells and tissues of the body.

STRUCTURE AND FUNCTION OF THE HEART

The heart consists of four chambers: a right and left atrium and a right and left ventricle. The walls of these chambers are cardiac muscle, or **myocardium.** Lining these chambers is a smooth delicate membrane, the **endocardium,** that is continuous with the lining of the blood vessels. The heart is enclosed in a double membranous sac, the **pericardium.** Figure 7–1 shows these tissues of the heart, any of which can become diseased.

A partition, or septum, separates the right and left sides of the heart. Between the atria and the ventricles are valves that assure a one-way blood flow, the **atrioventricular valves,** or AV valves. The valves are delicate but very strong and are continuous with the endocardium. The valve between the left atrium and left ventricle has two flaps, or cusps, that meet when the valve is closed and is called the **bicuspid** or **mitral** valve. The valve between the right atrium and right ventricle has three cusps and is called the **tricuspid** valve. Figure 7–2 shows these valves in the closed position. Valves are frequently damaged by rheumatic fever and endocarditis, diseases that will be explained.

At the entrance to the great vessels leaving the heart, the aorta and pulmonary

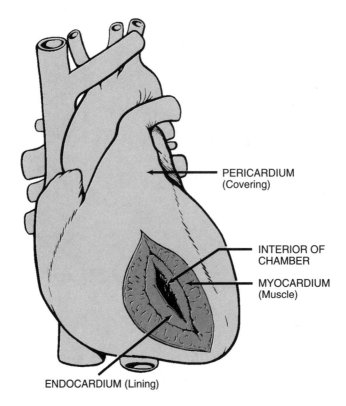

PERICARDIUM
(Covering)

INTERIOR OF
CHAMBER

MYOCARDIUM
(Muscle)

ENDOCARDIUM (Lining)

Figure 7–1. Tissues of the heart.

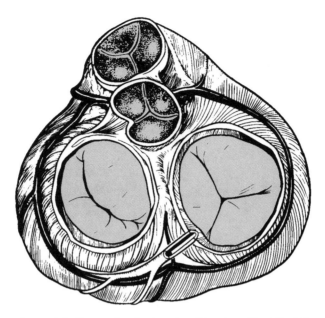

Figure 7–2. Heart valves in closed position viewed from the top.

artery, is another set of valves, the semilunar valves. The function of all the valves is to prevent the backflow of blood. The atria are the receiving chambers for blood returning from the body and the lungs; the ventricles serve as pumps sending blood throughout the body and to the lungs.

The ventricles alternately contract and relax, and when the ventricles are contracting, the atria are relaxing and filling with blood. This filling period is the **diastole,** or the diastolic phase, of the atria. The atria then contract and the ventricles relax and fill in their diastolic phase. The contracting phase of each is the **systole,** or systolic phase. The alternate contraction and relaxation of atria and ventricles comprises the **cardiac cycle.**

The heart muscle itself needs a good blood supply, which is provided by the coronary arteries that course over the surface of the heart (Fig. 7–3). These are the small vessels that frequently become blocked, causing a heart attack.

An understanding of the blood flow pattern through the heart and lungs will make the various diseases of the heart more meaningful. Valve defects, septal defects, heart attacks, and more will be considered in the light of the disease's interference with heart action.

THE RELATIONSHIP BETWEEN HEART AND LUNGS

Blood that has circulated throughout the body has given up most of its oxygen and has picked up waste products of cellular metabolism, particularly carbon dioxide.

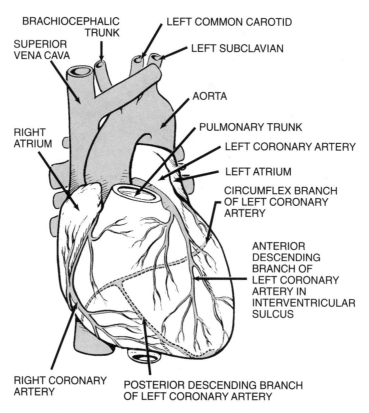

Figure 7–3. Coronary arteries and major blood vessels.

This blood enters the right atrium from the vena cavae and flows through the tricuspid valve to the right ventricle. It is then pumped into the pulmonary artery, which branches to the right and left lung. Figure 7–4 shows this path of blood flow.

At the lungs, carbon dioxide is given off and a fresh supply of oxygen is acquired by the hemoglobin. The oxygenated blood enters the left atrium through pulmonary veins and flows through the mitral valve to the left ventricle. From here the blood is pumped into the aorta, which distributes it to all parts of the body. Figure 7–5 shows the return of oxygenated blood to the left side of the heart.

INFLUENCE OF THE AUTONOMIC NERVOUS SYSTEM

Unlike other muscles, cardiac muscle can contract continuously and rhythmically without nerve stimulation. A small patch of tissue in the right atrial wall initiates the beat, and the impulse for contraction spreads over the atria and ventricles.

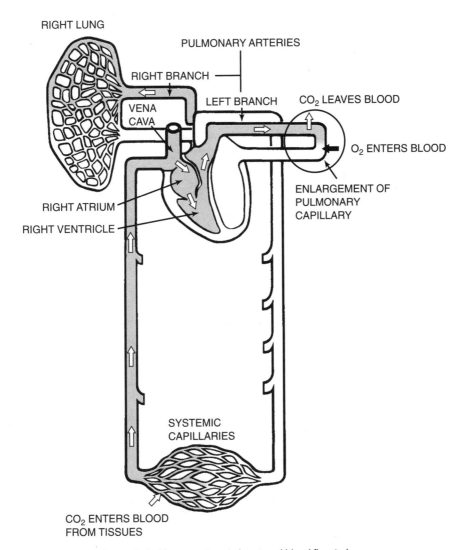

Figure 7–4. Venous return to heart and blood flow to lungs.

This specialized patch of tissue, the **sinoatrial node,** is called the **pacemaker.** A bundle of fibers, known as the *bundle of His,* conducts the impulse from the atria to the ventricles and terminates in the Purkinje fibers, which ramify through the ventricles. This conduction system is illustrated in Figure 7–6.

Although the heart muscle is not dependent on nerve stimulation for contraction, it is influenced by nerves of the autonomic nervous system for its rate of beating, the pulse rate. Two sets of nerves work antagonistically to each other, one slowing the heart, the other accelerating it. The vagus nerve slows heart action by

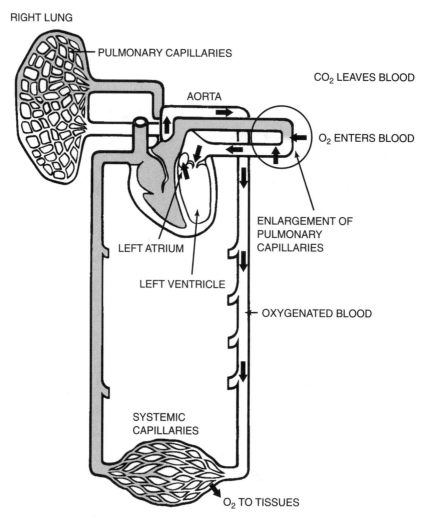

Figure 7–5. Return of oxygenated blood to heart and entry into aorta (white = oxygenated blood, red = deoxygenated blood).

means of a chemical it transmits, acetylcholine. This vagus nerve action is important because it prevents the heart from overworking by slowing it down during rest and sleep. The cardiac accelerator nerve of the sympathetic portion of the autonomic nervous system speeds up the action of the heart during periods of stress, strenuous physical activity, and excitement, when the body needs a greater blood flow. The sympathetic system triggers (or stimulates) the release of epinephrine into the blood stream. As this reaches the pacemaker of the heart, the speed of contraction is increased.

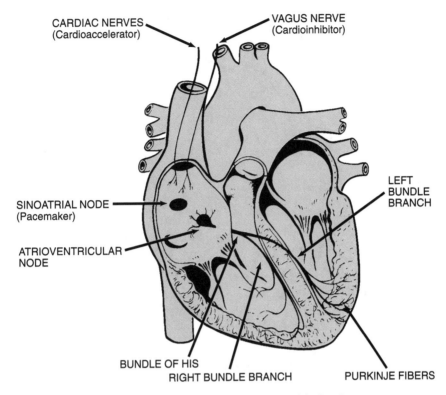

Figure 7–6. Conducting system of the heart.

DISEASES OF THE HEART

■ Coronary Artery Disease

The importance of the coronary arteries in supplying oxygenated blood to the myocardium, the heart muscle, has already been explained. Unfortunately, these small vessels can become blocked (occluded). This results when a blood clot forms on the inner wall of a coronary artery, causing a **coronary thrombosis,** or from a narrowing of the lumen, the opening within the vessel.

The narrowing of the lumen is due to deposits of fatty material, *plaque,* on the inner arterial wall, the condition termed **atherosclerosis** (Chapter 8). Figure 7–7A illustrates possible means of occlusion or blockage. **Ischemia,** a deficiency of blood supply to the heart muscle, results in a heart attack. Cardiovascular diseases are the leading cause of death in the United States.

If the lumen of the coronary artery narrows slowly, some heart muscle cells die and are replaced by scar tissue. When an area of the myocardium is suddenly deprived of blood due to occlusion of the coronary artery, that tissue dies and the dead muscle is called an **infarct.** This is a true heart attack or **myocardial infarction.** Severe chest pains generally accompany the attack, but the pain may be re-

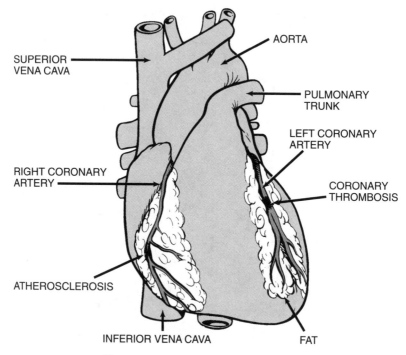

Figure 7–7A. Blockage of coronary arteries.

ferred to the neck or left arm, and the patient may feel nauseous or clammy.

The prognosis for the patient with a myocardial infarction depends on many factors. The speed with which medical attention is given is very important. Thus, CPR **(cardiopulmonary resuscitation)** can be of great assistance while waiting for an emergency care unit to arrive. Figure 7–7B shows a myocardial infarction.

The size of the coronary artery that is occluded and the extent of heart muscle damage, which is indicated by the level of certain blood enzymes, are also factors in the prognosis. If a collateral circulation is established—that is, if blood from a surrounding area channels into the damaged tissue—recovery will be better.

The damaged area can repair itself with scar tissue, but it will never serve as heart muscle again. There will be a tendency for blood clots to form or for a weakened area to rupture. Rest is needed for the repair period, but after this time, controlled exercise is advised to maintain circulation. In today's society the predisposing causes of coronary artery disease are generally well known: obesity, hypertension, smoking, a sedentary life-style, and a high-cholesterol diet.

Remarkable advances have been made in recent years in the treatment of heart disease. Severe damage to heart muscle following a heart attack has been greatly reduced by early administration of **thrombolytic** (blood clot dissolving) **drugs.** Such drugs commonly used are TPA **(tissue plasminogen activator)** and streptokinase. Other anticoagulants—aspirin and heparin—are used in conjunction with the thrombolytic drugs.

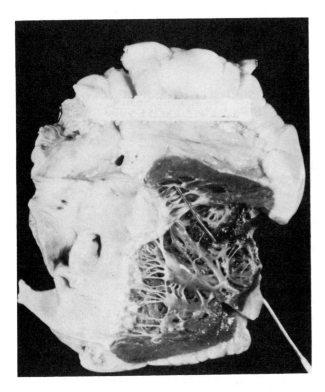

Figure 7–7B. Myocardial infarction. (*Courtesy of Dr. David R. Duffell.*)

Treatment of a myocardial infarction may require coronary bypass surgery in which a portion of the patient's vein, usually the saphenous, is used to replace the occlusion. When obstruction to blood flow is less severe, **angioplasty** may be performed. In this procedure a balloon-tip catheter is inserted into the coronary arteries and expanded to break and crush the plaques. Laser techniques have also been used to reduce the plaques.

Angina pectoris is caused by a temporary oxygen insufficiency. The patient experiences severe chest pains, which may radiate to the neck, jaw, and left arm. There is a feeling of tightness or suffocation. Attacks of angina may follow strenuous exercise, a heavy meal, exposure to severe cold, or emotional stress. **Nitroglycerin** is generally administered for angina to dilate the coronary arteries, permitting adequate blood flow. A person who experiences recurring attacks of angina should control exercise carefully.

■ Hypertensive Heart Disease

This condition is caused by long-standing high blood pressure or **hypertension.** The heart is overworked as it continues to pump against great resistance. The resistance is narrow blood vessels that result from hypertension. The **hypertensive heart** is enlarged and the left ventricle, which does the most work, hypertrophies in an attempt to meet its demands for pumping action. The ventricle finally **di-**

lates, the chamber enlarges, and it becomes exhausted, unable to pump adequately, and fails.

■ Cor Pulmonale

Cor pulmonale is a serious heart condition in which the right side of the heart fails as a result of chronic lung disease. **Pulmonary hypertension** develops as the lung blood vessels become diseased, impairing blood flow to the lungs. This hypertension overworks the right ventricle, causing it to dilate and hypertrophy. Treatment is aimed at relieving the causative lung disease by administration of bronchodilators and the use of a ventilator.

■ Congestive Heart Failure

Congestive heart failure means that the heart is pumping inadequately to meet the needs of the body. Pressure builds within the pulmonary or systemic veins, leading to distention and edema as fluid oozes into the adjacent tissues. Congestive heart failure usually develops gradually and is not necessarily life-threatening. It often follows myocardial infarctions but may also occur in other advanced heart diseases.

Congestive heart failure may involve either the right or the left side of the heart. Right-heart failure causes edema in the ankles, distention of the neck veins, and enlargement of the liver and spleen due to congestion in veins that cannot empty properly into the heart. Left-heart failure causes shortness of breath due to excessive fluid accumulation in the lungs, **pulmonary edema.** Figure 7–8 shows the effect of each type of congestive heart failure.

■ Congenital Heart Disease

The tremendous accomplishments in open heart surgery have drastically reduced the mortality rate of children born with heart defects. Most of the **congenital** abnormalities are in the septum that separates the right and left side of the heart. An opening in this septum allows a mixing of deoxygenated and oxygenated blood that causes the heart to overwork.

Septal defects may be large or small, with the smaller defects causing no problem. An example of a small septal defect is failure of the foramen ovale to close after birth. The **foramen ovale** is a small opening that allows blood from the right side of the heart to enter the left directly, bypassing the nonfunctional fetal lungs. Failure of this opening to close is the most common but least serious septal defect.

The septal defect may be in the wall between the two atria, atrial septal defect (ASD), or between the ventricles, ventricular septal defect (VSD), and it may be large. Because blood pressure is higher on the left side than on the right side of the heart, blood is generally shunted through the opening in a left-to-right direction. This factor alone would not be significant for oxygenation of the blood. Blood from the left side is already oxygenated, and blood from the right side is on its way to the lungs, but the right side of the heart is overworked. It receives blood as usual from the vena cava but also from the left side of the heart. To accommodate this blood volume, the right side dilates. Because it is required to pump more

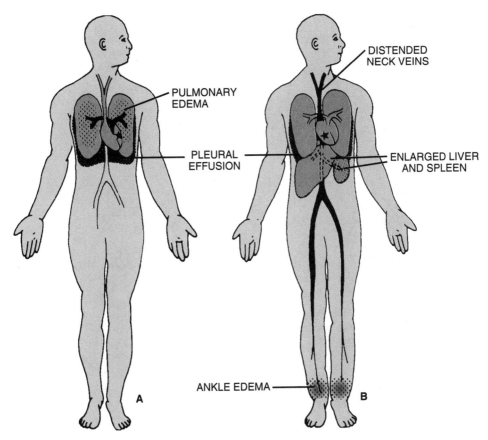

Figure 7–8. (A) Left-sided congestive heart failure. **(B)** Right-sided congestive heart failure. (*From Kent, Hart.* Introduction to Human Disease, *Appleton & Lange, 1987.*)

blood to the lungs, the right ventricle enlarges **(hypertrophies).** The left ventricle is overworked if a ventricular septal defect is large. Blood is shunted to the right ventricle, yet the left ventricle must pump enough blood into the aorta. This ventricle can become exhausted and fail.

Cyanosis, a blue color in the tissues, does not occur if the shunt of blood through the septal defect remains left to right. If the pressure becomes greater in the right ventricle than in the left, the shunt reverses and cyanosis does occur. The deoxygenated blood from the right side of the heart then enters the general circulation; the blue color is due to deoxygenated hemoglobin. Figure 7–9 illustrates the routine shunt and that which causes cyanosis.

Tetralogy of Fallot is one of the most serious of the congenital defects and consists of four (*tetra*) abnormalities. The victim of this condition is the true "blue baby"; it is born cyanotic, with all the tissues a definite blue; cyanosis is due to poorly oxygenated blood. The union of oxygen with hemoglobin gives normal arterial blood its bright red color.

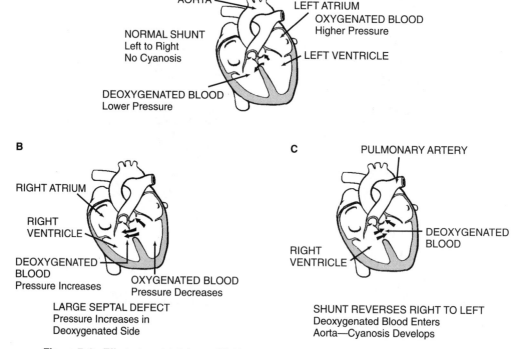

Figure 7–9. Effect of septal defects. **(A)** Normal shunt—no cyanosis. **(B)** Increased pressure in right ventricle. **(C)** Shunt reverses—cyanosis develops.

The first cause of the cyanosis is **pulmonary stenosis.** Remember, a valve leads into the pulmonary artery. **Stenosis** of a valve means that the opening is too small. Because of the narrow opening, an inadequate amount of blood reaches the lungs to be oxygenated and all body tissues suffer from this lack of oxygen.

Second, accompanying the pulmonary stenosis is a large ventricular septal defect, the seriousness of which has already been discussed. Third, a misplaced aorta overrides the ventricular septum. Normally, only oxygenated blood from the left ventricle enters the aorta, but in this case the right ventricle also feeds into the aorta, permitting the mixing of oxygenated and deoxygenated blood. Last, because of the increased strain on the right ventricle attempting to pump through a stenotic valve, the ventricle hypertrophies.

In addition to cyanosis, other signs accompany the disease. There is secondary polycythemia, a disease described in Chapter 6 as a compensatory mechanism. The inadequate oxygen supply stimulates erythropoiesis, and an excessive number of red blood cells are formed.

The fingers are clubbed and fingernails curled due to poor oxygenation of tissues at the fingertips. The child experiences **dyspnea** following any exertion, even crying. The child may assume a squatting position after exercise, which provides some relief from the breathlessness. Surgery can be performed quite successfully by bypassing the narrow opening to the lungs. Figure 7–10 shows the four abnormalities in the tetralogy of Fallot.

Patent ductus arteriosis (PDA) is a common congenital disease. The ductus arteriosis is a fetal blood vessel connecting the pulmonary artery and the aorta, shunting the blood from the nonfunctional lungs. Figure 7–11 shows this vessel diagrammatically. Soon after birth it normally closes, but if it remains open (patent), blood flows from the aorta to the pulmonary artery, where pressure is lower. This blood is oxygenated, so there is no cyanosis, but a danger is bacterial

TETRALOGY OF FALLOT

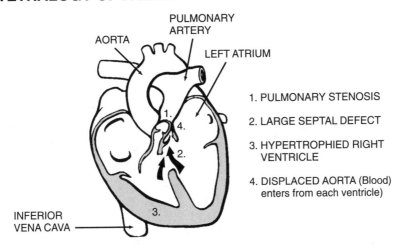

1. PULMONARY STENOSIS

2. LARGE SEPTAL DEFECT

3. HYPERTROPHIED RIGHT VENTRICLE

4. DISPLACED AORTA (Blood) enters from each ventricle)

NORMAL ANATOMY OF HEART

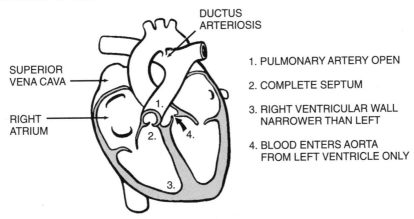

1. PULMONARY ARTERY OPEN

2. COMPLETE SEPTUM

3. RIGHT VENTRICULAR WALL NARROWER THAN LEFT

4. BLOOD ENTERS AORTA FROM LEFT VENTRICLE ONLY

Figure 7–10. Tetralogy of Fallot **(top)** compared to normal anatomy **(bottom).**

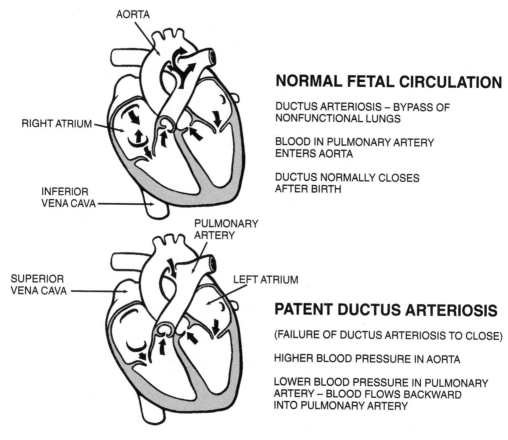

AORTA

NORMAL FETAL CIRCULATION

DUCTUS ARTERIOSIS – BYPASS OF
NONFUNCTIONAL LUNGS

BLOOD IN PULMONARY ARTERY
ENTERS AORTA

RIGHT ATRIUM

DUCTUS NORMALLY CLOSES
AFTER BIRTH

INFERIOR
VENA CAVA

PULMONARY
ARTERY

SUPERIOR
VENA CAVA

LEFT ATRIUM

PATENT DUCTUS ARTERIOSIS

(FAILURE OF DUCTUS ARTERIOSIS TO CLOSE)

HIGHER BLOOD PRESSURE IN AORTA

LOWER BLOOD PRESSURE IN PULMONARY
ARTERY – BLOOD FLOWS BACKWARD
INTO PULMONARY ARTERY

Figure 7–11. Patent ductus arteriosis.

infection at the site of the lesion, a common problem with all congenital heart defects. The open ductus can be corrected surgically by dividing the connection between the pulmonary artery and the aorta.

Coarctation of the aorta is a narrowing, or stricture, of the artery that provides blood to the entire body. The stricture occurs beyond the branching of blood vessels to the head and arms, so the blood supply to the upper part of the body is adequate. Little blood, however, flows through the constricted area to the abdomen and legs. Blood pressure is very low in the legs but is high in the arms. Many collateral blood vessels develop to compensate for this poor blood supply. This is comparable to the collateral circulation that develops after a myocardial infarction. The coarctation can be corrected surgically by cutting out (excising) the narrow segment and sewing the good ends of the aorta together. Coarctation of the aorta is pictured in Figure 7–12A as compared with the normal branching of the aorta (Fig. 7–12B).

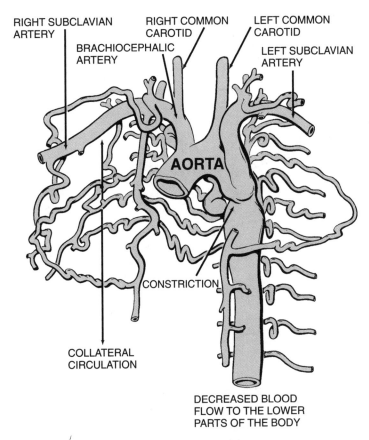

Figure 7–12A. Coarctation of the aorta.

■ Valvular Diseases

The valves assure a unidirectional flow of blood through the heart. Closed, they allow a heart chamber to fill with blood; open, they let blood flow forward.

Valves can malfunction in one of two ways. The opening may be too small **(stenotic)** for sufficient blood flow, or it may be too large to prevent backflow, **valvular insufficiency.** Valve defects cause **heart murmurs** with characteristic sounds that indicate the nature of the defect. If a valve problem is particularly serious, it can be corrected surgically by reconstruction or replacement. Some of the various valve defects and the effect they have on the heart are considered below.

In **mitral stenosis** the mitral valve opening is too small and the cusps that form the valve, normally flexible flaps, become rigid and fuse together. A deep funnel-shaped valve is formed, and much pressure is required to force enough blood through the narrow opening. Mitral stenosis often follows rheumatic fever and is more common in women than in men. Rheumatic heart disease will be described in the next section.

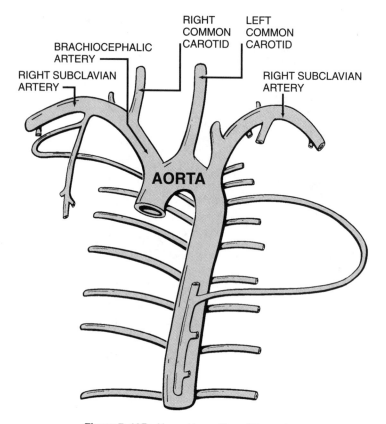

Figure 7–12B. Normal branching of the aorta.

What is the effect of mitral stenosis on the heart? The chambers that contain blood that must pass through this valve become greatly dilated. Keeping in mind the blood flow path through the heart, one can see that the left atrium and right side of the heart would be affected. This is illustrated in Figure 7–13. The left atrium also becomes hypertrophied because of overwork in pumping blood through the stenotic valve.

One of the complications of any valve defect is the tendency for a thrombus, or clot, to form on the affected area. As blood flows over the malfunctioning valve, clotting elements of the blood are deposited. If the thrombus becomes detached, it will travel as an embolism and possibly occlude a blood vessel to the brain, kidney, or other vital organ.

The damming up of blood behind the stenotic mitral valve causes a congestion in the veins. The veins, attempting to empty into the right atrium, do so with difficulty. The veins in the neck stand out prominently. As the congestion builds in the veins, fluid from the blood leaks out into the tissue spaces, causing edema.

Poor circulation causes cyanosis because an inadequate amount of oxygen is

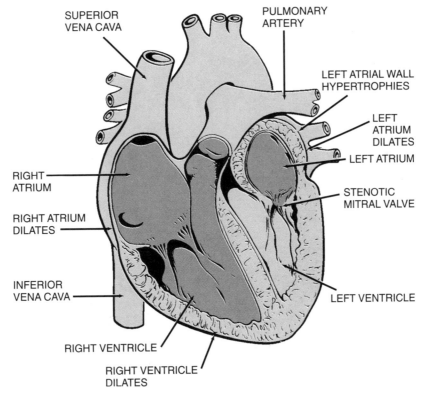

SUPERIOR
VENA CAVA

PULMONARY
ARTERY

LEFT ATRIAL WALL
HYPERTROPHIES

LEFT
ATRIUM
DILATES

LEFT ATRIUM

RIGHT
ATRIUM

STENOTIC
MITRAL VALVE

RIGHT ATRIUM
DILATES

INFERIOR
VENA CAVA

LEFT VENTRICLE

RIGHT VENTRICLE

RIGHT VENTRICLE
DILATES

Figure 7–13. Effect of mitral stenosis on the heart.

reaching the tissues. The backup of blood and congestion cause the heart to become exhausted, and **congestive heart failure** can result.

Mitral insufficiency, or incompetence, means that the opening in the mitral valve is too large and cannot close completely. This can occur if the cusps become hardened, **sclerotic,** and retract. Another cause is the failure of specialized muscles, called *papillary muscles,* in the ventricle. These are attached to the underside of the cusps by means of little cords and normally prevent the cusps from swinging up into the atria when the ventricles contract. If the papillary muscles fail to contract, the cusps open toward the atria under the force of ventricular blood.

Aortic stenosis, the narrowing of the valve leading into the aorta, occurs more often in men than in women and most frequently in men over 50. It may result from rheumatic fever but not as frequently as does mitral stenosis. Sometimes it is a congenital defect or it may occur with hardening of the arteries; the cusps become rigid and adhere together. Masses of hard, calcified material are deposited giving a warty appearance to the valve. Because the left ventricle of the heart must pump through this valve into the aorta, this chamber hypertrophies greatly through overwork. This condition is shown in Figure 7–14. An inadequate amount of blood may be pumped into the aorta to meet the requirements of the body. An

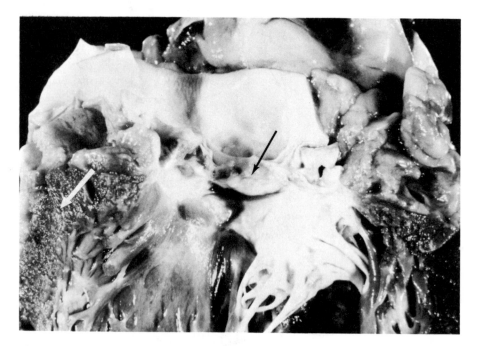

Figure 7–14. Calcified aortic stenosis **(black arrow).** Left ventricle is greatly hypertrophied **(white arrow).** (*Courtesy of Dr. David R. Duffell.*)

insufficient blood supply to the brain can cause **syncope** (fainting). This valve defect, like others, can be corrected surgically.

In **aortic insufficiency** the valve does not close properly. During diastole, blood flows back into the left ventricle from the aorta. This condition of the valve can result from an inflammation within the heart, **endocarditis.** It may also be due to a dilated aorta, where the ring around the valve is too large. Because of the backflow of blood, the left ventricle becomes greatly dilated. The left ventricle also hypertrophies because of overwork.

■ Rheumatic Heart Disease

Rheumatic heart disease is a peculiar disease that results from a streptococcal infection, although the organisms are no longer present when the disease presents itself. Rheumatic fever develops from a throat or ear infection caused by **Group A hemolytic streptococci.** The symptoms are fever, inflamed and painful joints, and sometimes a rash. There is a latent period of a few weeks between the infection and the development of rheumatic fever. The disease usually strikes children or very young adults.

Rheumatic fever is an **autoimmune disease.** It results from a reaction between streptococcal antigens and the patient's own antibodies against them. All parts of the heart may be affected, but most frequently it is the mitral valve that is damaged. The exact mechanism that causes the valve lesion is not known. There seems to be an attraction of the antigen–antibody complex for the mitral valve. The aortic semilunar valve is also affected at times.

The valves become inflamed as a result of the infection, and clotting elements are deposited by blood flowing over the valves. Small nodular structures called **vegetations** form along the edge of the cusps (Fig. 7–15). The normally delicate cusps thicken and adhere to each other. Later, fibrous tissue develops, which has a tendency to contract.

If the adhesions of the cusps seriously narrow the valve opening, the mitral valve becomes stenotic. The effects of mitral stenosis are described in this chapter (see Valvular Diseases). An inadequate amount of blood flows from the left atrium to the left ventricle. **Stasis,** or slowed blood flow, frequently causes thrombus formation.

It is possible for the cusps to retract to the extent that they fail to meet and the valve cannot close. The mitral valve is then insufficient, or incompetent, and there is a backflow of blood, regurgitation, from the left ventricle to the left atrium. Fortunately, rheumatic fever is not as common today as it once was. This is because of the widespread use of antibiotics in treating streptococcal infections.

■ Infectious Endocarditis

Infectious endocarditis is a disease that was once considered fatal but that now responds well to antibiotics if treated early. The endocardium is the inner lining of the chambers of the heart and covers the valves. Endocarditis is an inflammation of this lining caused by a strain of streptococcus bacteria. These organisms can en-

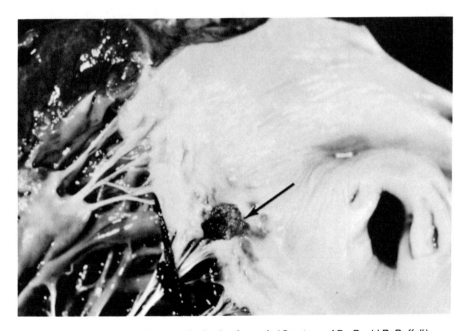

Figure 7–15. Vegetations on mitral valve **(arrow).** (*Courtesy of Dr. David R. Duffell.*)

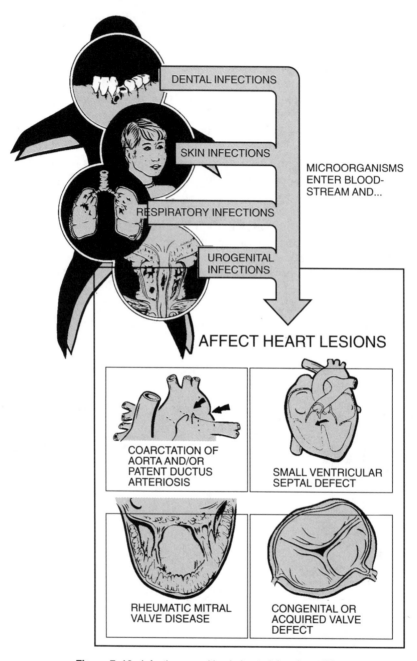

Figure 7–16. Infections resulting in bacterial endocarditis.

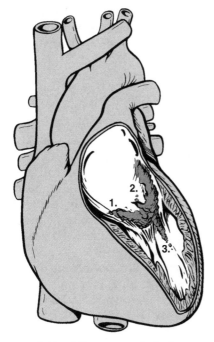

1. Vegetations cover mitral valve
2. Extend to atrial wall and on to
3. Cords which support valve

Figure 7–17. Bacterial endocarditis.

ter the bloodstream from an infected tooth, a skin infection, urinary tract infection, or other infections. Frequently this inflammation occurs on a rheumatic fever lesion, an already damaged valve, or on a congenital heart defect. Various routes of bacterial invasion are illustrated in Figure 7–16.

The nodules or vegetations that form in endocarditis are larger than those of rheumatic fever. They are also **friable,** tending to break apart easily and enter the bloodstream. The vegetations are filled with bacteria, unlike rheumatic fever vegetations. Typical lesions of endocarditis are shown in Figure 7–17. As fragments of the vegetations break apart, they enter the bloodstream to form emboli, which can travel to the brain, kidney, lung, or other vital organs, causing a variety of symptoms. The emboli can lodge in small blood vessels of the skin or other organs and cause the blood vessels to rupture. These small hemorrhages produce tiny red spots called **petechiae.**

SYMPTOMS OF HEART DISEASE

Some heart diseases, such as myocardial infarction and angina pectoris, cause severe chest pain or referred pain in the arm or neck. Dyspnea is a common symptom of many heart diseases; the lack of oxygen in the tissues stimulates the respiratory center, causing the patient to experience difficulty in breathing or shortness of breath. Fainting or loss of consciousness occurs when the brain is deprived of an adequate blood supply. Cyanosis may also develop.

ABNORMALITIES OF HEART ACTION

In reviewing the anatomy and physiology of the heart, a specialized patch of tissue, the pacemaker, was mentioned as establishing heart rate. Normally, the impulse for contraction then spreads over the atria and is conducted to the ventricles through a conduction bundle. This conduction system can fail and if the impulse does not spread from the atria to the ventricles, the pulse is drastically reduced; this failure in passage of the impulse is known as **heart block.** Heart block can result from scar tissue interfering with the conduction bundle, and it may be necessary to implant an electric pacemaker if the block is complete.

At times, the impulse for contraction spreads over the atria in an uncoordinated fashion. Because the heart muscle fibers are not working as a unit, atrial contraction is uncoordinated and ineffective, the condition known as **atrial fibrillation.** As a result of the uncoordinated contraction of the atria, the ventricles receive irregular input. They also begin to beat faster, but again in an uncoordinated and less efficient fashion. A medication such as lanoxin can be administered to slow the conduction of the impulse through the bundle of His to the ventricles. This allows the ventricles to fill properly before contraction.

Ventricular fibrillation is far more serious than atrial fibrillation. If the impulse for contraction spreads over the ventricles irregularly, they will twitch rather than contract. They fail to pump blood, which can lead to **cardiac arrest,** the sudden stoppage of heart action. Immediate attempts at **resuscitation** must be made or death will ensue. Permanent damage to other organs, particularly the brain, results when an inadequate blood supply reaches them. A machine called a **defibrillator** is used when available, which gives electrical shocks to the heart enabling it to re-establish its normal beat.

Heart beat rhythm may become irregular and is known as **cardiac arrhythmia.** Beats may be skipped or come in prematurely; these beats are called **premature ventricular contractions (PVCs).** The heart rate may increase significantly, **tachycardia,** or be abnormally slow, **bradycardia.**

DIAGNOSTIC PROCEDURES FOR HEART DISEASES

Modern medicine provides many techniques for diagnosing and treating heart problems. **Auscultation**—listening through a stethoscope for abnormal sounds—and the electrocardiogram provide valuable information regarding heart condition. The **electrocardiogram** (ECG) is an electrical recording of heart action and aids in the diagnosis of coronary artery disease, myocardial infarction, valvular heart disease, and some congenital heart diseases. It is also useful in diagnosing arrhythmias and heart block. **Echocardiography** (ultrasound cardiography) is also a non-invasive procedure that utilizes high-frequency sound waves to examine the size, shape, and motion of heart structures. It gives a time-motion study of the heart, which permits direct recordings of heart valve movement, measurements of the heart chambers, and changes that occur in the heart chambers during the cardiac cycle. Color Doppler echocardiography explores blood flow patterns and changes in velocity of blood flow within the heart and great vessels. It enables the cardiologist to evaluate valvular stenosis or insufficiency.

Another valuable procedure is **cardiac catheterization** in which a catheter is passed into the heart through appropriate blood vessels to sample the blood in each chamber for oxygen content and pressure. The findings can indicate valvular disorders, abnormal shunting of blood, and aids in determining cardiac output (Fig. 7–18).

X-rays of the heart and great vessels, the aorta and pulmonary artery, can be taken by means of **angiocardiography** in which a contrast indicator (dye) is injected into the cardiovascular system. A blockage is indicated by an area in which the dye fails to penetrate; coronary bypass surgery may be indicated by this procedure. **Coronary arteriography** employs selective injection of contrast material

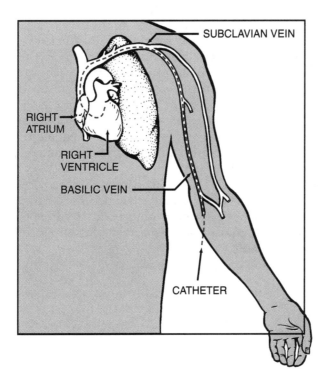

Figure 7–18. Cardiac catheterization.

into coronary arteries for a film recording of blood vessel action, and it too is valuable for possible indication of coronary bypass surgery.

CHAPTER SUMMARY

After reviewing the normal structure and function of the heart, heart diseases such as coronary artery disease, myocardial infarction, and angina pectoris were discussed. Myocardial infarction and angina pectoris cause severe chest pain or referred pain in the arm or neck. Dyspnea is a common symptom of many heart diseases; the lack of oxygen in the tissues stimulates the respiratory center, causing the patient to experience difficulty in breathing or shortness of breath. Fainting or loss of consciousness occurs when the brain is deprived of an adequate blood supply. All of the tissues and organs are affected by poor circulation. Cyanosis occurs when blood is not properly oxygenated and fluid accumulates in the tissues, causing edema when veins become congested.

Hypertensive heart disease develops from long-standing hypertension and cor pulmonale results from chronic lung disease. Congestive heart failure means that the heart is pumping inadequately to meet the needs of the body.

Congenital heart diseases, tetralogy of Fallot, patent ductus arteriosis, and coarctation of the aorta were explained. It was noted that a congenital defect is frequently the site of a bacterial infection.

Valvular diseases, valves that are stenotic or insufficient, cause heart murmurs. The abnormal sounds result from blood being forced through a stenotic valve or being regurgitated through an insufficient valve. Rheumatic heart disease is a common cause of valvular disease.

Abnormalities of heart action, heart block, fibrillation, and arrhythmia were described. Diagnostic procedures include auscultation, electrocardiography, ultrasound cardiography (echocardiography), and cardiac catheterization. The condition of coronary arteries and the great vessels can be evaluated through angiocardiography and coronary arteriography.

Advances in open heart surgery have made possible the correction of congenital heart defects, valve replacement, and electric pacemaker implantation. Antibiotics have reduced the danger of endocarditis and the frequency of rheumatic heart disease. Coronary bypass surgery and angioplasty reduce heart damage by increasing coronary circulation.

■ Self-Study

True or False

_____ 1. In the tetralogy of Fallot oxygenated and unoxygenated blood are mixed.

_____ 2. The left atria hypertrophies and dilates when the mitral valve is stenotic.

_____ 3. Pain of a myocardial infarction is relieved by nitroglycerin.

_____ 4. Tachycardia refers to a decreased heart rate.

_____ 5. The aorta is misplaced in patent ductus arteriosis.

_____ 6. Nitroglycerin slows the impulse for contraction between the atria and ventricles.

_____ 7. In stenosis of a valve there is a regurgitation of blood.

_____ 8. Aortic insufficiency causes back flow of blood from aorta to ventricle.

_____ 9. Failure of the foramen ovale to close is called patent ductus arteriosis.

_____ 10. Thrombolytic drugs are used to treat angina pectoris.

Multiple Choice

_____ 11. Congestive heart failure involving the _____ of the heart causes shortness of breath due to pulmonary edema.
   a. right side
   b. left side

_____ 12. Which defects are part of the tetralogy of Fallot?
   1. mitral insufficiency
   2. hypertrophy of right ventricle
   3. atrial septal defect
   4. pulmonary stenosis
   5. aortic stenosis
   6. ventricular septal defect
   7. misplaced aorta

8. hypertrophy of left ventricle
   a. 1, 2, 4, 8
   b. 3, 5, 7, 8
   c. 2, 3, 5, 7
   d. 2, 4, 6, 7
   e. 1, 3, 5, 8

_____ 13. _____ causes cyanosis.
   a. Failure of the foramen ovale to close
   b. Failure of the ductus arteriosis to close
   c. Pulmonary stenosis

_____ 14. _____ utilizes high-frequency sound waves to examine the heart.
   a. Angiocardiography
   b. Echocardiography
   c. Electrocardiography

_____ 15. Angioplasty may be performed for _____.
   a. valve disease
   b. congestive heart failure
   c. coronary artery disease

_____ 16. _____ requires immediate attempts at resuscitation to prevent cardiac arrest.
   a. Atrial fibrillation
   b. Ventricular fibrillation

_____ 17. Hypertension in a patient's arms but no femoral pulse indicates _____.
   a. tetralogy of Fallot
   b. coarctation of the aorta
   c. patent ductus arteriosis
   d. failure of the foramen ovale to close

_____ 18. Enlargement of the walls of the heart is _____.
   a. dilatation
   b. hypertrophy

_____ 19. Blood would flow from left ventricle to left atria in _____.
   a. mitral stenosis
   b. mitral insufficiency

_____ 20. In congenital heart disease there is a tendency toward _____.
   a. anemia
   b. polycythemia

(Answers on page 449)

Chapter 8

Diseases of the Blood Vessels

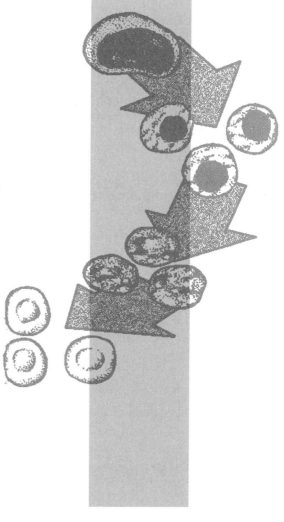

Chapter Outline

- Blood Vessels and Circulation
- Structure and Function of the Blood Vessels
- Diseases of the Arteries
- Diseases of the Veins
- Hypertension
- Shock
- Chapter Summary
- Self-Study

*T*he heart is an effective pump only if the blood vessels
through which it distributes blood are clear.

BLOOD VESSELS AND CIRCULATION

The importance of a well-functioning heart acting as a pump to provide blood to
all parts of the body has been discussed. Another factor essential to this distribution of blood, is a good vascular system, that is, healthy blood vessels.

The cardiovascular system is also called the *circulatory system* because of the distribution of blood from the heart, through the body, and back to the heart. This is accomplished by the arrangement of blood vessels in a circular fashion.

Two circulatory systems function concurrently: the systemic circulation and the pulmonary. The systemic circulation distributes oxygenated blood from the heart to all parts of the body, and it returns unoxygenated blood to the heart. The pulmonary system carries unoxygenated blood to the lungs to be oxygenated and returns the blood to the heart for systemic distribution (Fig. 8–1). A partition in the heart maintains the separation of oxygenated from deoxygenated blood (see Chapter 7).

Blood vessels that carry blood away from the heart are the arteries, the largest of which is the **aorta.** The aorta branches, sending blood to the head through the

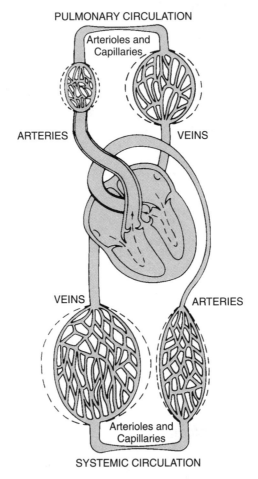

Figure 8–1. Pulmonary and systemic circulation. (*From Jackle & Halligan.* Cardiovascular problems: A Critical Care Nursing Focus, *Brady Media, 1980.*)

carotid arteries, to the upper extremities and throughout the body. These arteries continue to divide into smaller and smaller vessels called *arterioles*. Arterioles lead into capillaries, the connecting links between arteries and veins. Blood then flows into the smallest veins, venules, and then into veins. Veins return blood to the heart.

STRUCTURE AND FUNCTION OF THE BLOOD VESSELS

The structure of different blood vessel types varies. The walls of arteries are thick and strong with considerable elastic tissue and are lined with endothelium, which comprises the intima. Arterioles are not only smaller in diameter but their walls are thinner, consisting mostly of smooth muscle fibers arranged circularly; arterioles are also lined with endothelium. Capillaries are minute vessels about 1/2 to 1 mm long with a lumen as wide as a red blood cell. Their wall consists of a layer of endothelium. Veins have walls much thinner than their companion arteries but the lumen is considerably larger. Veins tend to collapse when empty.

Arterioles can change their diameter, that is, they constrict and dilate, which alters blood flow to the tissues as needed. This is controlled by the autonomic nervous system.

Capillaries, the thinnest-walled vessels, allow for the exchange of oxygen and carbon dioxide between the blood and tissues. Nutrients and waste products of cellular metabolism are also exchanged through capillary walls by diffusion.

Veins, particularly those of the legs, contain valves that help to return blood upward to the heart against gravity. The largest veins are the inferior vena cava, from the lower part of the body, and the superior vena cava, from the upper part, both of which empty into the heart.

DISEASES OF THE ARTERIES

■ Arteriosclerosis
Arteriosclerosis, or hardening of the arteries, is a degenerative condition that affects most people to some extent in the process of aging. There is a diffuse thickening of the inner lining, the **intima,** of the blood vessels. The vessels become brittle and are susceptible to rupture.

■ Atherosclerosis
One form of arteriosclerosis that is extremely serious, and frequently the cause of death, is **atherosclerosis.** Fatty deposits called **plaques** develop in the intima, narrowing the opening, or lumen, of the blood vessel, in some instances completely occluding it. This lipid material consists mostly of cholesterol. The aorta and its branches can be affected as seen in Figure 8–2, but so can small arteries such as the coronary and cerebral arteries. Occlusion of these vessels interferes

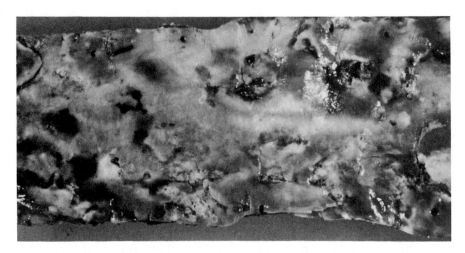

Figure 8–2. Atherosclerosis of the aorta. Inner surface should be smooth. (*Courtesy of Dr. David R. Duffell.*)

with blood flow to the heart muscle, causing a **myocardial infarction,** and to the brain, causing a stroke or **cerebral vascular accident (CVA).** Lack of blood to any organ is called **ischemia** and promotes tissue damage.

The cause of atherosclerosis is not completely known, but it does have a hereditary basis. Atherosclerosis is a common complication of diabetes, also a disease with a hereditary tendency. A low-cholesterol diet and regular exercise should reduce the risk of developing atherosclerosis. Figure 8–3 summarizes the possible effects of artery disease on the heart and brain.

■ Thrombosis and Embolism

One of the body's protective devices is the blood-clotting mechanism. When there is injury to tissues and blood vessels, excessive bleeding is prevented as the blood starts to clot. This same mechanism can function within the intact blood vessels, and this intravascular clotting produces a thrombus.

Several factors lead to **thrombosis,** the forming of blood clots on blood vessel walls. Clots tend to form where blood flow is slower. Since blood flows more slowly in veins than in arteries, veins are the more common site of thrombus formation. Clots are also likely to form where there is turbulence in the bloodstream, as there is over the heart valves. A diseased valve is a likely site for a clot formation.

Platelets, which normally initiate the blood-clotting mechanism, are deposited on the inner wall of a blood vessel or on a heart valve. Normally, these surfaces are very smooth, and platelets do not adhere. But when they are injured or diseased, the platelets stick and the clot begins to form. Atherosclerosis and rheumatic heart disease are predisposing causes of thrombus formation. Thrombosis in an atherosclerotic aorta is seen in Figure 8–4. Clots frequently form in coronary and cerebral arteries and in the legs when circulation is poor. Figure 8–5

HYPERTENSION AND ARTERY DISEASE

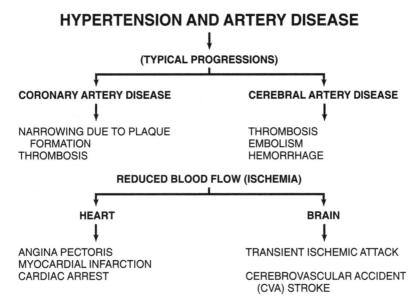

Figure 8–3. Possible effects of artery disease on the heart and brain.

illustrates thrombus formation. Changes in the blood itself can cause thrombosis. The blood may become too viscous or the platelet count may be excessively high.

Anticoagulant medications may be administered to prevent intravascular clotting. These medications can interfere with the person's normal ability to stop bleeding, and a small injury or cut may then cause undue bleeding.

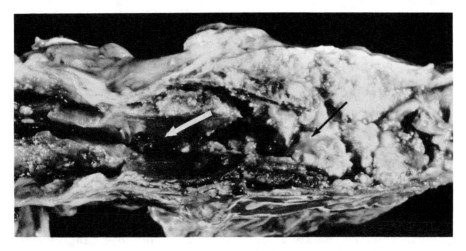

Figure 8–4. Thrombus **(white arrow)** in an atherosclerotic aorta. **Black arrow** indicates plaque. (*Courtesy of Dr. David R. Duffell.*)

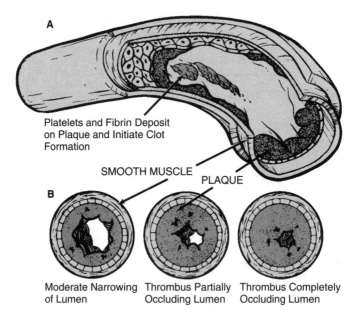

Figure 8–5. Thrombus formation in an atherosclerotic vessel. Depicted are the initial clot formation **(A)** and the varying degrees of occlusion **(B).**

The thrombus may retract and allow blood to flow, or it may permanently occlude the vessel. The thrombus can become detached and travel in the bloodstream as an embolus. Infected tissue around the thrombus can cause this detachment as can sudden movement.

Let us imagine a thrombus in a leg vein and follow its course as it travels as an **embolism.** Veins become larger as they approach the heart, so the clot travels easily to the heart. Vessels become smaller as they leave the heart; the embolus can then get stuck in a pulmonary artery and even occlude it. A pulmonary embolus is illustrated in Figure 8–6.

A damaged mitral valve which often results from rheumatic heart disease is a potential site for thrombus formation. A clot formed on this valve can break loose and enter the aorta. It then may travel to the brain, kidney, or some other organ. Figure 8–7 shows an embolus traveling to the brain through the carotid artery.

An embolism may contain infected material from pyogenic bacteria and is then called a **septic embolism.** This sometimes results from a lack of sterile technique during labor and delivery or an abortion. Substances other than blood can comprise an embolism. Air introduced into a vein during surgery producing air bubbles, fat globules, and groups of cancer cells can all travel in the blood as emboli with the potential of closing a blood vessel.

Lack of blood due to a closed blood vessel causes tissue death, an **infarct.** Bacteria can enter the **necrotic,** or dead, tissue and cause **gangrene** or gangrenous necrosis. The localized tissue death distal to the clot is called *coagulation necrosis.*

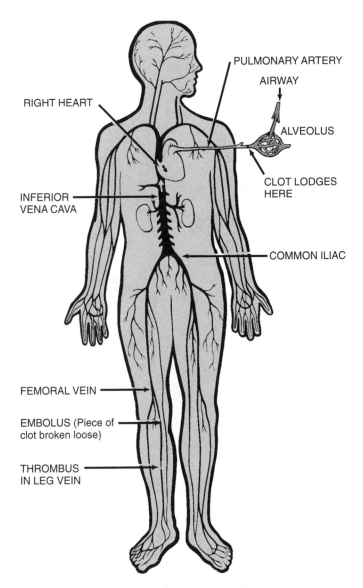

Figure 8–6. Pulmonary embolism.

If this occurs in the foot, a greenish color develops that turns to black, and the condition spreads up the leg.

■ Aneurysms

A weakening in the wall of a blood vessel due to disease, a congenital defect, or physical injury can cause a localized dilation or saclike formation known as an **aneurysm.** Aneurysms usually produce no symptoms and may be detected on an

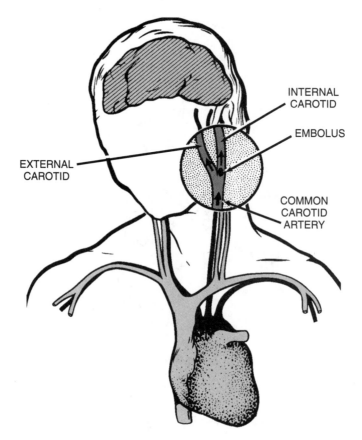

INTERNAL
CAROTID

EMBOLUS

EXTERNAL
CAROTID

COMMON
CAROTID
ARTERY

Figure 8–7. Embolus traveling to the brain.

X-ray taken for another purpose. Ultrasound techniques can now diagnose and measure asymptomatic aneurysms. MRI is beginning to be useful in visualization of vessels. The danger of an aneurysm is its tendency to increase in size and rupture, resulting in a hemorrhage, possibly in a vital organ such as the heart, brain, or abdomen. An aneurysm can be likened to a worn spot on a tire which can lead to dilation and then a blowout. An abdominal aortic aneurysm is seen in Figure 8–8. Atherosclerosis is a common cause of aneurysm formation. Early detection prevents the rupture.

Surgical procedures have been very successful in repairing blood vessels affected by aneurysm formation. The diseased area of the vessel is removed and replaced with a plastic graft or segment of another blood vessel. This procedure reduces the risk of hemorrhage and thrombus formation.

■ Hemorrhages

The rupture of blood vessels with subsequent bleeding is discussed in several contexts throughout the text. A large loss of blood in a short period of time, either in-

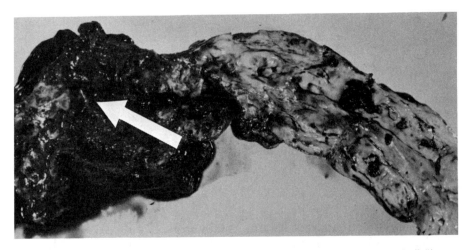

Figure 8–8. An abdominal aortic aneurysm (arrow). (*Courtesy of Dr. David R. Duffell.*)

ternally or externally, is termed a **hemorrhage.** Aneurysms, just described, head injuries (Chapter 5), and bleeding diseases (Chapter 6), are often causes of hemorrhage. The size and location of the ruptured blood vessels determine the result. Minute blood vessels that rupture in the skin cause tiny red or purple spots called petechiae (Chapter 6). Small hemorrhages into the tissue beneath the skin or mucous membranes are termed purpura. Trauma to underlying blood vessels which causes discoloration of an area is an ecchymosis or bruise. The colors of a bruise or "black and blue" spot are the result of the breakdown of hemoglobin when blood vessels are damaged.

■ Raynaud's Disease

Raynaud's disease is a problem of poor blood flow to the fingers or toes causing numbness, discoloration, and at times pain. An attack is usually brought on by ex-

On the Practical Side

COLORS IN A "BLACK AND BLUE" MARK

Trauma may injure soft tissue without breaking the skin. Tiny blood vessels are ruptured and blood flows into the tissue spaces. The bruise is red at first, then becomes purple, blue, green, and yellow before fading. The changes in color are due to the rupture of red blood cells with the release of hemoglobin. The breakdown of hemoglobin produces the colored molecules of the bruise.

posure to cold or as a reaction to stressful events. Blood vessels in the fingers or toes temporarily constrict and blood flow decreases. Lack of blood causes the fingers to turn white, then blue as venous blood remains without flowing, and finally red or purple as blood flow returns.

The condition can usually be controlled very well by protection from cold. Smoking should definitely be avoided as it constricts blood vessels. Relaxation techniques can help reduce stress which may bring about an attack.

DISEASES OF THE VEINS

■ Phlebitis

Phlebitis is an inflammation of a vein, usually in the leg. Veins are both superficial and deep. It is only when the deep veins are affected that the condition is considered potentially serious. Several factors may cause phlebitis: injury, general infection, poor circulation, and obesity to name a few.

The greatest danger in the deep veins is thrombus formation, and the condition is then called **thrombophlebitis.** If a vein becomes occluded by a clot, edema develops. The blood cannot return properly to the heart, the veins become congested with blood, and fluid seeps out into the tissues. It is important that the clot does not become dislodged and travel as an embolism. Anticoagulants may be administered to prevent further clot formation, and antibiotics, to prevent infection. Surgery is sometimes required to remove the thrombus.

■ Varicose Veins

Varicose veins generally develop in the superficial veins of the leg, most commonly the greater saphenous, near the medial side of the leg. The veins become swollen, painful, and appear knotty under the skin. The condition is caused by stagnation of blood in the veins that can result from several factors.

Development of varicose veins can be an occupational hazard for someone who stands or sits still for long periods of time. Normally the action of the leg muscles helps move the blood upward from one valve to the next. In the absence of this "milking action" of the muscles, the blood exerts a pressure on the closed valves and thin walls of the veins. The veins then dilate to the extent that the valves are no longer competent. The blood then collects, becomes stagnant, and the veins become more swollen.

Pregnancy or a tumor in the uterus can also cause varicose veins. The return flow of blood from the legs encounters resistance and a back pressure of blood results, breaking down more and more valves. Heredity often plays a part in the development of varicose veins as does obesity. Figure 8–9 illustrates normal veins and the flow of blood upward through the valves and varicose veins where the valves have become incompetent. Ulcers tend to develop because of poor circulation. The slowing blood flow **(stasis)** often causes infection. The distended veins can rupture, causing hemorrhage into the surrounding tissues.

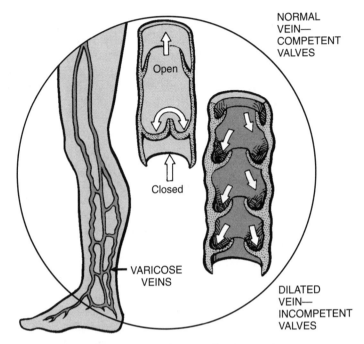

Figure 8–9. Development of varicose veins.

Treatment varies with the severity of the symptoms. At times an elastic bandage or support hose is adequate. Walking, elevating the legs when seated, and weight control can lessen the severity. A surgical procedure called "stripping the veins" is very successful. The superficial veins are tied off, **ligated,** and removed. A collateral circulation to the deep veins takes over. Small, dense, red networks of veins called **spider veins** can be effectively treated with laser. The light overheats and scars the tiny superficial veins which closes them off to blood flow.

Another treatment is **compression sclerotherapy** in which a strong saline solution is injected into specific sites of the varicose veins. The irritation causes scarring of the inner lining and fuses the veins shut. The procedure is followed by uninterrupted compression for several weeks to prevent reentry of blood. A daily walking program during the recovery period is required to activate leg muscle venous pumps.

Hemorrhoids are varicose veins of the rectum and cause pain, itching, and bleeding. Like varicose veins in the leg, hemorrhoids can develop from pressure on the veins. Straining due to constipation, pressure on the veins from a pregnant uterus, or a tumor may promote their development (see Chapter 10).

Esophageal varices, or varicose veins of the esophagus, frequently accompany cirrhosis of the liver. They result from pressure that develops within the veins as they try to empty. Because of blocked blood vessels within the damaged liver, there is a backup of blood and general congestion. A fatal hemorrhage from these varices can occur.

A relatively new procedure for treating esophageal varices is called **endo-scopic sclerotherapy.** In this procedure a retractable needle is guided into the esophagus by means of a fiber-optic endoscope. The gastroenterologist punctures the varicosities and injects a caustic **sclerosing** (hardening) solution to occlude the swollen veins. This prevents engorgement, rupture, and hemorrhage or stops a hemorrhage that has already begun.

HYPERTENSION

Hypertension, or high blood pressure, is a condition with which most people are familiar. Called the "silent killer," it is the leading cause of strokes and congestive heart failure. Warnings of the factors that can aggravate this disease are well publicized: smoking, obesity, excessive salt and lipid intake, and lack of exercise. The exact cause of hypertension is not known. It is thought to be a hereditary disease, but the site of the defective mechanism is not clear.

What determines blood pressure? It is a function of cardiac output, the amount of blood pumped per minute by the heart, and the resistance the blood meets from the walls of the blood vessels, total peripheral resistance. Hypertension results from persistent arterial resistance as atherosclerosis.

A blood pressure reading has two parts, corresponding to the two phases of heart activity: the **systolic pressure** and **diastolic pressure.** A normal adult has an average arterial pressure of 120 **millimeters of mercury** over 80 **millimeters of mercury** (120/80 mm Hg). The 120 mm Hg, or systolic pressure, is the highest pressure in the arteries due to the force of contraction of the heart. The 80 mm Hg, or diastolic pressure, is the pressure in the arteries when the ventricles are relaxing and filling.

■ Control Mechanisms

In the normal person, several mechanisms function to control blood pressure. Changing from a reclining to a standing position temporarily decreases blood flow to the head. Reflexes within the nervous system bring about constriction of blood vessels, increase peripheral resistance, and blood pressure to the head increases.

After a severe hemorrhage, blood pressure decreases and, again, a nerve reflex constricts blood vessels and pressure is elevated. On the other hand, if blood pressure is excessively high, specialized nerve receptors sense this and cause dilation of the arterioles of the kidney. This stimulates increased blood flow through the kidney and increased urine formation. With the loss of fluid, the blood volume is reduced, which decreases blood pressure. The kidneys are highly responsive to changes in blood pressure. When pressure is high, large quantities of water and salt are lost in the urine. When blood pressure is low, salt and water, and therefore blood volume, are retained.

Another means of reducing blood pressure by reducing blood volume, is the **capillary fluid shift mechanism.** The pressure within the capillaries is higher than that of the tissue fluid outside. The high pressure within forces fluid through the walls of the capillaries into the tissue spaces, thus reducing blood volume and pressure.

■ Hypertension and Kidney Disease

A close relationship exists between hypertension and kidney disease. Hypertension can contribute to kidney disease, and kidney disease can contribute to hypertension. Decreased function of the kidneys leads to water and salt retention, causing increased blood volume and elevated blood pressure levels. Long-standing hypertension causes arteriosclerosis of the renal artery that reduces blood flow to the kidneys and damages them.

■ Primary and Secondary Hypertension

A distinction is made between primary and secondary hypertension. **Primary** or essential **hypertension** is also called *idiopathic*, meaning that the cause is unknown. The hypertension may have a gradual onset and continue for a long time, or it may be malignant, with a sudden onset, and run its course very quickly. The latter type is quite rare but will end in death if not treated.

Secondary hypertension is high blood pressure that results from another disease. It may be a complication of malfunctioning kidneys or a tumor of the adrenal gland, the gland that regulates salt retention.

■ Effects of Hypertension

High blood pressure over a long period of time has several adverse effects on the body. It overworks the heart, causing the left ventricle to greatly enlarge, but the blood vessels to the hypertrophied heart muscle do not correspondingly increase. This means an inadequate blood supply going through the heart, and the patient is likely to experience attacks of angina pectoris (see Chapter 7). High blood pressure affects all the arteries of the body, including the coronary arteries. The risk of a coronary occlusion is very great.

All of the blood vessels become hard (sclerotic), and this is a frequent cause of thrombus formation. Weakened blood vessels can rupture and bleed due to the high pressure within, causing local tissue damage in the brain, kidney, or other organ.

■ Treatment of Hypertension

Medications, many of which are diuretics, are very effective in reducing blood pressure by reducing blood volume through the kidneys. Because salt holds water within the body, restricting salt intake lessens body fluids and blood volume. Exercise improves circulation, decreasing the progress of arteriosclerosis. This means less **peripheral resistance** to increase blood pressure. Hypertension overworks the heart and damages the arteries, causing them to become sclerotic. The converse is also true; sclerotic arteries cause hypertension by increasing peripheral resistance.

SHOCK

Shock is a vascular change resulting from assault or injury to the body. Any condition that reduces the heart's ability to pump effectively or decreases venous return can cause shock. **Hypovolemic shock** (hemorrhagic) results from fluid volume loss after severe hemorrhage or loss of plasma in burn patients. Treatment includes administration of plasma or whole blood. **Neurogenic shock** is due to generalized vasodilation, resulting from decreased vasomotor tone. The reduced blood pressure causes poor venous return to the heart and hence poor cardiac output. The decreased vasomotor tone may be due to spinal anesthesia, spinal cord injury, or certain drugs. **Anaphylactic shock** accompanies a severe antigen–antibody reaction such as occurs in an incompatible blood transfusion. **Cardiogenic shock** is the result of extensive myocardial infarction. It is often fatal, but drugs to combat it are sometimes effective. The types of shock are summarized in Figure 8–10.

DIAGNOSTIC PROCEDURES FOR VASCULAR DISEASE

Great advances have been made in non-invasive diagnostic techniques for peripheral vascular disease. This reduces the need for invasive angiography for many people. **Carotid phonoangiography (CPA),** also called **carotid audiofrequency analysis,** is an extension of auscultation. Special microphones are placed over areas of abnormal sounds that are heard with a stethoscope. The sound is pictured on an oscilloscope and photographed. Sound-frequency patterns can then be analyzed by computers, and the degree and location of carotid stenosis can be documented.

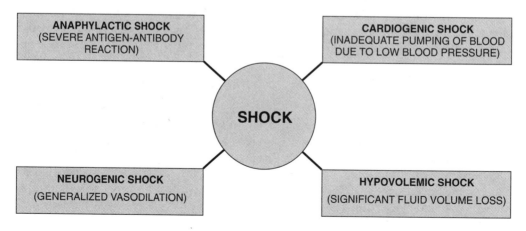

Figure 8–10. Various types of shock.

Ultrasound arteriography can show the anatomy of arteries, particularly the carotid bifurcation and the internal carotid artery. The **Doppler imaging** instrument uses echoes of moving blood columns to produce images of the vessel wall outline. The velocity of the blood is measured and the degree of carotid stenosis can be determined. The non-invasive test is very useful for patients who have had strokes or transient ischemic attacks.

CHAPTER SUMMARY

Healthy blood vessels are essential to adequate distribution of blood to all the tissues of the body. The condition of arteriosclerosis makes vessels susceptible to rupture and the roughened inner lining a site for clot formation. In atherosclerosis the fatty deposits that build up in the intima of the arteries narrow the lumen, greatly reducing blood flow. These lipid plaques can actually occlude the opening.

Although clotting within blood vessels does not normally occur, certain factors can promote it. Rough or diseased surfaces provide a site for thrombus formation. The clot may become detached and travel as an embolism, possibly lodging and blocking a critical artery. Veins may become congested with blood and distended to the extent that the valves cannot function. The stagnation of blood causes the infection and ulceration associated with varicose veins.

Hypertension is the leading cause of strokes and congestive heart failure. Its causes, effects, and treatment were described. Non-invasive procedures for diagnosing vascular disease were explained.

■ Self-Study

Multiple Choice

_____ 1. The depositing of fatty patches within the arteries is called _____.
      a. arteriosclerosis
      b. atherosclerosis

_____ 2. Hemorrhoids are _____.
      a. aneurysms
      b. varicose veins

_____ 3. Phlebitis is an inflammation of the _____.
      a. veins
      b. arteries

_____ 4. A bubble-like protrusion of an arterial wall is a/an _____.
      a. hematoma
      b. petechia
      c. aneurysm

_____ 5. Ultrasound arteriography is _____ procedure to show the anatomy of arteries.
      a. an invasive
      b. a non-invasive

_____ 6. An embolus traveling from the leg to the heart would be more likely to block the _____.
      a. aorta
      b. pulmonary artery

_____ 7. Heparin _____ intravascular clotting.
      a. prevents
      b. causes

_____ 8. Varicose veins generally affect the _____ veins of the leg.
      a. superficial
      b. deep

_____ 9. Varicose veins develop more from _____.
      a. excessive exercise
      b. long periods of no exercise

_____ 10. The highest pressure in a blood pressure reading indicates _____.
      a. systolic
      b. diastolic pressure

True or False

_____ 11. Long-standing hypertension causes the left ventricle to hypertrophy.

_____ 12. Ultrasound techniques can help diagnose and measure asymptomatic aneurysms.

_____ 13. An embolism in the brain may result from a thrombus on the mitral valve.

_____ 14. Neurogenic shock results from severe fluid volume loss.

_____ 15. After a severe hemorrhage, blood pressure increases.

Match

_____ 16. aneurysm   a) lipid deposit

_____ 17. plaque   b) inflammation of the vein

_____ 18. phlebitis   c) cerebral vascular accident

_____ 19. hemorrhoids   d) bulging of arterial wall

_____ 20. stroke   e) varicose veins

(Answers on page 449)

Chapter 9

Diseases of the Excretory System

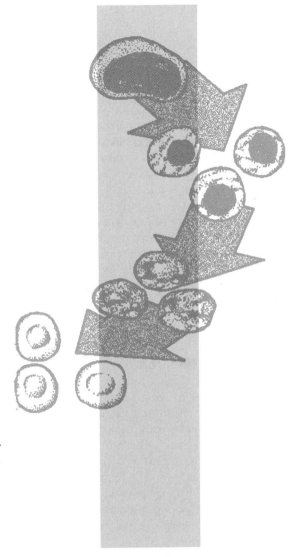

Chapter Outline

- Functions of the Kidney
- Diseases of the Kidney
- Diseases of the Urinary Bladder and Urethra
- Diagnostic Tests
- Chapter Summary
- Self-Study

*T*he kidneys are very interesting and complex organs. Not only do the kidneys remove waste products from the body, but they also conserve body fluids, nutrients, and salts.

FUNCTIONS OF THE KIDNEYS

The kidneys play an essential role in maintaining **electrolyte** (salt) **balance,** a factor essential to normal nerve and muscle physiology. The proper balance of salts like sodium, potassium, and calcium is required for normal heart activity.

Another kidney function is to help maintain the correct pH, or acid-base balance, of blood and body fluids. The body tolerates a very limited pH range of 7.35 to 7.45. If the pH of blood is lower than this, the blood is too acidic, and a condition called **acidosis** develops. The effect of acidosis will be discussed with diabetes mellitus because it is a complication of this disease. If the pH of blood is higher than 7.45 the blood is too alkaline, and the condition is called **alkalosis.** Death can result from either of these extremes. The kidneys help regulate body pH by excreting an acid urine when blood and body fluids are too acidic, and an alkaline urine when the pH is abnormally high. The kidneys also produce a hormone, erythropoietin, that stimulates red blood cell production. When kidneys become diseased, the hormone is not secreted and severe anemia develops. Specialized cells within the arterioles leading to the functional kidney area comprise the **juxtaglomerular apparatus.** These cells secrete **renin,** which is converted to angiotensin, an enzyme to help elevate blood pressure.

■ The Nephron

The functional unit of the kidney is the **nephron.** There are about a million nephrons in each kidney. It is the work of these minute structures to filter waste products from the blood, to reabsorb water and nutrients such as glucose and amino acids from the tubular fluid, and to secrete excess substances from the body fluids.

Each nephron consists of a **Bowman's capsule,** a proximal convoluted tubule, loop of Henle, and a distal convoluted tubule that leads to a collecting tubule. Urine is formed in the nephron. Figure 9–1 illustrates the parts of the nephron. As the various kidney diseases are considered, the effect of the malfunction of these parts will become clear.

■ Formation of Urine

Blood to be filtered is carried to a tuft of capillaries called the **glomerulus,** which is situated inside Bowman's capsule. These capillary walls are very thin. Their surface area is large, and the blood pressure within them is higher than the pressure in Bowman's capsule. These factors cause the filtration of fluid into Bowman's capsule. This fluid is initial urine and is equivalent to protein-free plasma. In a healthy nephron, neither protein nor red blood cells pass through the filter into Bowman's capsule.

In the proximal convoluted tubule, most of the nutrients and a large amount of water are reabsorbed and taken back into blood capillaries surrounding the tubules. Salts, particularly sodium and chloride, are selectively reabsorbed according to the body's needs. Water is also reabsorbed with the salts.

The nitrogen-containing waste products of protein metabolism, urea and crea-

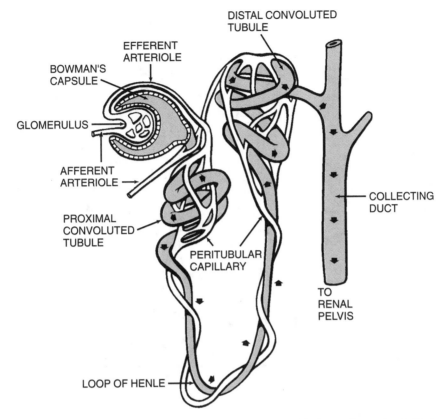

Figure 9–1. A nephron—the kidney's functional unit—shown with the capillary network (Red—nephron; White—capillary network).

tinine, pass on through the tubules to be excreted in the urine. Substances that are in excess in the body fluids, such as hydrogen ions if the fluid is too acidic, are secreted into the distal tubules to be excreted.

Two hormones play a very important role in the regulation of salt and water reabsorption. They are aldosterone, secreted by the adrenal glands, and antidiuretic hormone, secreted by the posterior pituitary gland. More will be said of these hormones when the diseases of the endocrine glands are discussed (Chapter 13).

Final urine from all the collecting ducts empties into the **renal pelvis,** the juncture between the kidneys and the **ureters.** It then moves down the ureters to be stored in the urinary bladder, which empties to the outside through a single tube called the **urethra.** Figure 9–2 illustrates the urinary system.

An obstruction along this path can set the stage for infection. The obstruction may be a kidney stone; an enlarged prostate gland, the male gland that surrounds the urethra, or a tumor. Any blockage causes stasis and a diminished flow of urine, and bacteria thrive in the stagnant fluid.

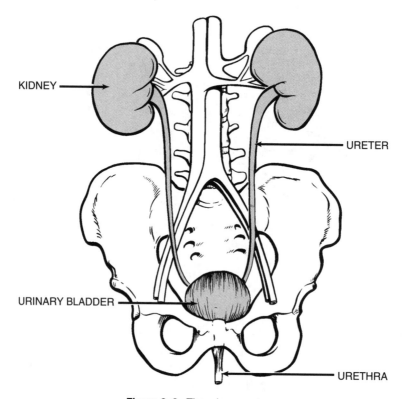

Figure 9–2. The urinary system.

DISEASES OF THE KIDNEY

■ Glomerulonephritis

Acute Glomerulonephritis. Acute **glomerulonephritis** is a common disease primarily affecting children and young adults. It usually results from a previous streptococcal infection: strep throat, scarlet fever, or rheumatic fever. The symptoms are chills and fever, loss of appetite, and a general feeling of weakness. There may be **edema,** or puffiness, particularly in the face and ankles. A urinalysis shows **albuminuria,** the presence of the plasma protein albumin in the urine. **Hematuria,** blood in the urine, is also commonly found. **Casts,** which are molds of kidney tubules consisting of coagulated protein and blood, are present. The signs and symptoms of acute glomerulonephritis are presented in Figure 9–3.

The presence of blood, albumin, and casts in the urine indicates that the glomeruli are diseased. Glomerulonephritis is a degenerative inflammation of the glomeruli. It is **nonsuppurative,** that is, no pus formation is associated with it, nor are any bacteria found.

Glomerulonephritis is a type of allergic disease caused by an antigen–antibody

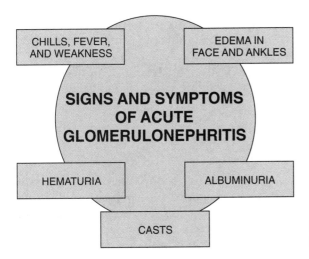

Figure 9–3. Signs and symptoms of acute glomerulonephritis.

reaction. One to 4 weeks before the onset of the kidney inflammation, the strep infection triggers antibody production against the strep antigen. The antigen–antibody complexes become trapped in the glomeruli, blocking them and causing the inflammatory response. Numerous neutrophils crowd into the inflamed loops of the glomeruli, and blood flow to the nephrons is reduced. Less filtration into Bowman's capsule occurs, and less urine is formed.

Many glomeruli degenerate along with the nephrons they serve. This causes a shrinking of the kidney tissue. The remaining glomeruli become extremely permeable, allowing albumin and red blood cells to enter the nephrons and appear in the urine.

The prognosis for acute glomerulonephritis is generally good. Normal kidney function is restored after a period of time. Repeated attacks of acute glomerulonephritis can lead to the chronic condition.

Chronic Glomerulonephritis. Chronic glomerulonephritis may persist for many years with periods of remission and exacerbation. Hypertension generally accompanies this disease. The relationship between high blood pressure and kidney disease was discussed in Chapter 8. As more and more glomeruli are destroyed, the work of filtering the blood is accomplished by the remaining ones. Elevated blood pressure makes this possible.

A significant test to determine the extent of kidney function is to measure the specific gravity of a urine specimen. **Specific gravity** indicates the amount of dissolved substances in a sample compared with distilled water. Distilled water has a specific gravity of 1.000. The normal range for specific gravity of urine is 1.015 to 1.025, with variations throughout the day.

In advanced chronic glomerulonephritis, the specific gravity is low and fixed. This indicates that the kidney tubules are unable to concentrate the urine.

After a long period of this disease, the kidneys shrink severely and are referred to as **granular contracted kidneys.** They gradually atrophy, dry up, and cease functioning.

Uremia, a toxic condition of the blood, is the end result of kidney failure. Waste products not excreted by the kidney accumulate to a poisonous level in the blood.

RENAL FAILURE

Several factors can cause the renal system, or kidneys, to stop functioning. Lack of blood flow to the kidneys due to severe hemorrhage, various poisons, and severe kidney diseases are some causes of renal failure. The kidneys are unable to clear the blood of **urea** and **creatinine,** which are nitrogen-containing waste products of protein metabolism. Urea is formed in the liver and is the primary method of nitrogen excretion from the body. If the kidneys are unable to excrete urea normally, it accumulates in the blood and a toxicity develops. The urea nitrogen can be analyzed as **blood urea nitrogen,** or **BUN.** An increase in the BUN is referred to as **azotemia** and the condition is known as **uremia.**

Measurement of the glomerular filtration rate (GFR) is used to assess the severity of renal disease or to follow its progress. Glomerular filtration rate is evaluated through clearance tests, most commonly clearance of the waste product, creatinine. Serum creatinine level rises and creatinine clearance rate falls when the GFR is impaired.

$$\text{Creatinine clearance} = \frac{\text{Urine creatinine concentration (mg\%)} \times \text{Urine volume (ml/min)}}{\text{Plasma creatinine concentration (mg\%)}}$$

■ Acute Renal Failure

Acute renal failure is a condition that develops suddenly and that can usually be treated successfully. The cause is often decreased blood flow to the kidneys resulting from surgical shock, shock after an incompatible blood transfusion, or severe dehydration. Kidney disease or trauma can also cause renal failure.

There is a sudden drop in urine volume, or **oliguria,** or even a total stoppage of urine production known as **anuria.** The patient experiences headache and gastrointestinal distress. The breath has the odor of ammonia due to accumulation in the blood of nitrogen-containing substances. An excess of potassium, **hyperkalemia,** causes muscle weakness and can slow the heart to the point of cardiac arrest.

If proper treatment is administered the prognosis is good. The condition causing the kidney failure must be corrected, and restoration of the patient's blood volume to normal is very important. Oral fluid intake should be restricted, allowing the kidneys to rest and the nephrons to regenerate. A dialysis machine, an artificial kidney, may be used temporarily to clear the patient's blood of toxic substances.

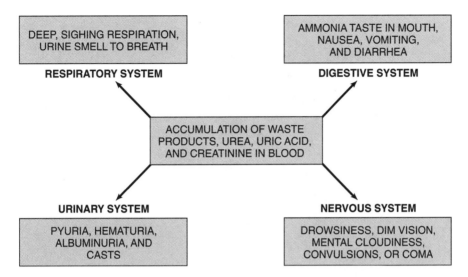

Figure 9–4. Effects of chronic renal failure—azotemia, accumulation of nitrogen-containing compounds in the blood.

■ Chronic Renal Failure

Chronic renal failure is a very serious disease generally ending in death. The condition develops slowly; there is no sudden drop in urinary output as there is in acute renal failure. Chronic renal failure can be the result of long-standing kidney disease such as chronic glomerulonephritis, hypertension, or **diabetic nephropathy,** a kidney disease resulting from diabetes mellitus.

The poisonous substances accumulate in the blood with adverse effects on all the systems. Urea is converted to ammonia, which acts as an irritant in the gastrointestinal tract to produce nausea, vomiting, and diarrhea. The nervous system is affected; vision becomes dim, mental ability is decreased, and convulsions or coma may ensue. Manifestations of chronic renal failure are summarized in Figure 9–4.

Dialysis—the artificial cleansing of the blood—may be used, but in advanced chronic renal failure it is not very successful. Although kidney transplants involve many problems, great success has been achieved in recent years. Improved antirejection medications with fewer side effects have contributed significantly to the success of transplants.

PYELONEPHRITIS

Pyelonephritis is a suppurative inflammation of the kidney and renal pelvis. The renal pelvis is the cavity in the center of the kidney formed by the expanded, upper

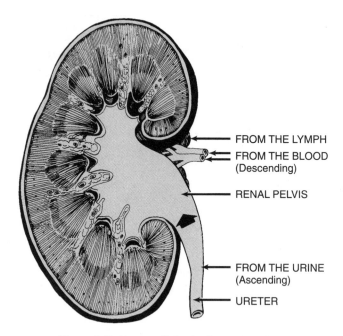

Figure 9–5. Routes of infection for pyelonephritis.

portion of the ureter which fits into it. Pyelonephritis is caused by pyogenic (pus-forming) bacteria. *Escherichia coli,* streptococci, and staphylococci are examples of such bacteria. Interstitial tissue, the kidney tissue between the tubules, is the site of the inflammation.

The infection may be an ascending one that originates in the lower urinary tract, possibly the bladder, and spreads up into the kidneys, or it may be a descending infection carried by the bloodstream or lymph. Figure 9–5 shows the possible routes of infection. Any obstruction of the urinary tract—a congenital defect, a kidney stone, or an enlarged prostate gland—paves the way for an infection due to stagnation of the urine.

Abscesses frequently form and rupture. Pus can then enter the renal pelvis and appear in the urine. This condition is called **pyuria.** The abscesses can fuse until the whole kidney is filled with pus. Renal failure occurs and uremia develops.

If the infection is less severe, healing can occur, but scar tissue will form. Fibrous scar tissue tends to contract, and as it does, the kidney shrinks and becomes a granular contracted kidney.

The symptoms of pyelonephritis are chills, high fever, and sudden back pain that spreads over the abdomen. Painful urination, **dysuria,** is experienced. Microscopic examination of the urine reveals numerous pus cells and bacteria. Hematuria is also common. Antibiotics are prescribed to counteract the infection.

PYELITIS

Pyelitis is an inflammation of the renal pelvis, the juncture between the ureter and the kidney. Pyelitis, like pyelonephritis, is caused by *E. coli* or other pyogenic bacteria. It can result from a bladder infection, or the organism can be carried by the blood.

Pyelitis occurs commonly in young children, particularly girls because the urethra in females is shorter than that of males. Microorganisms from fecal material can enter from the outside and travel easily to the bladder. The infection can then spread up the ureter to the renal pelvis. Painful urination as well as frequency and urgency are common symptoms of pyelitis. A urinalysis will reveal numerous pus cells.

This disease responds well to treatment with antibiotics. Early diagnosis and treatment are important in preventing the spread of the infection into the kidney tissue, thus becoming pyelonephritis.

RENAL CARCINOMA

Carcinoma of the kidney, also called **hypernephroma,** causes enlargement of the kidney and destroys the organ. The tumor may not manifest itself for a long time. Painless hematuria will eventually become the chief symptom. When the tumor has become large, an abdominal mass may be felt. This mass can then be detected on an x-ray as a tumor of the kidney.

Metastasis to other organs often occurs before the presence of the kidney tumor is known. The malignancy frequently spreads to the lungs, the liver, bones, and the brain. Sites of metastasis from the male urogenital tract are illustrated in Figure 9–6.

Late symptoms include pain, loss of appetite, weight loss, anemia, and an elevated white blood cell count. Surgical removal is the best treatment.

A malignant tumor of the kidney that develops in very young children is **Wilms' tumor.** The tumor grows very fast and spreads through the blood and lymph vessels. The symptoms are the same as those described in renal carcinoma of an adult. Prognosis for this fast-growing cancer has improved in recent years.

KIDNEY STONES

Urinary calculi, or kidney stones, may be present and cause no symptoms until they become lodged in the ureter. The stones then cause intense pain that radiates from the kidney area to the groin.

Calculi are formed when certain salts in the urine form a precipitate, that is, come out of solution, and grow in size. Small stones are often passed spontaneously in the urine, but larger stones may require surgery or other treatment. A stone may become so large that it fills the renal pelvis completely, blocking the

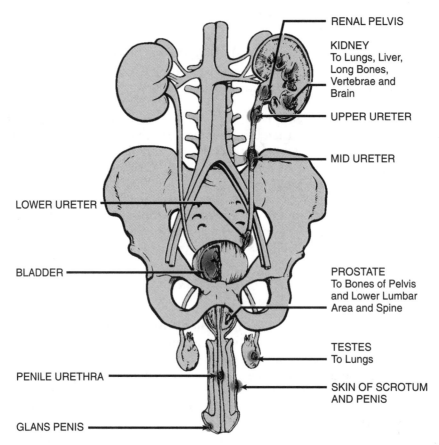

RENAL PELVIS

KIDNEY
To Lungs, Liver,
Long Bones,
Vertebrae and
Brain

UPPER URETER

MID URETER

LOWER URETER

BLADDER

PROSTATE
To Bones of Pelvis
and Lower Lumbar
Area and Spine

TESTES
To Lungs

PENILE URETHRA

SKIN OF SCROTUM
AND PENIS

GLANS PENIS

Figure 9–6. Sites of tumors and metastases in the male urogenital system, with surrounding lymph nodes affected at each site.

flow of urine. A stone of this type, named for its shape, is the **staghorn calculus** illustrated in Figure 9–7. A kidney containing numerous small calculi is also shown. Calcium excess often leads to stone formation. Hyperactive parathyroid glands can cause the excess of circulating calcium, thus promoting urinary calculi formation.

Stones can also form in the urinary bladder. The presence of stones causes urinary tract infections as they frequently obstruct the flow of urine. The converse is also true; urinary tract infections can lead to stone formation.

Urinary calculi are sometimes partially dissolved by medication and then passed in the urine. **Lithotripsy,** the crushing of kidney stones, is now the preferable procedure to remove them, replacing the need for surgery. Laser beams have been effectively used in crushing stones, either with the patient immersed in a tank of water, a procedure called **hydrolithotripsy** or performed out of water, **nephrotripsy.** In the newest technique, the patient is immersed in a tank of water to which acoustic shock waves from a lithotripter are admitted. These shock waves

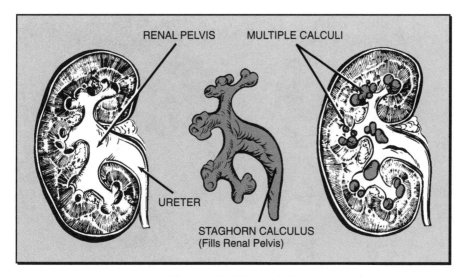

Figure 9–7. Urinary calculi.

shatter the hard stones into sand-sized particles that are eliminated through the urine. Recovery from the procedure is very rapid, and the patient usually requires only two to three days of hospitalization. Drugs that prevent new stones from forming are a significant advance in treating urinary calculi, as some patients tend to develop stones repeatedly.

HYDRONEPHROSIS

As a result of urinary calculi, a tumor, an enlarged prostate gland, congenital defect, or other obstruction of the renal pelvis, the kidney can become extremely dilated with urine. This condition is called **hydronephrosis.** The ureters above the obstruction are dilated from the pressure of urine that is unable to bypass the obstruction and are called **hydroureters.** Figure 9–8 shows this dilated condition. A **ureterocele** can cause hydronephrosis. In this condition the terminal portion of the ureter **prolapses** or slips into the bladder. When detected by tests (see Diagnostic Tests), it can be corrected surgically.

The degree of pain accompanying hydronephrosis depends on the nature of the blockage. Hematuria is generally present. If an infection develops because of the stagnation of urine, pyuria may be detected. Fever would then be a symptom too. Figure 9–9 depicts hydronephrosis of the kidney.

POLYCYSTIC KIDNEY

Polycystic kidney is a congenital anomaly, an error in development. Both kidneys are usually involved in this hereditary disease. The multiple cysts are dilated kid-

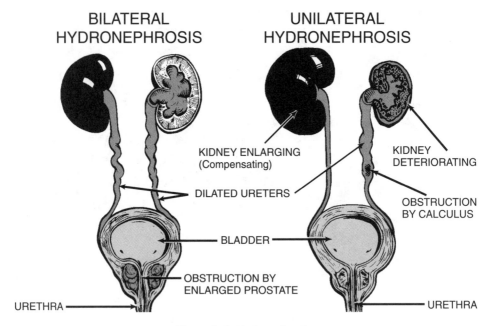

BILATERAL HYDRONEPHROSIS

UNILATERAL HYDRONEPHROSIS

KIDNEY ENLARGING (Compensating)

DILATED URETERS

BLADDER

OBSTRUCTION BY ENLARGED PROSTATE

URETHRA

KIDNEY DETERIORATING

OBSTRUCTION BY CALCULUS

URETHRA

Figure 9–8. Hydronephrosis.

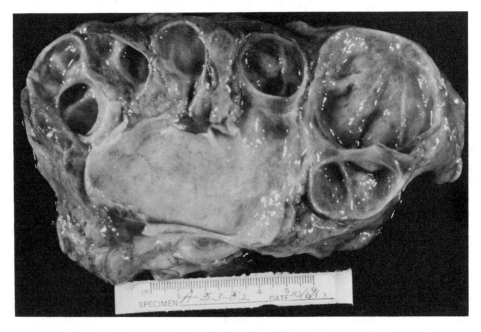

Figure 9–9. Hydronephrosis. (*Courtesy of Dr. David. R. Duffell.*)

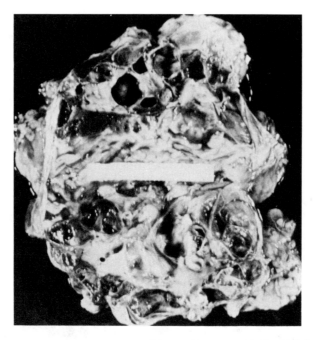

Figure 9–10. A cut view of polycystic kidney. (*Courtesy of D. David R. Duffell.*)

ney tubules that do not open into the renal pelvis as they should. The cysts enlarge, fuse, and usually become infected. As the cysts enlarge they compress the surrounding kidney tissue. Figure 9–10 illustrates the polycystic kidney of an adult. Hypertension develops as a result of this long-standing kidney disease. The kidneys eventually fail, and death is caused by uremia.

DISEASES OF THE URINARY BLADDER AND URETHRA

■ Cystitis

Cystitis is an inflammation of the urinary bladder. Commonly called a "bladder infection," it is more common in women than in men due to their shorter urethra. The chief causative agent is one present in fecal material, *Escherichia coli*, which can reach the urinary opening and travel upward to the bladder. Cystitis can also develop from sexual intercourse when infecting organisms around the vaginal opening spread to the urinary opening.

The symptoms are urinary frequency, urgency, and a burning sensation during urination. Microscopic examination of the urine reveals bacteria, pus, and casts. As in any inflammation, leukocytes are present.

■ Carcinoma of the Bladder

Certain chemicals used in industry have been linked to carcinoma of the urinary bladder. The tumor may grow, sending fingerlike projections into the lumen of the bladder. These tumors can be seen with a **cystoscope** and removed, but they tend to recur. A more invasive pattern of growth develops where the tumor infiltrates the bladder wall. Surgery is then required to remove the malignant section (Fig. 9–11).

■ Urethritis

Any part of the urinary tract can become inflamed, and the urethra is no exception. This inflammation is called **urethritis.** In males the infecting organism is usually a gonococcus, although other bacteria, viruses, or chemicals can cause this disease. The symptoms of urethritis include a discharge of pus from the urethra, an itching sensation at the opening of the urethra, and a burning sensation during urination. In females urethritis frequently accompanies cystitis. An obstruction at the urinary opening is sometimes responsible for the inflammation in women.

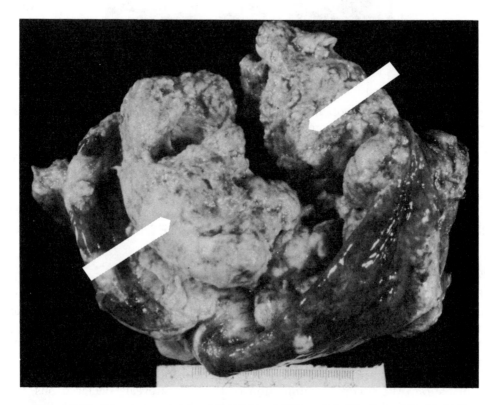

Figure 9–11. Advanced carcinoma of the bladder **(white arrow).** (*Courtesy of Dr. David R. Duffell.*)

On the Practical Side

INCONTINENCE

Lack of voluntary control over urination is normal in infants about 2 years old and younger because nerve control of the bladder is not completely developed. Training at the proper time overcomes the incontinence.

Involuntary urination or incontinence can occur in an adult as a result of damage to the spinal nerves controlling the bladder, unconsciousness, or disease of the urinary bladder. Irritation due to a urinary infection or irritating substance in the urine can also cause incontinence. The problem is often one of aging.

DIAGNOSTIC TESTS

Kidney disease symptoms such as pain, dysuria (painful urination), blood or pus in the urine, or edema indicate that specific diagnostic tests should be performed. Edema is caused by the loss of protein from the blood, resulting in hypoproteinemia. Normally these blood proteins have a water-holding power within the blood vessels. With their depletion, fluid moves out of the capillaries and into the tissues, causing swelling or puffiness. Significant information can be obtained by a simple diagnostic tool, a **urinalysis,** which examines a urine specimen physically, chemically, and microscopically. Physical observation gives the color, pH, and specific gravity of a urine specimen.

Chemical tests reveal the presence of abnormal substances: protein, specifically albumin, glucose, and blood. For microscopic examination a urine sample is centrifuged to obtain the sediment. Urine is normally yellow or amber, but hematuria (blood in the urine) can darken the color to a reddish brown. The degree of color depends on the amount of water the urine contains. Urine is pale in the case of diabetics, whose water output is large. In long-standing kidney diseases, the ability of the tubules to concentrate the urine is lost. As a result the urine is dilute and pale. Specific gravity is low in this case.

The pH of urine has a broad range. The ability of the kidneys to excrete an acid or an alkaline urine is a mechanism for maintaining the narrow range of pH tolerated by the blood. Urine specimens should be examined when fresh as they tend to become alkaline on standing due to bacterial contamination. Urine from a cystitic patient tends to be alkaline for the same reason.

Albuminuria indicates inflammation of the urinary tract, particularly of the glomeruli. The inflammation increases the permeability of blood vessels, allowing the protein, albumin, to enter the nephrons and appear in the urine. This loss reduces the level of protein in the blood, causing the condition called **hypoproteinemia.**

The presence of sugar (glucose) in the urine usually indicates diabetes mellitus. This is not a disease of the kidneys but of the endocrine glands of the pancreas. Diabetes over a period of time does affect the kidneys adversely.

Hematuria may be obvious to the naked eye or require microscopic determination. Any serious disease of the urinary tract may give this symptom: glomerulonephritis, kidney stones, tuberculosis, cystitis, or tumors. If the passage of urine is accompanied by pain, a stone or tuberculosis may be the cause. Painless hematuria indicates the possibility of a malignant tumor in the urinary system.

Pyuria results from a suppurative inflammation caused by pyogenic bacteria, and pus causes the urine to appear cloudy. Microscopic examination of the urine reveals numerous pus cells, or polymorphs, engaged in fighting the infection. Diseases such as pyelonephritis, pyelitis, tuberculosis, and cystitis show pus in the urine.

Casts are cylindrical rods, molds of kidney tubules. They consist of coagulated protein, a substance not normally present in kidney tubules. Casts can include various kinds of blood cells, as well as epithelial cells from the lining of the urinary tract. Casts always indicate inflammation.

Microscopic examination determines the presence or absence of bacteria. Bacteria are found in tuberculosis of the kidney, pyelonephritis, and frequently, cystitis. For microscopic examinations a urine sample may be removed from the bladder by catheterization to ensure that no external contamination occurs.

A **cystoscopic examination** enables the physician to view the inside of the bladder and urethra. The cystoscope is a long, lighted instrument resembling a hollow tube. Tumors, stones, or inflammations may be identified with this device. Using an additional instrument, small tumors may be removed or biopsied. Stones in the bladder can be crushed and removed.

The **intravenous pyelogram (IVP)** allows the visualization of the urinary system by means of contrast dyes injected into the veins followed by x-ray examination. When these dyes concentrate in the urinary system, it is possible to note tumors, obstructions, or other deformities.

CHAPTER SUMMARY

The importance of kidney function was reviewed to show the seriousness of kidney disease. Although acute glomerulonephritis generally has a good prognosis, repeated attacks can lead to chronic glomerulonephritis. This chronic disease, possibly persisting for many years, is one that often ends with kidney failure. Kidney failure can be acute due to a newly developed condition. If the cause of the kidney failure is treated, renal function is restored to normal. Chronic renal failure does not respond to treatment and generally ends with uremia. Pyelonephritis is a destructive, suppurative inflammation of the kidney. Abscesses usually form and pus appears in the urine. If not treated, renal failure results. Various other urinary tract infections were considered: cystitis, pyelitis, and urethritis. These infections frequently follow some obstruction of the flow of urine. Urinary calculi, tumors, and congenital anomalies can cause such blockages. Symptoms of kidney disease may include pain, painful urination, and blood or pus in the urine. Edema is also a sign of certain kidney diseases. An abnormal mass may be felt when a tumor of the kidney or bladder is large. This is a late sign of malignancy, and metastases have probably already occurred. Interpretations of abnormal conditions of the urine were also discussed along with certain diagnostic procedures.

■ Self-Study

True or False

_____ 1. A sudden drop in urine volume indicates chronic renal failure.

_____ 2. Glomerulonephritis is often an ascending infection.

_____ 3. In acute uremia, fluid intake should be decreased.

_____ 4. Both kidneys are always involved in pyelonephritis.

_____ 5. Albuminuria leads to hypoproteinemia.

_____ 6. Painful and frequent urination accompanies tuberculosis of the bladder.

_____ 7. Numerous abscesses are found in pyelonephritis.

_____ 8. Excretion of urine increases as blood pressure decreases.

_____ 9. Bacteria are not found in acute glomerulonephritis.

_____ 10. Pyelonephritis is a suppurative disease.

_____ 11. Pyelitis affects females more than males.

_____ 12. A specific gravity of 1.000 for a urine sample would be in the normal range.

_____ 13. Acute renal failure can be treated successfully.

_____ 14. Absence of urine formation is anuria.

_____ 15. Crushing of kidney stones is called cystoscopy.

Match

_____ 16. cystitis

_____ 17. diabetes mellitus

_____ 18. congenital cystic kidney

_____ 19. tuberculosis

_____ 20. urinary calculi

a) glycosuria

b) series of cavities in kidney

c) inflammation of the bladder

d) both kidneys usually involved

e) causes stasis of urine

Multiple Choice

_____ 21. Which of the following would cause chronic uremia?
   a. surgical shock
   b. severe dehydration
   c. complications of pregnancy
   d. diabetes mellitus
   e. severe burns

_____ 22. An inflammation of the interstitial tissue of the kidney is _____.
   a. acute uremia
   b. polycystic kidney
   c. hydronephrosis
   d. diabetic nephropathy
   e. pyelonephritis

_____ 23. Inflammation of the renal pelvis is _____.
   a. pyelonephritis
   b. glomerulonephritis
   c. pyelitis
   d. congenital cystic kidney
   e. tuberculosis

_____ 24. Breath has an ammonia-like odor of urine in _____.
   a. glomerulonephritis
   b. pyelonephritis
   c. tuberculosis
   d. uremia
   e. cystitis

_____ 25. A severe transfusion reaction would cause _____ uremia.

(Answers on pages 449–450)

Chapter 10

Diseases of the Digestive System

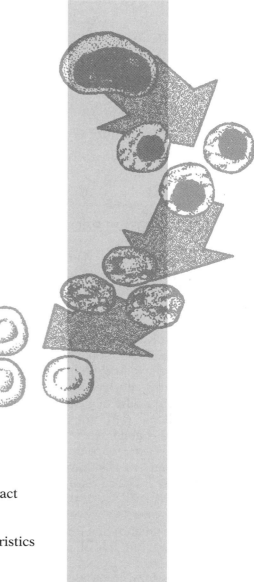

Chapter Outline

- The Digestive Process
- Diseases of the Mouth
- Diseases of the Esophagus
- Diseases of the Stomach
- Diseases of the Intestines
- General Disorders of the Digestive Tract
- Diagnostic Procedures for the Digestive Tract
- Diseases Indicated by Stool Characteristics
- Chapter Summary
- Self-Study

*F**ood would be of no value to us if it were not broken down into units small enough to be absorbed out of the gastrointestinal tract and into the bloodstream. The digestive system accomplishes this by breaking down carbohydrates to glucose and other simple sugars, proteins to amino* *acids, and lipids or fats to fatty acids and glycerides. Once these small units are absorbed by the blood, they are distributed to all the cells and tissues of the body. It is only in the cells that these units are metabolized—that is, used for production of energy—and converted into other material needed by the cells.*

THE DIGESTIVE PROCESS

Digestion begins in the mouth with chewing, the mechanical breakdown of food. Salivation, the secretion of saliva, moistens the food and provides an enzyme for initial digestion of starch. The food is then swallowed and passes through the pharynx, or throat, and into the esophagus.

The moistened food moves down the esophagus to the stomach, where the digestion of proteins, large complex molecules, begins. A sphincter muscle at the juncture of the esophagus and stomach prevents regurgitation. The stomach secretes gastric juice that contains enzymes—biological catalysts—that act on protein. Gastric juice also contains hydrochloric acid, which activates these enzymes. The high acidity of gastric contents would be very irritating to the stomach lining if the lining were not protected by a thick covering of mucus. A great deal of moistening and mixing occurs within the stomach.

The next part of the gastrointestinal tract is the small intestine. The entrance to this intestine is guarded by a sphincter muscle, the **pyloric sphincter.** This sphincter is closed until it receives nerve and hormonal signals to relax and open. The moistened food, referred to as chyme at this stage, is propelled along its course by rhythmical smooth muscle contractions called **peristalsis.**

The greatest amount of digestion occurs in the first part of the small intestine, the duodenum. Intestinal juice contains mucus and is rich in enzymes. Here digestive substances from other organs enter by means of ducts. The pancreas secretes enzymes for the digestion of protein, lipid, and carbohydrate. It also secretes an alkaline solution for the neutralization of acid carried into the small intestine from the stomach. This pancreatic juice enters the duodenum through the pancreatic duct.

Bile, secreted by the liver and stored in the gallbladder, enters the duodenum through the common bile duct. Bile is not an enzyme but an emulsifier, a substance that allows the mixing of fat and water much like the action of soap. The action of bile enables the lipid enzymes to digest fat into small, absorbable units.

When digestion is complete, the nutrients are absorbed into blood capillaries and lymph vessels in the intestinal wall. The inner surface of the small intestine is arranged to provide the greatest amount of surface area possible for digestion and absorption. This mucosal surface contains numerous fingerlike projections called villi, each of which contains blood capillaries and lymph vessels for absorption (Fig. 10–1).

Material not digested passes into the large intestine, or colon. The first part of the colon is a blind sac, the cecum to which the appendix, a nonfunctional structure is attached. Water and minerals are absorbed from the large intestine, and the remaining matter is excreted as feces. Figure 10–2 illustrates the complete digestive tract.

Diseases of the gastrointestinal tract are caused by a variety of factors. Tumors or malformations can produce obstructions, the mucous membrane lining can become ulcerated, and cells can fail to function in their secretory or absorptive action.

In this chapter the diseases of each part of the digestive tract will be described. These include diseases of the mouth, esophagus, stomach, and small and

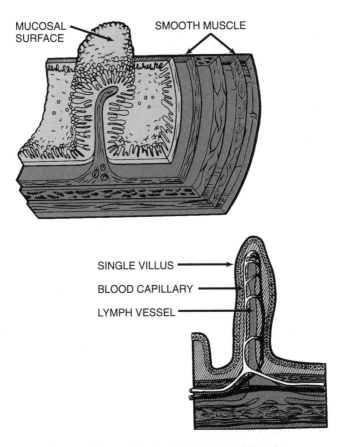

Figure 10–1. Mucosal surface of the small intestine.

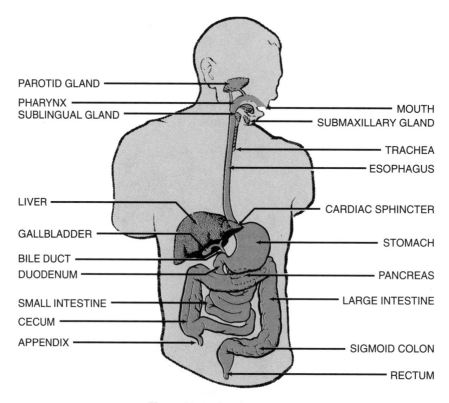

Figure 10–2. The digestive tract.

large intestines. In the next chapter, diseases of the accessory organs of digestion—the pancreas, liver, and gallbladder—will be covered.

DISEASES OF THE MOUTH

It would be impossible in a book this size to cover oral pathology, or diseases of the teeth and gums, adequately. This study will be limited to the diseases that directly affect the digestive system.

■ Cancer of the Mouth

Neoplasms can develop in any part of the mouth: gums, cheeks, or palate. A common malignant tumor is carcinoma of the lip. It occurs more often in men than in women and generally affects the lower lip. It may be related to pipe smoking. This malignancy may develop from a chronic lesion, a sore or crack that does not heal. It is a type of cancer that responds well to treatment such as radiation or surgery. If it is not treated, it will spread.

A malignant tumor can develop on the tongue, usually at the edge. Carcinoma of the tongue may be caused by a chronic irritation from a tooth or denture. This cancer spreads rapidly and is more difficult to treat than cancer of the lip.

DISEASES OF THE ESOPHAGUS

The **esophagoscope** is the endoscope used to view the inside of the esophagus. It may be used in combination with a microscopic study of the cells of the esophagus. Malignant tumors tend to shed cells, as was mentioned in Chapter 3. Washings from the esophagus can be examined for the presence of cancer cells.

■ Cancer of the Esophagus

A malignant tumor of the esophagus narrows the lumen causing the principal symptom, difficulty in swallowing, or **dysphagia.** The obstruction causes vomiting, and the patient may experience a bad taste in his or her mouth or bad breath. There is accompanying weight loss because of the inability to eat.

The carcinoma spreads into adjacent organs and to remote sites through the lymph vessels. It frequently metastasizes before it is detected. Prognosis for cancer of the esophagus is poor.

■ Esophageal Varices

Varicose veins sometimes develop in the esophagus and are called esophageal varices. They result from pressure within the veins. This pressure develops when venous return to the liver is obstructed. The veins appear very dilated and knotty. Esophageal varices are frequently a complication of cirrhosis of the liver. The destruction of liver tissue interferes with drainage of the portal vein. Congestion then builds within the veins, and those of the esophagus are unable to empty. The most serious danger in esophageal varices is that of hemorrhage.

■ Esophagitis

The most common cause of **esophagitis,** inflammation of the esophagus, is a **reflux**—a back flow of the acid contents of the stomach. This is caused by an incompetent **cardiac sphincter.** The acid of the stomach is an irritant to the lining of the esophagus and stimulates an inflammatory response. The various causes of esophagitis are illustrated in Figure 10–3.

The patient experiences burning chest pains, which can resemble the pain of heart disease. The pain may follow eating or drinking, and some vomiting of blood **(hematemesis)** may occur.

Treatment includes a nonirritating diet and antacids. Frequent small meals are recommended. Alcohol is an irritant to the inflamed mucosal lining and should be avoided.

■ Hiatal Hernia

A hernia is the protrusion of part of an organ through a muscular wall or body opening. A **hiatal hernia** is the protrusion of part of the stomach through the di-

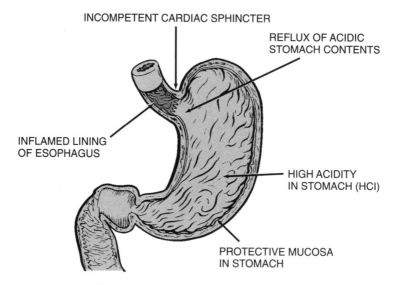

Figure 10–3. Various causes of esophagitis.

aphragm at the point where the esophagus joins the stomach. Figure 10–4 shows this condition.

The patient experiences indigestion and heartburn after eating and may feel short of breath. Avoidance of irritants such as spicy foods and caffeine and frequent small meals may be adequate treatment. If the patient is obese, weight loss

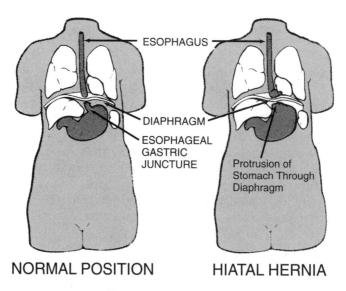

Figure 10–4. Hiatal hernia.

is recommended. Various kinds of supports can sometimes be worn to hold the organs in place. Surgery is often required to correct the defect.

DISEASES OF THE STOMACH

When a person experiences indigestion **(dyspepsia),** abdominal pain, or bleeding from the digestive tract, it is difficult to diagnose the exact cause as many gastrointestinal disorders have similar symptoms. Because of the arrangement of the abdominal nerves, there is sometimes referred pain. This pain is felt in one area but is caused in another.

Many excellent diagnostic procedures are available for abnormalities of the digestive system. In addition to barium x-ray films and fluoroscopy, which show the contour of the gastrointestinal tract, the endoscope is used to view the inside of the organs. The specific endoscope for the stomach is the **gastroscope.**

Washings from the stomach may reveal cancer cells. This procedure can distinguish between a malignant and benign tumor. Malignant tumors frequently ulcerate. Analysis of gastric juice, obtained by means of a stomach tube, reveals abnormalities of various secretions, and excessive secretion or the lack of secretion are very significant diagnostically.

■ Gastritis

Acute **gastritis** is an inflammation of the stomach caused by some agent that acts as an irritant, such as aspirin or excessive coffee, tobacco, or alcohol, or by an infection. Vomiting of blood frequently occurs as the principal symptom. **Gastroscopy** is extremely valuable in diagnosing this disease. A camera may be attached to the gastroscope and the entire inner stomach photographed. Gastritis cannot be seen on an x-ray, but it can be viewed well with this technique.

If bleeding of the mucous membrane is observed by gastroscopy, it can sometimes be stopped with the use of ice water, which constricts the small blood vessels. Acute alcoholism is a major cause of hemorrhagic gastritis. Alcohol stimulates acid secretion, which irritates the mucosa. If the bleeding cannot be controlled, surgery may be required.

■ Chronic Atrophic Gastritis

Lack of intrinsic factor as a cause of pernicious anemia was described in Chapter 6. In the absence of intrinsic factor, vitamin B_{12} cannot be absorbed. In cancer of the stomach neither intrinsic factor nor hydrochloric acid is secreted. This inability of the **mucosal** lining of the stomach to secrete its normal juices is due to chronic atrophic gastritis. Little can be done to treat the disease as the name, **atrophic** (wasting), suggests. It is a degenerative condition, and irritants such as alcohol, aspirin, and certain foods should be avoided.

■ Peptic Ulcers

Ulcers are lesions that can occur on any body surface where necrotic tissue forms as a result of inflammation and is sloughed off, leaving a hole. Ulcers of the stom-

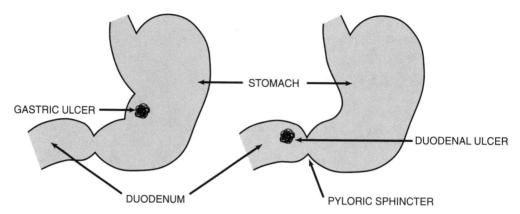

Figure 10–5A. Common sites of peptic ulcers.

ach and small intestine are termed **peptic ulcers.** They are due in part to the action of pepsin, a proteolytic enzyme secreted by the stomach. Figure 10–5A shows common sites of peptic ulcers. Figure 10–5B shows a peptic ulcer of the stomach.

Ulcer pain is caused by the action of hydrochloric acid on the raw surface of the lesion. Normally, the inner lining of the digestive tract is protected from the

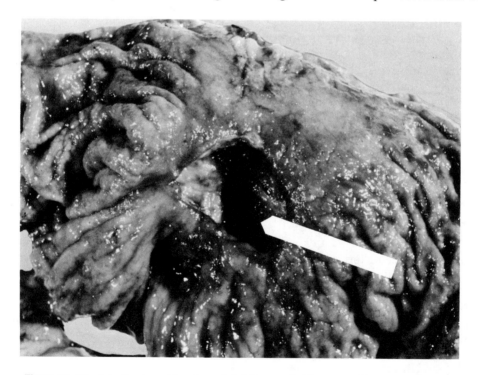

Figure 10–5B. A peptic ulcer of the stomach **(white arrow).** (*Courtesy of Dr. David R. Duffell.*)

acid by a thick layer of mucus. The muscular contractions of peristalsis also intensify the pain.

Abdominal ulcer pain is relieved by antacids and temporarily by food, which acts as a protection from the acid. Ulcers of the stomach are called **gastric ulcers** and those of the small intestine are called **duodenal ulcers.** The patient with a **gastric ulcer** experiences nausea, vomiting, and abdominal pain. The ulceration is thought to be caused by the hydrochloric acid and pepsin secretion of the stomach and by intestinal juice, including bile, that is regurgitated through the pyloric sphincter. The gastric mucosa becomes irritated by this bile-containing secretion and the lesion develops.

The patient with **duodenal ulcers** usually has an excessive secretion of hydrochloric acid. This acid secretion of the stomach is carried into the duodenum, where the ulceration develops. The mucous membrane becomes necrotic; the acid eats away the dead tissue, leaving a hole. The ulcer can erode through the pyloric sphincter. Hydrochloric acid secretion is under nerve and hormonal control. Stressful situations can affect the nerves that increase acid secretions.

New information suggests that bacteria called ***Helicobacter pylori*** may cause ulcers. Experimental treatment with antibiotics has been quite effective.

Several complications of a peptic ulcer are illustrated in Figure 10–6. At times bleeding from the ulcer occurs. A potential complication of any ulcer is hemorrhage; severe hemorrhage may even lead to shock. It is possible for a large artery

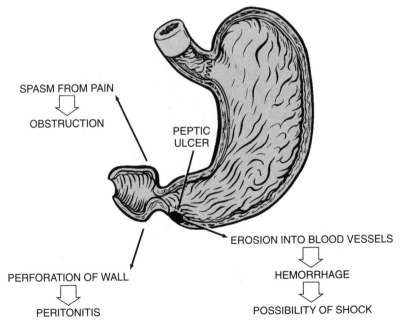

Figure 10–6. Complications of peptic ulcers.

at the base of the ulcer to rupture as the erosion of the lesion goes deeper into underlying tissues. Bleeding from the ulcer may appear as **hematemesis** or bloody vomitus. Blood from the upper part of the digestive tract gives the stools a dark, tarry appearance, which is referred to as **melena.** Iron pills and some antacids can also turn the stools dark.

Another danger in an ulcer patient is **perforation.** If an ulcer perforates, that is, breaks through the intestinal or gastric wall, there is sudden and intense abdominal pain. Surgery is required immediately. **Peritonitis,** inflammation of the lining of the abdominal cavity, usually results when the digestive contents enter the cavity, as this material contains numerous bacteria. The spread of peritonitis throughout the entire abdominal cavity is sometimes impeded by adhesions. The fibrous tissue of the adhesions can serve to localize the inflammation.

Obstruction of the gastrointestinal tract can result from an ulcer and the scar tissue surrounding it. This is most likely to occur in a narrow area of the stomach, such as the area of the pyloric sphincter. The pain of the ulcer can cause the sphincter to go into spasm, also resulting in obstruction.

Treatment of ulcers is aimed at reducing gastric acidity and healing the mucosal lining. Irritants such as aspirin, alcohol, and smoking should be avoided. Ulcers can usually be healed by medication, antacids, and proper diet such as the avoidance of gas producers, and fried foods. If the ulcer is stress- or tension-related, certain changes in the patient's life style might be advantageous. Even a change in the patient's psychological approach to the stressful situation can be beneficial.

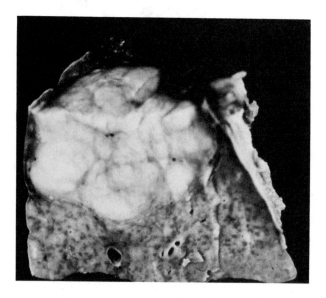

Figure 10–7. An infiltrating adenocarcinoma of the stomach invading the liver. (*Courtesy of Dr. David R. Duffell.*)

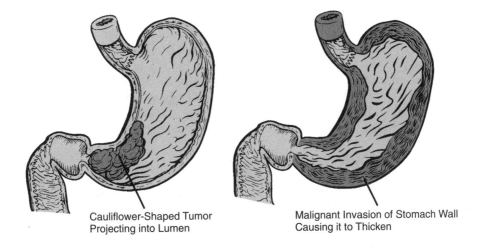

Cauliflower-Shaped Tumor
Projecting into Lumen

Malignant Invasion of Stomach Wall
Causing it to Thicken

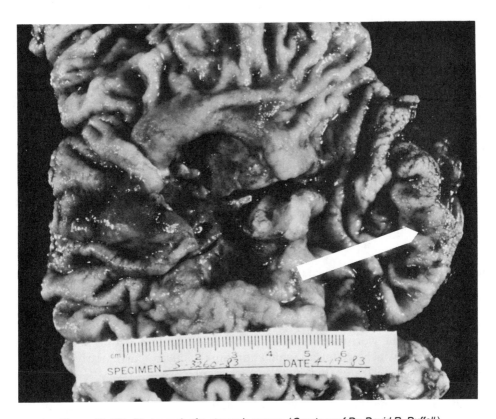

Figure 10–8B. Photograph of a stomach cancer. (*Courtesy of Dr. David R. Duffell.*)

Gastroenteritis

Gastroenteritis is an inflammation of the stomach and intestines. Symptoms include anorexia, nausea, vomiting, and diarrhea. The onset may be abrupt and violent with rapid loss of fluid and electrolytes.

Treatment replaces fluid and nutritional requirements including the lost salts. Antispasmodic medications can control the vomiting and diarrhea. Possible causes are bacterial or viral invasion, chemical toxins, lactose intolerance, or other food allergy, although the actual cause is not always clear.

Cancer of the Stomach

Pain is not an early sign of stomach cancer. Carcinoma of the stomach, which is more common in men than in women, may be very advanced before it is detected. It may even have spread to the liver and surrounding organs through the lymph and blood vessels. Figure 10–7 shows an infiltrating adenocarcinoma that has invaded the liver. Early symptoms are vague; loss of appetite, heartburn, and general stomach distress. Blood may be vomited or appear in the feces. Pernicious anemia generally accompanies cancer of the stomach, as in both diseases the gastric mucosa fails to secrete intrinsic factor. Gastric analysis by means of a stomach tube demonstrates the absence of hydrochloric acid, or **achlorhydria.** Biopsy of any lesions seen through the gastroscope is an essential diagnostic procedure for carcinoma of the stomach.

The malignancy may be a large mass projecting into the lumen of the stomach or it may invade the stomach wall, causing it to thicken. These patterns of growth are illustrated in Figure 10–8A. As the tumor grows, the lumen is narrowed to the point of obstruction. The remainder of the stomach becomes extremely dilated due to the blockage, and pain is experienced from the pressure on nerve endings. Infection frequently accompanies cancer, which causes additional pain. Figure 10–8B shows an actual photograph of a specimen of stomach cancer.

The etiology of this malignancy is not known but current research is investigating the relationship between food preservatives and cancer. Studies correlating dietary habits and the incidence of stomach carcinoma are also being made. Good prognosis for this disease depends on early detection and treatment.

DISEASES OF THE INTESTINES

Appendicitis

Appendicitis is an acute inflammation of the appendix usually caused by infection or obstruction. The wormlike shape of the appendix and its location on the cecum make it a trap for fecal material, which contains bacteria, particularly *Escherichia coli.* Figure 10–9 illustrates this potential site of infection.

The pain of appendicitis is not always typical. It often begins in the middle of the abdomen and shifts to the lower right quadrant. Nausea, vomiting, and fever are often symptoms. Leukocytosis is indicative of the inflammation. Perforated ul-

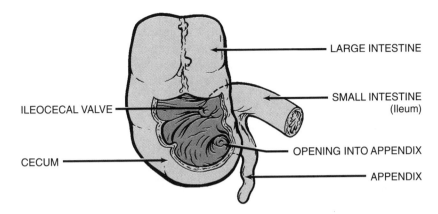

Figure 10–9. Appendix attached to cecum, into which the small intestine empties.

cer, kidney stones, pancreatitis, and other diseases have similar symptoms, making diagnosis difficult.

The inflamed appendix becomes swollen, red, and covered with an inflammatory exudate. Because the swelling interferes with circulation, it is possible for **gangrene** to develop. The appendix then becomes green and black.

The wall of the appendix can become thin and rupture. Fecal material then spills out into the peritoneal cavity, causing peritonitis. Before antibiotic treatment, peritonitis was almost always fatal. Rupture of the appendix tends to give relief from the pain, which is very misleading. Surgery should be performed before rupture occurs.

■ Malabsorption Syndrome

A person unable to absorb fat or some other substance from the small intestine is said to have **malabsorption** syndrome. Defective mucosal cells can account for this abnormality. Because fat cannot be absorbed from the intestine it passes into the feces, and the result is unformed, fatty, pale stools that have a terrible stench. The fat content causes the stools to float.

Many other diseases cause secondary malabsorption syndrome. A diseased pancreas or blocked pancreatic duct deprives the small intestine of lipases. In the absence of the enzymes, fat is not digested and cannot be absorbed.

Inadequate bile secretion, due to liver disease or a blocked bile duct, will also prevent lipid digestion and cause secondary malabsorption. One of the complications of the malabsorption syndrome is a bleeding tendency. Vitamin K, a fat-soluble vitamin that is essential to the blood-clotting mechanism, cannot be absorbed.

Treatment for malabsorption syndrome depends on its cause, and diet is carefully controlled. Supplements are administered, such as the fat-soluble vitamins A, D, E, and K, which are not being absorbed.

■ Diverticulosis

A **diverticulum** is a little pouch or sac that forms in the intestine as the mucosal lining pushes through the underlying muscle layer. If there are many of these pouches, and their number tends to increase with age, the condition is called **diverticulosis.** There are usually no symptoms, but the diverticula can be seen on x-rays.

■ Diverticulitis

Diverticulitis is an inflammation of the diverticula. The inflammation occurs when the sacs become impacted with fecal material and bacteria. The patient experiences low cramplike pain, usually on the left side of the abdomen. As inflammation spreads, the lumen of the colon is narrowed and an obstruction can develop. Abscesses frequently form. Antibiotic therapy, together with a controlled diet, is usually effective. Figure 10–10 shows an example of diverticulitis.

■ Regional Enteritis (Crohn's Disease)

Regional enteritis is an inflammatory disease of the intestine that affects most frequently young adults, particularly females. The intestinal walls become thick and rigid. As the wall thickens with the formation of fibrous tissue, the lumen is narrowed and a chronic obstruction can develop.

The cause of regional enteritis is not known, but there seems to be a psychogenic element involved; stress or emotional upsets are frequently related to the onset of relapse of the disease.

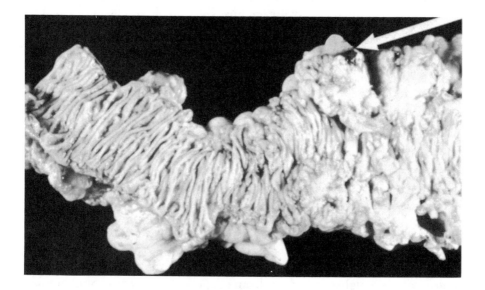

Figure 10–10. Diverticulosis with diverticulitis. Arrow indicates the thickened inflamed wall. (*Courtesy of Dr. David R. Duffell.*)

The pain of regional enteritis resembles that of appendicitis; it is in the lower right quadrant of the abdomen. A tender mass may be felt in this area and there is frequently an alternation between diarrhea and constipation. Melena, dark stools containing blood pigments, is common. The severe diarrhea can cause an electrolyte imbalance because of the large amount of water and salt lost in the stools.

Anorexia, nausea, and vomiting lead to a loss of weight. Periods of exacerbation and remission are common. In severe cases, hemorrhage or perforation is a threat.

Regional enteritis is usually treated with medication such as corticosteroids. Surgery is not performed unless complications demand it.

■ Chronic Ulcerative Colitis

Chronic ulcerative colitis is a serious inflammation of the colon, the origin of which is unknown. A **psychogenic factor** may be involved, as the condition is often aggravated by stress. Persons of high-strung, neurotic temperament are most prone to the disease. Hypersensitivity to certain foods may play a part in the course of the disease. Chronic ulcerative colitis may be an autoimmune disease in which the person's antibodies destroy the body's own tissue. Periods of remission and exacerbation are characteristic of ulcerative colitis.

There is extensive ulceration of the colon and rectum. Diarrhea with pus, blood, and mucus in the stools is the typical symptom. Cramplike pain is experienced in the lower abdomen. Anemia often accompanies ulcerative colitis because of the chronic blood loss through the rectum.

The colon of a chronic ulcerative colitis patient has a characteristic appearance on x-ray examination. The normal pouchlike markings of the colon, the haustra, are lacking. The colon appears straight and rigid, and is referred to as a **"pipe-stem" colon** (Figure 10–11A).

There is a high risk of a colon malignancy developing as a complication of long-standing ulcerative colitis, and the incidence of this is significant. Figure 10–11B shows a large polyp, which may become malignant.

Treatment of any chronic disease is limited, but the symptoms of chronic ulcerative colitis may be alleviated if certain stressful conditions are removed. Foods found to aggravate the disease should be avoided. Because the patient is usually of a very nervous temperament, mild sedation may be helpful and corticosteroids are sometimes administered.

If the patient does not respond to these treatments, surgery may be necessary, occasionally requiring a colostomy. A **colostomy** is an artificial opening in the abdominal wall with a segment of the large intestine attached. Evacuation of the feces is through this opening. A colostomy may be temporary or permanent depending on the nature of the colon surgery.

■ Salmonella (Food Poisoning)

One of the most common forms of food poisoning is caused by the bacteria, **salmonella.** Large numbers of the organisms ingested from contaminated food invade the mucosa of the gastrointestinal tract and cause the illness. The incubation

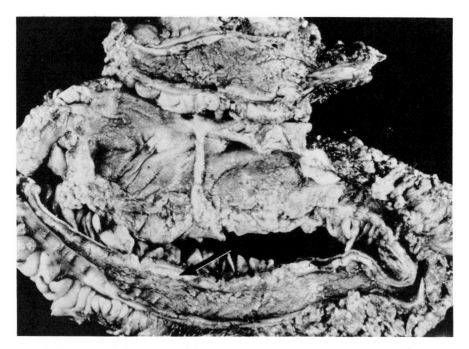

Figure 10–11A. Chronic ulcerative colitis. Arrow indicates the thickened rigid wall referred to as a "pipe-stem" colon. (*Courtesy of Dr. David R. Duffell.*)

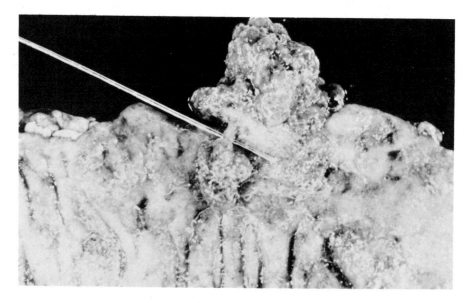

Figure 10–11B. Large polyp (seen over probe) in chronic ulcerative colitis. (*Courtesy of Dr. David R. Duffell.*)

period is 6 to 48 hours after eating the food. The infected individual experiences sudden, colicky abdominal pain, nausea and vomiting. Diarrhea, sometimes bloody, is accompanied by fever. A stool culture confirms the diagnosis. Symptoms can last up to two weeks with possible dehydration developing. There is no specific treatment. Salmonella infection can be prevented by proper refrigeration of food, thorough cooking, and strict handwashing precautions. Carriers harbor the infection and are the source of outbreaks.

On the Practical Side

PREVENTING PICNIC POISONING

Cold food must be kept cold and hot food, hot. Insulated coolers with ice or frozen packs on top of cold food work well as long as coolers are kept out of hot car trunks and/or sun. Hot foods can be kept in insulated containers. Covering food and utensils until serving time prevents flies and other insects from contamination with salmonella and other germs. Disposable hand towels are convenient to use before and after eating. Food should not be unrefrigerated longer than two hours.

■ Carcinoma of the Colon and Rectum

Carcinoma of the colon and rectum is a leading cause of death from cancer in the United States, yet it can be more easily diagnosed than many other cancers. The mass is often felt by rectal examination or seen with the protoscope or colonoscope, endoscopes used for viewing the rectum and colon. If detected early, it responds well to surgical treatment.

The symptoms vary according to the site of the malignancy. A change in bowel habits—diarrhea or constipation—is symptomatic. As the tumor grows there may be abdominal discomfort and pressure. Blood often appears in the stools, and continuous blood loss from the malignant tumor causes anemia.

The mass can partially or completely obstruct the **lumen** of the colon. As the tumor invades underlying tissue, the cancer cells spread through the lymph vessels and veins.

As in all cancers, early detection and treatment are essential to prevent its spread. Most malignancies of the large intestine are in the rectum or the sigmoid colon (see Fig. 10–2). This makes their detection and removal easier than malignant tumors in other areas of the digestive tract. A colostomy may be necessary.

There are two diseases that predispose to cancer of the colon: long-standing ulcerative colitis, which has been described, and familial polyposis of the colon. **Familial polyposis** is a hereditary disease in which numerous polyps develop in the intestinal tract. The polyps give no symptoms until a malignancy develops, but this is the usual outcome. An example of familial polyposis is seen in Figure 10–12.

■ Intestinal Obstructions

An obstruction can occur anywhere along the intestinal tract, and the contents within the tract are unable to move forward. **Obstructions** are classed as **organic** when there is some material blockage, or as **paralytic,** in which case there is a decrease in peristalsis preventing the propulsion of intestinal contents.

Tumors and hernias, both hiatal and inguinal, can cause organic obstructions. The intestine may be twisted on itself, a condition known as **volvulus** that may be unwound surgically. The intestine may be kinked, allowing nothing to pass. **Adhesions,** the linking together of two surfaces normally separate, can distort the tract. Abdominal adhesions sometimes follow surgery, when fibrous connective tissue grows around the incision. Adhesions also develop as a result of inflammation. Another type of organic obstruction is **intussusception,** in which a segment of intestine telescopes into the part forward to it. This occurs more often in children than in adults. Figure 10–13 shows various types of organic obstructions.

A paralytic obstruction can result from peritonitis. If a loop of small intestine is surrounded by pus from the infection, the smooth muscle of the intestinal wall cannot contract. Sphincters can go into spasm and fail to open as a result of intense pain.

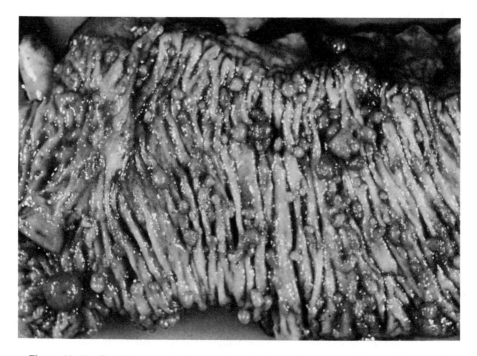

Figure 10–12. Familial polyposis. Note number of polyps. (*Courtesy of Dr. David R. Duffell.*)

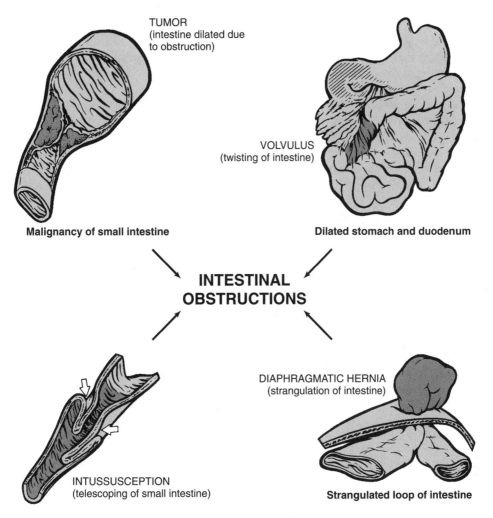

TUMOR
(intestine dilated due
to obstruction)

Malignancy of small intestine

VOLVULUS
(twisting of intestine)

Dilated stomach and duodenum

**INTESTINAL
OBSTRUCTIONS**

DIAPHRAGMATIC HERNIA
(strangulation of intestine)

INTUSSUSCEPTION
(telescoping of small intestine)

Strangulated loop of intestine

Figure 10–13. Organic obstructions of the intestinal tract.

If an acute organic obstruction develops, the patient experiences severe pain. The abdomen is distended and vomiting occurs. There is complete constipation; not even gas **(flatus)** is passed. This is a very serious condition, and the patient must be watched closely. Sometimes the obstruction can be relieved by means of a suction tube, but frequently surgery is required. If the obstruction is a strangulated hernia, a protrusion of intestine through the abdominal wall, surgery is required as the blood supply is cut off to the strangulated segment, and it can become gangrenous.

■ Spastic Colon (Irritable Bowel Syndrome)

Many of the symptoms described for diseases of the lower intestinal tract are also characteristic of a **spastic colon** or **irritable bowel.** These symptoms include diarrhea, constipation, abdominal pain, and gas. The difference between a spastic colon or irritable colon and the diseases already discussed is that the spastic colon has no lesion. There is no tumor or ulceration. It is a functional disorder of motility, the movement of the colon. The pain is probably caused by muscle spasms in the wall of the intestine.

Certain foods and beverages, particularly caffeine, alcohol, spicy foods, and concentrated orange juice, can irritate the bowel, and the patient with a spastic colon should avoid them. Fatty foods should also be avoided. Laxatives should not be used; adding fiber to the diet helps prevent constipation.

Emotional stress has an adverse effect on the digestive system. Digestion is very much affected by the nerves of the autonomic nervous system. For the patient with a spastic colon, emotional stress and upset are even more disruptive. If stressful situations can be alleviated, the colon will function more normally. Tension-relieving activities, sports, hobbies, or regular exercise (see Chapter 18) may help.

■ Dysentery

People often use the terms dysentery and diarrhea interchangeably, which is not accurate. Dysentery is a disease; diarrhea is a symptom. **Dysentery** is an acute inflammation of the colon, a colitis. It can be caused by bacteria, parasitic worms, and other microorganisms. Its major symptom is diarrhea in which the stools contain pus, blood, and mucus. Severe abdominal pain accompanies the diarrhea. Dysentery is principally a disease of the tropics, where sanitation is poor. Infective organisms enter the body through uncooked food and contaminated water. Organisms invade the wall of the colon and cause numerous ulcerations, which account for the pus and blood in the stools. Antibiotics can be effective depending on the causative organism.

GENERAL DISORDERS OF THE DIGESTIVE TRACT

The symptoms describing the diseases of the digestive system are common phenomena. Vomiting, diarrhea, and constipation are some of these symptoms. The physiologic basis of each symptom will be described briefly.

■ Vomiting

Vomiting is a protective mechanism, a means of ridding the digestive tract of an irritant or of alleviating overdistention. Sensory nerve fibers are stimulated by the irritant, and the message is conveyed to the vomiting center in the medulla of the brain. Motor impulses then stimulate the diaphragm and abdominal muscles. Contraction of these muscles squeezes the stomach. Normal peristalsis is reversed so movement of the stomach contents is upward. The sphincter at the base of the esophagus is opened, and the gastric contents are **regurgitated.**

A feeling of nausea often precedes vomiting. The cause of the nausea may be nerve factors other than a gastric or intestinal irritant. Motion sickness produces this effect. A very unpleasant smell or a sickening sight can cause nausea with possible subsequent vomiting.

■ Diarrhea

Diarrhea results when the fluid contents of the small intestine are rushed through the large intestine, causing watery stools. It was stated earlier that the main function of the large intestine is to reabsorb water and minerals. In an attack of diarrhea there is no time for this reabsorption. The smooth muscle in the walls of the intestine is so stimulated that peristalsis is intensified.

Nervous states can cause this increased motility of the large intestine, as most people have experienced. An infection such as food poisoning can bring about the same effect. If any area of the mucosal lining is infected, the glands pour out copious amounts of their mucous secretions. This helps to flush out the invading organisms and infection.

■ Constipation

The cause of constipation is the reverse of diarrhea. Feces remain in the colon too long, with excessive reabsorption of water; they then become hard and dry. Poor habits of elimination are a major cause of constipation. Defecation should be allowed to occur when the defecation reflexes are strong, usually in the morning after breakfast. A proper diet is also important, one that contains adequate amounts of fiber. Fiber is obtained from fresh fruits, vegetables, and cereals and is now thought to reduce the incidence of colon cancer. Various disorders of the digestive system cause constipation. Any obstruction of the lumen or interference with motility will result in this condition.

■ Hemorrhoids

Hemorrhoids, also called "piles," are enlarged (varicosed) veins in the lining of the rectum near the anus. Hemorrhoids may be internal or external. A physician can observe internal hemorrhoids with a **proctoscope,** a hollow tube with a lighted end. Straining to have a bowel movement can cause bleeding or cause the hemorrhoid to **prolapse,** i.e., come through the anal opening. External hemorrhoids can be seen with a hand-held mirror and appear blue because of decreased circulation. They can become red and tender if inflamed.

Causes of hemorrhoids include heredity, poor dietary habits, inadequate fiber, overuse of laxatives, and lack of exercise. Hemorrhoids frequently develop during pregnancy because of pressure from an enlarged uterus.

Treatment includes adding fiber and water to the diet to soften the stools and the use of medicated suppositories or anorectal creams.

DIAGNOSTIC PROCEDURES FOR THE DIGESTIVE TRACT

A combination of procedures enables the physician to view the inside of the digestive tract for malignancies, polyps, diverticulitis, bleeding, and inflammatory bowel disease. To visualize the upper gastrointestinal (GI) tract, esophagus, stomach, and small intestines under fluoroscopy, the patient swallows barium sulfate. The lumen and mucosa of the colon can be studied through x-ray following a barium or barium and air enema.

Barium is opaque to x-rays, so the rays do not pass through it. The silhouette produced shows tumors, malformations, or other obstructions that may be present. Motion pictures can even be taken of the movement of barium through the gastrointestinal tract. These pictures can show abnormalities of smooth muscle action or improperly functioning sphincters.

Certain lesions of the inner wall of the digestive tract do not show up on x-ray examination. To view this inner surface an instrument called an **endoscope** is used. It is a hollow tube with a lens and light system. There is an endoscope designed specially for each part of the digestive tract. It is possible with this technique to take a biopsy of a suspected malignant lesion. Gastric analysis is performed to determine if the patient is able to secrete acid and the rate of gastric secretion. Lack of gastric juice is significant in diagnosing pernicious anemia whereas a high rate of secretion suggests active peptic ulcer disease.

DISEASES INDICATED BY STOOL CHARACTERISTICS

In addition to the diagnostic procedures described for gastrointestinal disorders, examination of the stools is also important. Signs of several of the diseases discussed include blood in the stools. But blood appears differently, depending upon the site of bleeding.

Streaks of red blood can indicate bleeding hemorrhoids. **Hemorrhoids** are varicose veins of the rectum or anus. If the blood in the stools is bright red, the bleeding is from the distal end of the colon, the rectum. This symptom can indicate cancer of the rectum.

Dark blood may appear in the stools giving them a dark, tarry appearance; the condition of melena. This blood was altered as it passed through the digestive tract, so it is from the stomach or duodenum. A bleeding ulcer or cancer of the stomach may be indicated by melena. It should be mentioned here that certain medications, those containing iron, for instance, can also give this tarry appearance to the stools.

Blood may not be apparent to the naked eye, but a chemical test is required to show its presence. This is referred to as **occult blood.** It can indicate bleeding ulcers or a malignancy in the digestive tract.

If the stools are large and pale, appear greasy, and float on water, they contain fat. This is a symptom of the malabsorption syndrome. It may also indicate a diseased liver, gallbladder, or pancreas. Diseases of these organs will be discussed in the next chapter.

CHAPTER SUMMARY

The anatomy and physiology of the digestive system was reviewed to understand the diseases of each organ. The importance of such diagnostic procedures as barium x-rays, endoscopy, and microscopic cell study was stressed.

Certain diseases are characteristic of a particular organ, such as varicose veins of the esophagus, esophageal varices. Others occur in certain areas of the gastrointestinal tract; ulcers, for example, which develop in both the stomach and duodenum. Inflammation and cancer develop in all parts of the digestive system.

Some disorders result from anatomic abnormalities: A hiatal hernia, twisting of the intestine on itself (volvulus), and a kink in the intestine due to adhesions are of this type.

A psychogenic element, stress or emotional upset, is a factor in regional enteritis and chronic ulcerative colitis. Nervous states also aggravate duodenal ulcers and a spastic colon.

Any number of disorders—tumors, hernias, and gallstones—can cause an obstruction of the digestive tract. The motility of peristalsis can be inhibited by severe inflammation, as in the case of peritonitis. Motility can be increased in the colon, so that diarrhea results.

■ Self-Study

True or False

_____ 1. Esophageal varices are a complication of regional enteritis.

_____ 2. Hematemesis often occurs with peptic ulcer.

_____ 3. Amebic dysentery is a disease of the small intestine.

_____ 4. Numerous protrusions of mucous membranes through the intestinal wall are termed diverticulosis.

_____ 5. Intussusception is a disease of the stomach.

_____ 6. An acute intestinal obstruction requires immediate surgery.

_____ 7. A twist or kink in the small intestine could cause organic intestinal obstruction.

_____ 8. In acute organic obstruction there is no flatus.

_____ 9. Greasy, pale stools may indicate gallstones.

_____ 10. Chronic ulcerative colitis is caused by *E. coli,* staph, or strep organisms.

_____ 11. Corticosteroids may be used to treat Crohn's disease.

_____ 12. A hiatal hernia always requires surgery.

_____ 13. Colon cancer can be easily diagnosed.

_____ 14. "Pipe-stem" colon is characteristic of Crohn's disease.

_____ 15. Malabsorption syndrome causes black, tarry stools.

Multiple Choice

_____ 16. _____ is also called Crohn's disease.
    a. Regional enteritis
    b. Chronic ulcerated colitis

_____ 17. _____ would be the most likely cause of peritonitis.
    a. Gastritis
    b. Ulcer
    c. Cancer

_____ 18. Achlorhydria in gastric juice would suggest _____.
  a. peritonitis
  b. stomach cancer
  c. peptic ulcer

_____ 19. _____ causes pain in the lower abdomen.
  a. Diverticulitis
  b. Diverticulosis

_____ 20. Small area of mucous membrane becomes necrotic in _____.
  a. cancer of the stomach
  b. gastritis
  c. peptic ulcer

_____ 21. Hematemesis may accompany _____.
  a. Crohn's disease
  b. esophagitis

_____ 22. Absence of lipid enzymes causes _____ malabsorption.
  a. primary
  b. secondary

_____ 23. Peritonitis may cause _____ obstruction.
  a. paralytic
  b. organic

_____ 24. Pain is relieved by food in _____.
  a. gastritis
  b. ulcer
  c. cancer of the stomach

_____ 25. Cancer of the stomach is more common in _____.
  a. men
  b. women

(Answers on page 450)

Chapter 11

Diseases of the Liver, Gallbladder, and Pancreas

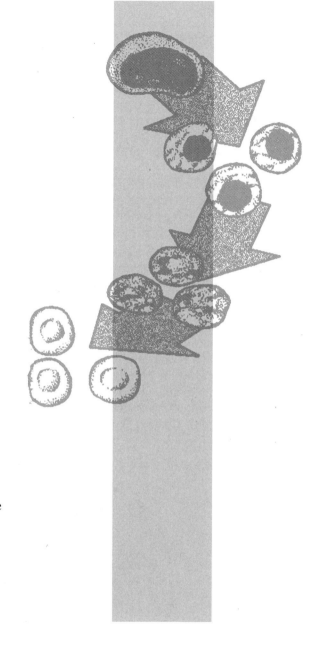

Chapter Outline

- Functions of the Liver
- Diseases of the Liver
- Diseases of the Gallbladder
- Structure and Function of the Pancreas
- Diseases of the Pancreas
- Diagnostic Procedures
- Chapter Summary
- Self-Study

*T*he complex process of digestion requires more than a well-functioning gastrointestinal tract. The liver, gall-bladder, and pancreas play essential roles.

FUNCTIONS OF THE LIVER

The liver is the largest glandular organ of the body, and it is unique in several ways. It has great powers of **regeneration;** it can replace damaged or diseased cells. The liver has countless functions essential to life, and even a small part of this organ can carry out these functions. The liver has a dual blood supply: It receives oxygenated blood from the hepatic artery and blood rich in nutrients from the portal vein. Figure 11–1 shows the arrangement of blood vessels associated with the liver.

The blood reaching the liver through the portal vein comes from the stomach, intestines, spleen, and pancreas. Blood from the small intestines carries absorbed nutrients such as simple sugars and amino acids. One of the functions of the liver is to store any of these substances that are in excess. The liver plays an important role in maintaining the proper level of glucose in the blood. It acts as a buffer, taking up excess glucose and storing it as **glycogen.** When the level of circulating glucose falls below normal, the liver releases glucose. Iron and vitamins are also stored by the liver.

Another function of the liver is to synthesize various proteins. These proteins include enzymes necessary for various cellular activities. One means of evaluating liver function is to determine the level of these enzymes in the blood. The liver also synthesizes blood proteins. Albumin is the blood protein that has a water-holding power within the blood vessels. If the albumin level is too low, plasma seeps out of the blood vessels and into the tissue spaces, causing edema. The development of this condition in certain kidney diseases, in which albumin is lost in the urine, was explained in Chapter 9. Other essential blood proteins synthesized by the liver are

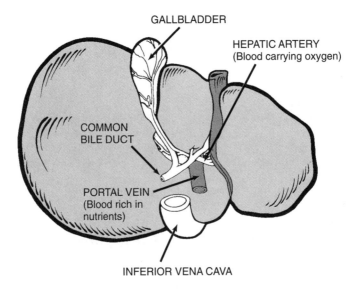

GALLBLADDER

HEPATIC ARTERY
(Blood carrying oxygen)

COMMON
BILE DUCT

PORTAL VEIN
(Blood rich in
nutrients)

INFERIOR VENA CAVA

Figure 11–1. Liver viewed from below showing dual blood supply.

those required for blood clotting, fibrinogen and prothrombin. If the liver is seriously diseased or injured and is unable to make these proteins, a bleeding tendency will result.

The liver can **detoxify** various substances, i.e., make poisonous substances harmless. Ammonia, which results from amino acid metabolism, is converted to urea by the liver. The urea then enters the bloodstream and is excreted by the kidneys. Certain drugs and chemicals are also detoxified by the liver. Specialized cells called **Kupffer's cells** line the blood spaces within the liver. These cells engulf and digest bacteria and other foreign substances, thus cleansing the blood.

Bile, necessary for fat digestion, is secreted by the liver. As mentioned in the previous chapter, bile is an emulsifier, acting on fat in such a way that the lipid enzymes can digest it. The end product of lipid digestion can then be absorbed by the walls of the small intestine. In the absence of bile, the fat-soluble vitamins A, D, E, and K cannot be absorbed. Various functions of the liver are shown in Figure 11–2.

Bile consists of water, bile salts, cholesterol, and bilirubin, which is a colored substance resulting from the breakdown of hemoglobin. It is bilirubin that gives bile its characteristic color of yellow or orange.

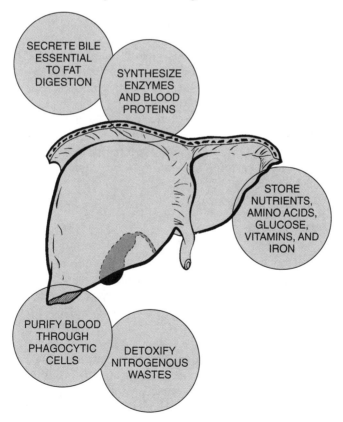

Figure 11–2. Functions of the liver.

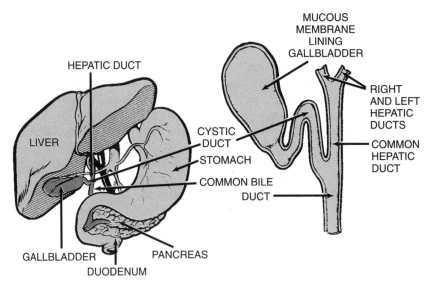

Figure 11–3. Bile duct system of the liver and gallbladder.

Bile is secreted continuously by the liver and channeled into the hepatic duct. The body is very conservative. The bile is sent into the small intestine only as needed, when there is fat to be digested. Until it is needed, bile is stored in the gallbladder, a small saclike structure on the undersurface of the liver. The gallbladder releases the bile into the cystic duct when it receives neural and hormonal signals to do so. Bile is concentrated in the gallbladder, with water and salts being absorbed out of it. Figure 11–3 shows the relationship between the liver and gallbladder, as well as the duct system. The common bile duct empties into the duodenum.

DISEASES OF THE LIVER

If the liver is injured by a virus or a chemical agent such as alcohol, the cells become necrotic. If the injury is slight, the dead cells are removed and replaced with new ones. If the damage is extensive, however, fibrous connective tissue replaces normal cells. When this occurs, the functioning of the liver is impaired.

■ Jaundice

One sign frequently associated with liver disease is jaundice. **Jaundice** is a yellow or orange discoloration of the skin and tissues, and the whites of the eyes frequently show this pigmentation. It is caused by a build-up of bilirubin, the pigment normally secreted in the bile and removed from the body in the feces, in the blood.

Causes of Jaundice. The liver may be normal and secreting bile as usual, but an obstruction may cause the bile to back up. The obstruction might be a tumor, a gallstone in the duct system, or a congenital defect. Since the bile cannot move forward, it leaks into the blood, with bilirubin coloring the plasma. When the blood reaches the kidneys, the bile filters into the glomeruli and appears in the urine, giving it a dark color. Since the bile is unable to reach the duodenum, because of the obstruction, the stools are light in color. They are usually described as clay-colored.

Complications can result from this blockage to bile flow. Any condition of **stasis,** a stagnation, can lead to infection. Lack of bile interferes with fat digestion and absorption which means that the fat-soluble vitamins are not being absorbed. In the absence of vitamin K, bleeding tendencies will develop. The obstruction can also cause liver damage.

Jaundice can also occur if the liver is diseased. If the cells are unable to function normally in secreting bile, bilirubin escapes into the blood. This condition will be discussed in more detail under hepatitis and cirrhosis.

Hemolytic jaundice has an entirely different cause, or etiology. This symptom accompanies the hemolytic anemias explained in Chapter 6. The condition may be congenital or acquired. In these anemias, the red blood cells hemolyze, and an excess of bilirubin results from the breakdown of released hemoglobin. Abnormal discoloration follows. Figure 11–4 illustrates the causes of jaundice and the complications of inadequate bile secretion.

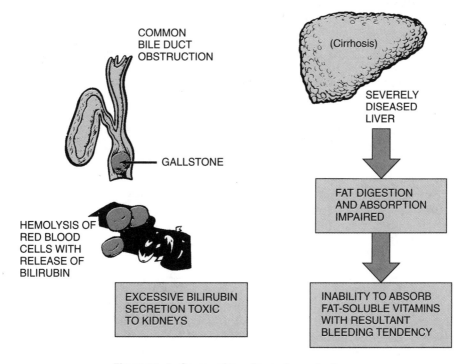

Figure 11–4. Causes of jaundice and complications.

■ Viral Hepatitis

Hepatitis, or inflammation of the liver, is caused by a number of factors. Certain viruses have been identified as causing three particular forms of hepatitis. They are hepatitis virus type A, hepatitis virus type B, and hepatitis virus type C.

Hepatitis virus type A, formerly called *infectious hepatitis,* is the least serious form and can develop as an isolated case or in an epidemic. Contaminated water or food is the usual source of the infection, which spreads under conditions of poor sanitation. The virus is excreted in the stools and urine, infecting soil and water.

The incubation period, the time from exposure to the development of symptoms, is from 2 to 6 weeks. The symptoms include anorexia, nausea, and mild fever. The urine becomes dark in color, and jaundice appears in some cases. On examination, the liver may be found to be enlarged and tender.

Hepatitis virus type A is usually mild in children; it is sometimes more severe in adults. Prognosis is usually good, with no permanent liver damage resulting. **Immunoglobulin** injections provide temporary protection against hepatitis virus type A for people exposed to it. Once a person has had either type of hepatitis, he or she is immune to that particular type for life.

Hepatitis virus type B, formerly called *serum hepatitis,* is a more serious disease. It can lead to chronic hepatitis or cirrhosis of the liver. Hepatitis virus type B can be transmitted by blood or serum transfusions in which the donated blood contains the virus. (Today, blood donations are routinely screened to minimize this risk; see below). It also is transmitted through the use of contaminated needles or syringes used by drug addicts and as a sexually transmitted disease.

The symptoms are similar to those of hepatitis virus type A but develop more slowly. The incubation period is long, lasting from 2 to 6 months. The severity of the disease varies greatly. A person's physical condition at the onset of the disease makes a difference in the seriousness of the infection. A person with poor nutritional status, for example, will be more adversely affected by hepatitis.

Occasionally a **fulminating** case of hepatitis virus type B develops, and it is fatal. This form has a sudden onset and progresses rapidly. The patient becomes delirious, then becomes comatose, and dies.

Let us relate the functions of the liver previously described to the failure of these functions, causing death. In the fulminating case, the liver becomes necrotic, so the cells stop functioning. They no longer produce the blood proteins necessary for blood clotting, so hemorrhage results. The liver cells are not able to detoxify poisonous substances, and as these molecules accumulate in the blood they affect the brain. This causes delirium and coma. Bilirubin is no longer secreted in the bile. Instead, it is carried to the kidneys in large amounts.

A specific blood test, which identifies the presence of a viral antigen in an infected person's blood, is used to screen all blood and plasma products for hepatitis virus type B. Blood is also routinely tested for antibodies to the virus.

Hospital personnel must be well informed of the hazards that can lead to acquiring hepatitis. Great precautions must be taken by nurses, laboratory technicians, dialysis workers, and blood bank personnel to prevent becoming infected. See Precautions for Health Care Providers (Chapter 2 under AIDS).

A vaccine called **Hepatavax B** is now available that provides immunity for viral type B hepatitis. Hepatitis B vaccination must be made available at no cost, on a voluntary basis to all employees who are at risk of occupational exposure. Employees who decline vaccination must sign a statement to that effect to comply with the directive of OSHA (Occupational Safety and Health Administration).

Hepatitis C is caused by an RNA virus and has an incubation period of 2 weeks to 6 months. Manifestation of the disease is similar to the other types of hepatitis and is spread much like hepatitis B. The virus for hepatitis C can now be identified and therefore the screening of blood and serum should reduce the risk of post-transfusion infection.

■ Cirrhosis of the Liver

Cirrhosis of the liver is a very serious disease. There are several types of cirrhosis, but the symptoms for each are similar. Most people associate cirrhosis of the liver with chronic alcoholism, which is the leading cause, but severe chronic hepatitis can develop into cirrhosis. A chronic inflammation of the bite ducts can also have the same effect. Certain drugs and toxins can cause necrosis of the liver cells, which is the first step in the development of cirrhosis.

Cirrhosis is chronic destruction of liver cells and tissues with a nodular, bumpy regeneration. In the normal liver there is a highly organized arrangement of cells, blood vessels, and bile ducts. A cirrhotic liver loses this organization and as a result the liver cannot function. Figure 11–5 illustrates the normal arrangement of liver cells, bile ducts, and blood vessels.

As the liver cells are damaged by excessive alcohol, drugs, or viral infection, they die, and are replaced by fibrous connective tissue and scar tissue. This tissue has none of the liver cell functions. At first the liver is generally enlarged due to regeneration but then becomes smaller as the fibrous connective tissue contracts. The surface acquires a nodular appearance. This liver, sometimes referred to as a "hobnailed" liver, is pictured in Figure 11–6.

Alcoholic cirrhosis, the most common type of cirrhosis, is the one that will be described in detail. This disease is also called portal, Laennec's, or fatty nutritional cirrhosis. An accumulation of fat often develops within the liver. Cirrhosis is more common in males than in females. The exact effect of excessive alcohol on the liver is not known, but it may be related to the malnutrition that frequently accompanies chronic alcoholism, or the alcohol itself may be toxic. Rather than name the symptoms of cirrhosis as a dull list to be memorized, each symptom will be related to the malfunctioning liver to be more meaningful.

The important **portal vein** passes through the liver and empties into the vena cava, returning blood to the heart. This vein becomes obstructed because of the disorganization, destruction, and nodular regeneration of the liver tissue. The blood backs up, affecting the organs drained by the portal vein: the stomach, intestines, spleen, and pancreas. Frequently the spleen becomes greatly enlarged, a condition known as **splenomegaly.**

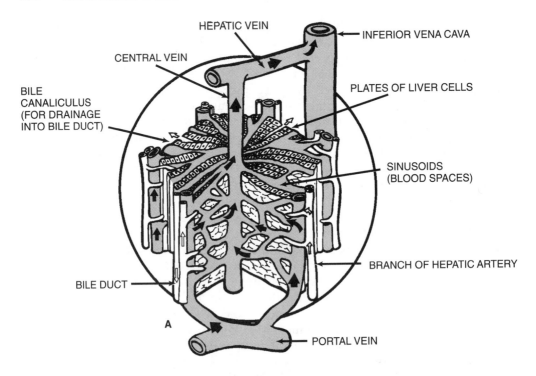

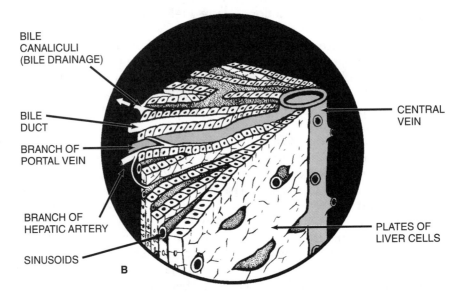

Figure 11–5. Arrangement of liver cells, bile ducts, and blood vessels in a liver lobule.

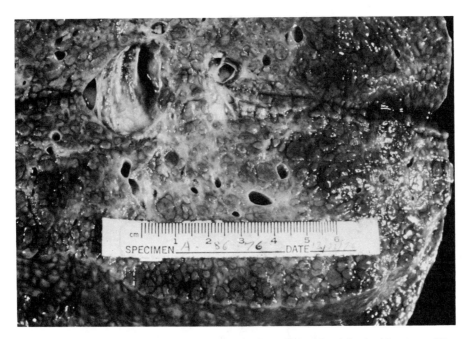

Figure 11–6. Typical "hobnailed" appearance of a liver affected by cirrhosis. (*Courtesy of Dr. David R. Duffell.*)

Unable to flow through the portal vein, blood seeks alternative routes to bypass the liver, forming a **collateral circulation.** These large dilated veins become prominent on the abdominal wall in the area of the navel.

Pressure builds within the veins of the esophagus as a result of blockage of the portal vein and **esophageal varices,** described in Chapter 8, develop. These varices tend to rupture, causing severe hemorrhages that can lead to shock and even death.

Hemorrhage can also occur in the stomach and intestines, and **hematemesis,** vomiting of blood, is often the first symptom of cirrhosis. The bleeding occurs because damaged liver cells fail to secrete the blood proteins essential to the blood-clotting mechanism. Alcohol, which causes the liver damage, is an irritant to the inner surface of the digestive tract, and as a result, the lining becomes inflamed. Another disease, acute hemorrhagic gastritis, often accompanies cirrhosis.

A relatively new procedure for treating esophageal varices is called **endoscopic sclerotherapy.** In this procedure a retractable needle is guided into the esophagus by means of a fiber-optic endoscope. The gastroenterologist punctures the varicosities and injects a caustic sclerosing (hardening) solution to occlude the swollen veins. This prevents engorgement, rupture, and hemorrhage or stops a hemorrhage that has already begun. Figure 11–7 shows the site of the back pressure that develops within the esophageal veins.

A characteristic symptom of cirrhosis is distention of the abdomen due to the accumulation of fluid in the peritoneal cavity. This fluid is called **ascites** and de-

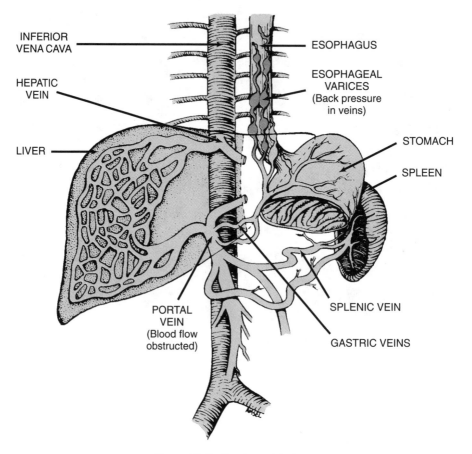

INFERIOR
VENA CAVA

ESOPHAGUS

ESOPHAGEAL
VARICES
(Back pressure
in veins)

HEPATIC
VEIN

STOMACH

SPLEEN

LIVER

PORTAL
VEIN
(Blood flow
obstructed)

SPLENIC VEIN

GASTRIC VEINS

Figure 11–7. Esophageal varices.

velops as a result of liver failure. The pressure within the obstructed veins forces plasma into the abdominal cavity, as illustrated in Figure 11–8. This fluid often has to be drained.

One function of the liver cells is to produce an important blood protein, albumin. When an albumin deficiency **(hypoalbuminemia)** develops, fluid leaks out of the blood vessels and causes edema. Since the necrotic cells of the cirrhotic patient fail to produce albumin, ascitic fluid develops, as does edema, particularly in the ankles and legs.

Jaundice usually results from obstruction of the bile ducts. The blockage of these ducts, like that of the blood vessels, follows the disorganization of the liver. Bile accumulates in the blood, giving the characteristic yellow coloration, and since bile is not secreted into the duodenum, stools are clay-colored. The excess of bile, carried by the blood to the kidneys, gives a dark color to urine.

A group of signs are related to the fact that the diseased liver cannot perform its usual biochemical activities. Normally, the liver inactivates small amounts of

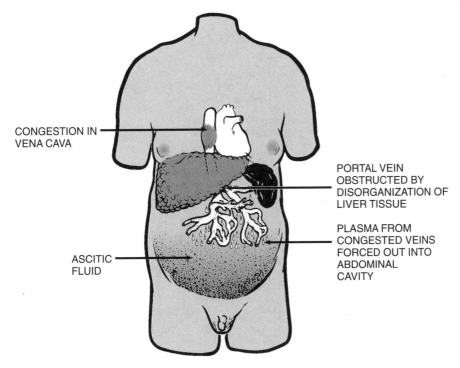

CONGESTION IN
VENA CAVA

PORTAL VEIN
OBSTRUCTED BY
DISORGANIZATION OF
LIVER TISSUE

PLASMA FROM
CONGESTED VEINS
FORCED OUT INTO
ABDOMINAL
CAVITY

ASCITIC
FLUID

Figure 11–8. Accumulation of ascitic fluid.

female sex hormones secreted by the adrenal glands in both males and females. Estrogens then have no effect on the male, but the cirrhotic liver does not inactivate estrogens. They accumulate and have a feminizing effect on males. The breasts enlarge, a condition known as **gynecomastia,** and the palms of the hand are red due to the estrogen level. Hair on the chest is lost, and a female-type distribution of hair develops. Atrophy of the testicles can also occur.

The necrotic liver cells are unable to carry out their normal function of detoxification, so blood is not cleansed by Kupffer's cells. As a result, ammonia and other poisonous substances accumulate in the blood and affect the brain, causing various neural disorders. The patient becomes confused and disoriented, even to the point of stupor, and a characteristic tremor or shaking develops. This shaking, together with hallucinations, is referred to as **delirium tremens,** or **DTs.** Somnolence, or abnormal sleepiness, may lead to **hepatic coma.** This is a possible cause of death in cirrhosis. The typical signs of cirrhosis are shown in Figure 11–9.

■ Carcinoma of the Liver

Hepatocarcinoma, or cancer of the liver, is sometimes a complication of cirrhosis. This is a primary malignancy of the liver which is rare. More often cancer detected in the liver is a result of metastasis from other organs such as the breast, the colon, or the pancreas. These tumors are secondary carcinomas.

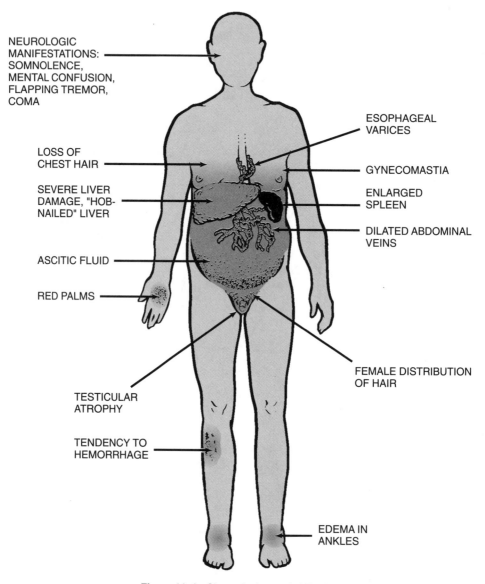

NEUROLOGIC
MANIFESTATIONS:
SOMNOLENCE,
MENTAL CONFUSION,
FLAPPING TREMOR,
COMA

LOSS OF
CHEST HAIR

SEVERE LIVER
DAMAGE, "HOB-
NAILED" LIVER

ASCITIC FLUID

RED PALMS

TESTICULAR
ATROPHY

TENDENCY TO
HEMORRHAGE

ESOPHAGEAL
VARICES

GYNECOMASTIA

ENLARGED
SPLEEN

DILATED ABDOMINAL
VEINS

FEMALE DISTRIBUTION
OF HAIR

EDEMA IN
ANKLES

Figure 11–9. Signs of advanced cirrhosis.

As mentioned in the chapter on neoplasia (Chapter 3), cancer spreads by way of the blood vessels and lymphatics. Because of the arrangement of these vessels through the liver, it is a frequent site of metastases. Cancer also spreads by invading surrounding tissue. A malignancy of the gallbladder or pancreas can grow into the liver. A high percentage of patients that die of cancer are found to have had liver metastases.

The symptoms of hepatocarcinoma vary according to the site of the tumor. If the tumor is obstructing the portal vein, ascites develops in the abdominal cavity, as it does in cirrhosis. If the fluid is found to contain blood, a malignancy is indicated. A tumor blocking the bile duct will cause jaundice, as a result of the escape of bile into the blood. General symptoms may include loss of weight, an abdominal mass, and pain in the upper right quadrant of the abdomen.

Prognosis for cancer of the liver is poor. Usually the malignancy has developed elsewhere and has spread to the liver. Techniques such as the liver scan and needle biopsy are used in diagnosing the condition.

DISEASES OF THE GALLBLADDER

The function of the gallbladder is to store and concentrate bile. The bile is sent to the duodenum when fat is present. This little muscular saclike structure does a lot of work. Like any organ it can become diseased or prevented from working by an obstruction.

■ Cholecystitis

Cholecystitis is an inflammation of the gallbladder. Note how meaningful the word is. The root word *chole* always refers to bile. A cyst is a sac. The gallbladder is a sac containing bile. The suffix, *itis,* indicates inflammation.

Cholecystitis is usually caused by an obstruction, a gallstone or tumor. Because of the blockage, bile cannot leave the gallbladder. The bile becomes more concentrated and irritates the walls of the gallbladder. The typical inflammatory response occurs, and the gallbladder becomes extremely swollen. Figure 11–10 illustrates various forms of bile obstruction. Pain is experienced under the right rib cage and radiates to the right shoulder. At this point the gallbladder can usually be felt (palpated). The patient experiences chills and fever; nausea and vomiting are also common symptoms.

Serious complications can result from cholecystitis. Lack of blood flow due to the obstruction brought about by the swelling can cause an infarction. With the death of the tissues, gangrene can set in. The acutely inflamed gallbladder, like an inflamed appendix, may rupture, causing peritonitis. A complication of chronic cholecystitis is that bile accumulates in the bile ducts of the liver. This causes necrosis and fibrosis of the liver cells lining the ducts. This is another form of cirrhosis, **biliary** (bile) **cirrhosis.** Possible complications of bile duct obstruction are summarized in Figure 11–11.

A patient with chronic cholecystitis experiences distress after eating fatty foods. The presence of fat in the duodenum stimulates the gallbladder to contract and release bile, and the contraction of the inflamed gallbladder causes pain. Nausea and indigestion, accompanied by belching, follow eating a heavy meal.

Prolonged inflammation causes the gallbladder to lose its ability to concentrate bile. The walls of the gallbladder may thicken, making it impossible for the gallbladder to contract properly.

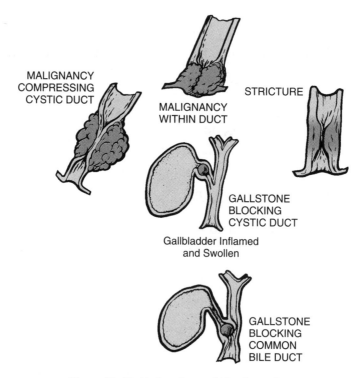

Figure 11–10. Various forms of bile obstruction.

■ Gallstones (Cholelithiasis)

Gallstones, also called **biliary calculi,** may be present in the gallbladder and give no symptoms. There may be one gallstone present or several hundred, which can be large or small. Small stones, referred to as gravel, are the ones that enter the cystic duct and cause an obstruction with excruciating pain. The formation or presence of gallstones is called **cholelithiasis;** the word element *lith(o)* refers to a stone.

Gallstones form when substances that are normally soluble precipitate out of solution. The stones consist principally of cholesterol, bilirubin, and calcium when

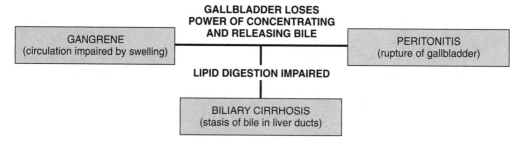

Figure 11–11. Complications of bile duct obstruction.

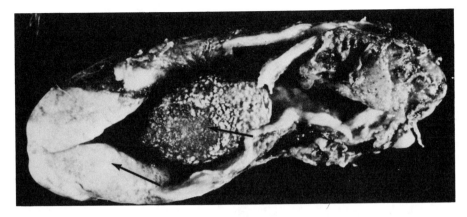

Figure 11–12. Gallbladder with chronic cholecystitis. Center arrow illustrates the gallstone. Left arrow points to the thickened inflamed wall. (*Courtesy of Dr. David R. Duffell.*)

in excess. Certain factors tend to stimulate gallstone formation such as obesity and pregnancy (because of an increased cholesterol level). The incidence of gallstones is higher in women.

The danger of gallstones is obstruction of the bile ducts, which causes inflammation. The converse is also true; inflammation of the gallbladder causes gallstone formation. Figure 11–12 shows a gallbladder with chronic cholecystitis and cholelithiasis. Stones can sometimes be dissolved by medication, depending on their chemical composition.

A new procedure, **extracorporeal shockwave lithotripsy (ESWL),** is now being used experimentally to shatter gallstones for removal without surgery. Lithotripsy was described in Chapter 9 for the removal of kidney stones. The position of the stones is one significant factor in determining feasibility of the procedure.

Gallstones can be located by sonography and x-ray. The usual treatment for cholecystitis and cholelithiasis is surgical removal of the gallbladder, a **cholecystectomy.** The cystic duct is then ligated and the common bile duct examined for stones. Occasionally undetected cholesterol stones are retained in the common bile duct following surgery. These stones have been successfully dissolved by administering a solubilizing agent through a catheter into the bile duct. This prevents the necessity of repeated surgery.

STRUCTURE AND FUNCTION OF THE PANCREAS

The pancreas is a unique organ, having glands of both internal and external secretion. The glands of internal secretion are located in patches of tissue called the islands of Langerhans. They make up the endocrine part of the pancreas. These glands secrete two important hormones, insulin and glucagon, which regulate the level of circulating blood glucose. **Endocrine glands** have no ducts but secrete

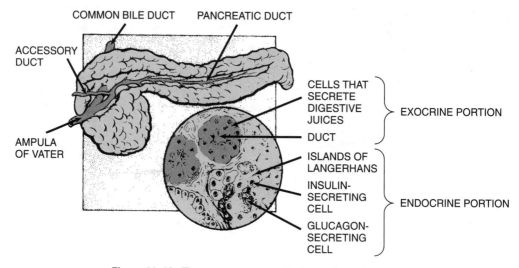

COMMON BILE DUCT   PANCREATIC DUCT

ACCESSORY
DUCT

CELLS THAT
SECRETE
DIGESTIVE
JUICES   } EXOCRINE PORTION

DUCT

AMPULA
OF VATER

ISLANDS OF
LANGERHANS

INSULIN-
SECRETING
CELL   } ENDOCRINE PORTION

GLUCAGON-
SECRETING
CELL

Figure 11–13. The pancreas—an endocrine and exocrine gland.

their hormones directly into the blood and lymph. Diseases of this part of the pancreas will be studied with those of other endocrine glands. Hormones of one endocrine gland often affect another gland. Figure 11–13 shows the structure of the pancreas.

The glands of external secretion comprise the exocrine part of the pancreas. These glands secrete the digestive enzymes and juices that are carried to the duodenum by the pancreatic duct. The pancreatic duct and the common bile duct generally enter the duodenum at a common point, the ampulla of Vater.

The pancreas is a fish-shaped organ extending across the abdomen behind the stomach. The head fits into the curve of the duodenum, and it is here the pancreatic duct empties. Figure 11–14 shows the relationship between the pancreas and other digestive organs.

The pancreas is one of the most important organs of digestion. It secretes enzymes specific for carbohydrate, protein, and fat digestion. **Amylase** breaks down carbohydrates, **trypsin** and **chymotrypsin** digest protein, and **lipase** breaks down lipid or fat. The proteolytic enzymes are in an inactive state until they reach the duodenum.

Diseases of the pancreas severely interfere with the digestive process. The great number of digestive enzymes contained within the pancreas make it a threat to itself, as will be explained in a particular disease condition.

DISEASES OF THE PANCREAS

■ Pancreatitis

Acute **pancreatitis** is a serious inflammation of the pancreas that can result in death. For some reason, the protein- and lipid-digesting enzymes become acti-

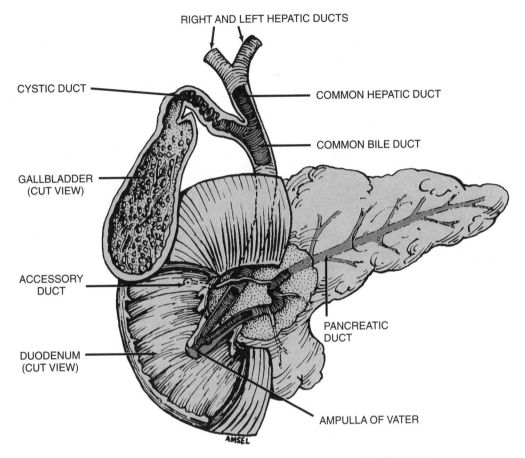

Figure 11–14. Relationship between pancreas and other digestive organs.

vated within the pancreas and begin to digest the organ itself. Severe necrosis and edema of the pancreas result. The digestion can extend into blood vessels, which, of course, causes bleeding; if hemorrhaging occurs, the patient may go into shock. When the condition becomes this severe, it is called acute hemorrhagic pancreatitis. This is shown in Figure 11–15.

Severe, steady abdominal pain of sudden onset is the first symptom. The intense pain radiates to the back, and it can resemble the sharp pain of a perforated ulcer. The patient feels some relief by drawing up the knees or assuming a sitting position. There may also be nausea and vomiting. Jaundice sometimes develops if the swelling of inflammation blocks the common bile duct.

Several factors can cause pancreatitis, but the most common one is excessive alcohol consumption. Inflammation of pancreatic ducts due to the presence of gallstones is another possible cause. Many cases of pancreatitis cannot be attributed to either of these causes. The etiology is said to be idiopathic, its cause is

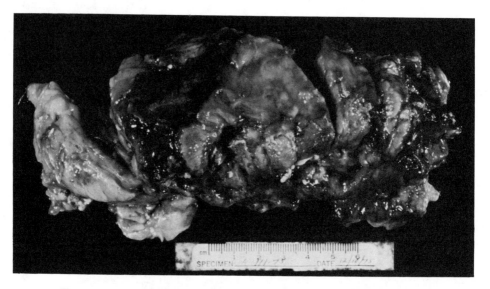

Figure 11–15. Acute hemorrhagic pancreatis. (*Courtesy of Dr. David R. Duffell.*)

unknown. Pancreatitis is more common in women than in men and usually occurs after age 40.

If a large area of the pancreas is affected, both endocrine and exocrine functions of the gland become inadequate. Digestion is severely impaired. In the absence of lipid enzymes from the pancreas, fat cannot be digested. Stools are then greasy and have a terrible stench. Secondary malabsorption syndrome develops, as fat that is not digested cannot be absorbed.

The most significant diagnostic procedures for pancreatitis are blood tests and urinalysis. High levels of pancreatic enzymes, particularly **amylase,** confirm the diagnosis of pancreatitis.

■ Cancer of the Pancreas

Cancer of the pancreas, an **adenocarcinoma** because the pancreas is a gland, has a high mortality rate. It occurs more frequently in males than in females. If the malignancy is in the head of the pancreas, it can block the common bile duct. This will give earlier symptoms than cancer in the body or tail, which can be very advanced before it is discovered.

Obstruction of the bile duct causes jaundice, as explained previously. Digestion is impaired if the pancreatic enzymes and bile cannot enter the duodenum. This causes malabsorption of fat and clay-colored stools. The patient cannot eat properly and loses weight. Great pain is experienced as the tumor grows, and the cancer usually metastasizes to the surrounding organs: the duodenum, stomach, and liver. Prognosis for cancer of the pancreas is poor and death occurs in a relatively short time.

DIAGNOSTIC TESTS

Liver function tests include those for serum and urine bilirubin, and serum enzyme assays. **Ultrasound** is used to evaluate the liver, biliary system, including the gallbladder, and pancreas. High-frequency sound waves are directed into the area to be examined. Through echoes converted into electrical energy, a pattern of spikes and dots appearing on an oscilloscope can depict organ size, shape, and position. Ultrasound has generally replaced the cholecystogram and cholangiogram, which are x-rays used in combination with radiopaque dyes to show the presence of gallstones, tumors, or a malfunctioning gallbladder. Computed tomography (CT) scans of the abdomen and pelvis visualize the liver, biliary system, and pancreas. This is a very significant test in diagnosing acute pancreatitis and cancer of the pancreas.

CHAPTER SUMMARY

The normal functions of the liver were reviewed, so that symptoms of liver disease would be meaningful. Liver cells become necrotic when injured, but the liver is able to regenerate new cells if the injury is slight. If the liver damage is extensive and liver cells are replaced by fibrous scar tissue, liver function fails.

Jaundice is frequently associated with liver disease because of abnormal bile production or release. Bile deficiency impairs digestion of fat and absorption of fat-soluble vitamins. In the absence of vitamin K, bleeding tendencies develop.

Hepatitis and cirrhosis are the serious liver diseases that were considered. Chronic hepatitis can lead to cirrhosis, but the most common cause of cirrhosis is alcoholism.

Cholecystitis, inflammation of the gallbladder, can cause gallstone formation, which in turn can cause inflammation. The most serious complication of gallstones is obstruction of the bile duct.

Inflammation of the pancreas, pancreatitis, is a serious disease in which enzymes intended for the digestive tract digest the pancreas itself. Carcinoma of the pancreas is a malignancy with a very poor prognosis.

■ Self-Study

True or False

_____ 1. Cirrhosis can lead to hepatic carcinoma.

_____ 2. Pancreatitis may be caused by a lodged gallstone.

_____ 3. Greasy, pale stools may indicate gallstones.

_____ 4. Incubation period is longer in virus type B hepatitis than in virus type A hepatitis.

_____ 5. Virus type B hepatitis may be caused by contaminated syringes.

_____ 6. Health professionals are encouraged to be vaccinated against virus type A hepatitis.

_____ 7. Stools are not infective in virus type A hepatitis.

_____ 8. Neural disorders can accompany serious liver disease.

_____ 9. A collateral circulation often develops in cirrhosis.

_____ 10. Virus type B hepatitis can be transmitted as a venereal disease.

Multiple Choice

_____ 11. Liver may excrete bile normally, yet jaundice may result in _____.
   a. hepatic jaundice
   b. obstructive jaundice

_____ 12. _____ is an infection of fecal origin.
   a. Virus type A
   b. Virus type B
   c. Toxic hepatitis

_____ 13. Formation of gallstones is called _____.
   a. cholelithiasis
   b. cholecystitis

_____ 14. "Hobnail" liver is associated with _____.
   a. cirrhosis
   b. hepatitis

_____ 15. Accumulation of fluid in the abdominal cavity is associated with
_____.
   a. hepatitis
   b. cirrhosis
   c. cholecystitis

_____ 16. Extracorporeal shockwave lithotripsy is a treatment for _____.
   a. biliary calculi
   b. esophageal varices
   c. cholecystitis

_____ 17. Cancer of the pancreas occurs more frequently in _____.
   a. females
   b. males

_____ 18. Pancreatitis is more common in _____.
   a. females
   b. males

_____ 19. Stools may be clay-colored in _____.
   a. cirrhosis
   b. peptic ulcers

_____ 20. Esophageal varices are a complication of
   a. cholelithiasis
   b. cholecystitis
   c. cirrhosis

(Answers on page 450)

Chapter 12

Diseases of the Respiratory System

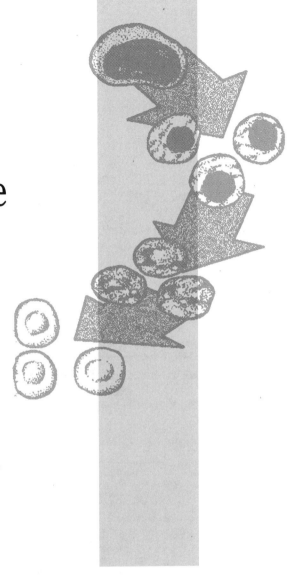

Chapter Outline

- Structure and Function of the Respiratory System
- Upper Respiratory Diseases
- Lower Respiratory Diseases
- Sudden Infant Death Syndrome
- Diagnostic Procedures for Respiratory Diseases
- Chapter Summary
- Self-Study

*W*e often use the familiar term "breath of life." What does this really mean? Every cell of the body is dependent on a fresh oxygen supply to utilize its nutrients with the production of energy.

The respiratory system provides oxygen to the circulatory system to distribute, so the two work hand in hand. A significant determination of pulmonary function is by blood gas analysis of the levels of oxygen and carbon dioxide.

STRUCTURE AND FUNCTION OF THE RESPIRATORY SYSTEM

The respiratory system consists of a tubular air passageway from the external environment to the lungs. Smooth muscle comprises the walls of these tubes, a significant factor in asthma. Air enters the nasal cavity, passes through the **pharynx,** or throat, to the **trachea,** the windpipe. The entrance to the trachea is the **larynx,** the voice box. The trachea branches out to the **bronchi,** one of each going to each lung. The bronchi continue to branch into smaller and smaller tubules called

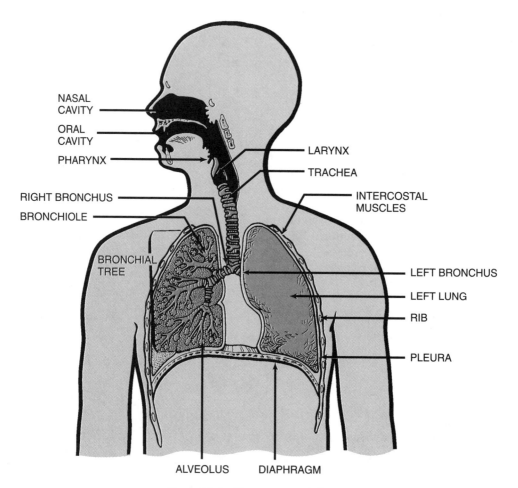

Figure 12–1. Air passageway to lungs.

On the Practical Side

HYPERVENTILATION

A story is told of a young babysitter whose infant charge fell out of bed. The panicked sitter ran down the stairs to phone the paramedics, up to check on the infant, and down again to unlock the door. When the paramedics arrived the baby was fine but the sitter had passed out. The cause? Hyperventilation brought on by acute anxiety. Overventilation causes expiration of excessive carbon dioxide (the stimulus to the respiratory center) so that breathing is reduced and inadequate oxygen reaches the brain. Constriction of cerebral blood vessels also occurs.

bronchioles. The structure resembles an inverted tree and is often called the "bronchial tree." The bronchioles terminate in the lungs as small air sacs called the **alveoli.** Figure 12–1 illustrates the air passageway.

The alveoli are very thin-walled sacs surrounded by blood capillaries where the exchange of gases occurs. Oxygen that is inspired, or inhaled, diffuses from the alveoli into the blood capillaries. The hemoglobin molecules of the red blood cells become saturated with oxygen. Carbon dioxide, a waste product of cellular metabolism, diffuses from the blood capillaries into the alveoli to be expired, or exhaled. This exchange of gases is illustrated in Figure 12–2. In obstructive respiratory disease, this exchange of gases is impaired.

Why does air move in and out of the lungs? The movement occurs constantly without your thinking about it. You can only hold your breath so long and are then forced to breathe. Respiration is controlled by a center in the medulla of the brain. The respiratory center is regulated by the level of carbon dioxide in the blood. The more carbon dioxide, the greater the need for oxygen. This center stimulates the muscles of inspiration—the **diaphragm** and the muscles between the ribs called **external intercostals** (*costa* means rib).

When the muscles of inspiration contract, the volume of the chest cavity increases. The pressure within the lungs decreases and air rushes in. The same muscles relax, the volume of the chest cavity decreases, and air is pushed out. There are also special muscles of expiration, the **abdominal** and **internal intercostal** muscles, but they are only needed in difficult breathing. These muscles are used in emphysema for example.

The lungs are encased by a double membrane consisting of two layers of **pleura.** One layer of this membrane covers the lungs, and the other lines the inner chest wall or thoracic cavity. There is only a potential space, the **pleural cavity,** between them, containing a small amount of fluid. This fluid lubricates the sur-

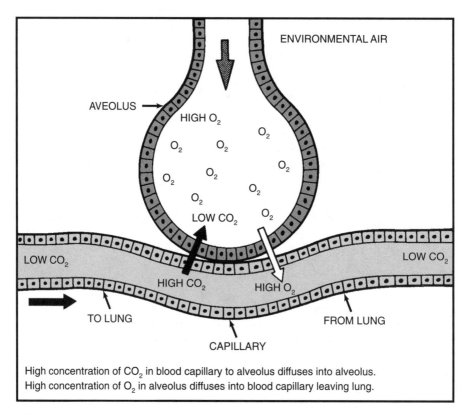

High concentration of CO_2 in blood capillary to alveolus diffuses into alveolus.
High concentration of O_2 in alveolus diffuses into blood capillary leaving lung.

Figure 12–2. Exchange of gases between lungs and blood. High concentration of CO_2 in blood capillary to alveolus diffuses into alveolus. High concentration of O_2 in alveolus diffuses into blood capillary leaving lung.

faces, preventing friction as the lungs expand and contract. The fluid also reduces surface tension, which helps to keep the lungs expanded. The airtight space between the lungs and the chest wall has a pressure slightly less than the pressure within the lungs. This difference in pressure acts as a vacuum and prevents the lungs from collapsing, as shown in Figure 12–3.

The lungs have a double blood supply. Unoxygenated blood is carried from the right ventricle of the heart through the pulmonary artery. Oxygenated blood is carried through the bronchial arteries to the lungs. Blood, rich in oxygen, returns to the left side of the heart to be distributed to the entire body. (See Chapter 7 for a review of heart–lung blood flow.)

The entire respiratory tract is lined with a mucous membrane, the **respiratory epithelium.** Numerous hairlike projections **(cilia)** are contained within this mucosa. When air is inspired, it is moistened and warmed as it passes to the lungs. The cilia exert a sweeping action, preventing dust and foreign particles from reaching the lungs. The breakdown of this mucous membrane paves the way for infection.

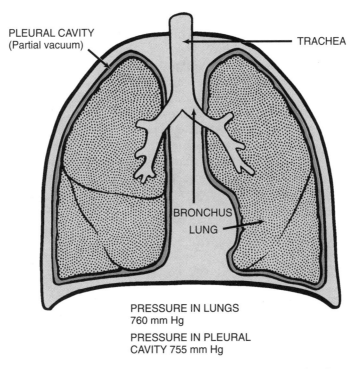

Figure 12–3. Air pressure difference between lungs and pleural cavity.

The lungs are in direct communication with the external environment because of the open air passageway. Bacteria and viruses, entering with inspired air, can set up various sites of infection along the respiratory tract. Diseases of the nose and throat are called **upper respiratory diseases.** Those of the trachea, bronchi, and lungs are **lower respiratory diseases.**

UPPER RESPIRATORY DISEASES

■ The Common Cold

The common cold is a disease that is within everyone's experience. The symptoms would not even have to be written. What causes the stuffed-up head, runny nose, watery eyes, and fever? Countless strains of a tiny virus are capable of causing this misery. The common cold is highly contagious. Unlike many other diseases, having had a cold provides no immunity. Another strain of virus is always ready to attack.

A cold is an acute inflammation of the mucous membrane lining the upper respiratory tract. The initial stuffed-up feeling is due to the swelling of the mucous membrane, which narrows the air passageway. Then the mucous glands begin their copious secretion.

Many people believe that you catch a cold by such actions, for example, as getting soaked in the rain, sleeping in a draft, or getting chilled. This is not true. It is a virus that causes a cold; however, these factors can lower your resistance, making you less able to fight off the viral attack.

There is no known cure for the common cold. The symptoms can be treated by using aspirin for the fever and antihistamines for relieving the congestion. Drinking fluids may help, but generally the disease has to run its course.

Very often with a viral disease, bacteria come in as secondary invaders. These are usually streptococci, staphylococci, or pneumococci. Bacterial infection frequently develops with the cold and may spread to the **paranasal sinuses,** spaces within the skull bones, or down the trachea. Many bacteria are pyogenic, and this accounts for the change in consistency of nasal secretion from watery to thick and yellow.

On the Practical Side

SNORING

The irritating sound of snoring is caused by vibration of the soft palate and back of the tongue when air flows through an open mouth. Sleeping on one's back can partially block the windpipe and thus cause snoring. Anything that interferes with air passage, nasal congestion, enlarged tonsils or adenoids, or a deviated septum can result in snoring. Drugs that depress the central nervous system reduce throat muscle tone and can prevent normal breathing. Sleeping on one's side and avoiding drugs such as tranquilizers, sleeping pills, and strong pain killers can often prevent snoring.

■ Hay Fever (Seasonal Allergic Rhinitis)

Hay fever, also called allergic rhinitis, is an allergic disease, and although it is not inherited, it does tend to run in families. A person does inherit a predisposition to become sensitive to certain foreign proteins called **antigens.** The most common offenders are the pollens of ragweed and grasses.

Chapter 2 discussed allergies in general. The allergic person has an abundance of antibodies called **reagins** or **immunoglobulins,** specifically **IgE.** These antibodies attach to the **mast cells** of the mucous membrane lining the nose and to the inner surface of the eyelids. When pollen, the antigen, contacts the antibodies, a complex is formed. This complex breaks down certain cells, causing the release of **histamine.** Histamine dilates small blood vessels that increase blood flow into the area. Histamine also makes the walls of blood vessels leaky. Fluid oozes out of the blood vessels into the surrounding tissue, causing edema. This accounts for the feeling of congestion in the nasal passages. Figure 2–7 is a diagrammatic representation of the allergic reaction.

The irritation of the mucosal cells stimulates an excessive secretion of mucus, causing the runny nose and watery eyes. Because the release of histamine causes these unpleasant effects, a substance that counteracts its action, an **antihistamine,** may give relief. Antihistamines do have side effects, such as drowsiness, dizziness, or muscular weakness. Antihistamines have a drying effect on the mucous membranes, and the mouth and throat tend to become dry. Because patients who use antihistamines can become drowsy, they are warned about driving or operating heavy machinery.

Many hay fever sufferers take allergy injections to **desensitize** them to pollen or other allergens. By administering small doses of antigen and gradually increasing the dosage, the patient produces antibodies against it. It is hoped that these antibodies can inactivate the pollen before it interacts with the reagins attached to the nasal mucosa.

■ Tonsillitis

The same bacteria that cause strep throat, the streptococci, can cause tonsillitis, or inflammation of the tonsils. The tonsils are patches of **lymph tissue** at the entrance to the throat (Fig. 12–4). Lymph tissue is very important, serving a protective function against disease. Lymph tissue, such as the tonsils, filters out bacteria and it then destroys them through the action of **phagocytic cells.** Antibodies produced to fight foreign antigens are also produced by lymph tissue (Chapter 2).

At times, too many strep organisms are trapped by the tonsils, and they themselves become infected. The tonsils become very enlarged and red. The opening to

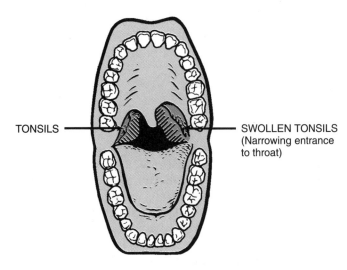

TONSILS

SWOLLEN TONSILS
(Narrowing entrance
to throat)

Figure 12–4. Tonsils—normal and enlarged.

the throat narrows because of the swelling, and swallowing is difficult. The throat is very sore, and a high fever develops owing to the strep toxins. The surface of the tonsils may become covered with pus. A blood count shows an elevated number of leukocytes, or leukocytosis, resulting from the infection.

Antibiotics are effective in counteracting the strep invasion. If the tonsillitis recurs frequently, it may be recommended that the tonsils be removed. This procedure used to be done routinely in children, but now that the protective function of tonsils is better understood, they are not removed unnecessarily.

A danger of strep infections, strep throat, or tonsillitis, is the onset of other diseases resulting from them. In Chapter 7, "Diseases of the Heart," it was explained that strep infections are the basis of rheumatic fever. The kidney disease glomerulonephritis also develops as the result of a strep infection.

■ Influenza

Influenza is a viral infection of the upper respiratory system. Everyone is familiar with the symptoms of the flu because it is so common. The onset of the disease is sudden. The patient experiences chills and a fever, a cough, sore throat, and runny nose. Chest pains, muscular aching, and gastrointestinal disorders may also be symptoms. Many different strains of viruses causing influenza are known. Recent epidemics have been classified as influenza A and influenza B, caused by viruses so named. Unfortunately, immunity for one strain does not protect against another.

There is a broad range in the severity of flu cases. It can be very mild, or it can lead to pneumonia and be life-threatening. Influenza is particularly serious in the elderly and chronically ill. The virus can destroy the respiratory epithelium, a strong line of defense against bacterial invasion. With the loss of the protective epithelium, bacterial infection can invade any part of the respiratory tract. Pneumococci, streptococci, and staphylococci are all capable of causing pneumonia.

There is no medication that cures influenza. Sometimes antibiotics are prescribed to ward off secondary bacterial infection. Bed rest, fluids, and aspirin to reduce fever are the usual treatments. Flu vaccines are only beneficial before onset of the disease, and these shots do not give immunity for all strains of the flu virus.

LOWER RESPIRATORY DISEASES

■ Chronic Obstructive Pulmonary Disease (COPD)

Chronic obstructive pulmonary disease (COPD), or chronic obstructive lung disease (COLD), includes a number of conditions in which the exchange of respiratory gases is ineffective. It includes, primarily, chronic bronchitis and emphysema. The respiratory control center of COPD patients is often affected.

These patients lose the normal respiratory response to elevated levels of carbon dioxide. When this occurs, the only stimulus for respiration is low oxygen tension. In this case, oxygen therapy can be fatal, as the effective stimulus on the respiratory control center to breathe is removed.

On the Practical Side

HOW LONG CAN YOU HOLD YOUR BREATH?

Only as long as the brain allows. Carbon dioxide builds up, stimulates the respiratory center of the brain, and one is forced to exhale.

During intensive study or reading, breathing is shallow. Again, carbon dioxide accumulates, stimulates the respiratory center, and a deep sigh follows.

One tends to hold one's breath while concentrating on a difficult physical task. Observe a basketball player about to make a free-throw and the intake of air that just precedes the throw.

Bronchitis. Bronchitis, inflammation of the **bronchi,** may be acute or chronic. The mucous membrane lining the bronchi becomes swollen and red, the typical inflammatory response. Irritants such as industrial fumes, automobile exhaust, viruses, or bacteria can cause acute bronchitis. If a **pyogenic organism,** a pus-forming bacteria such as streptococci, is the causative agent, pus can fill the lumen of the bronchi. The trachea as well as the bronchi may become inflamed, and the condition then is called **tracheobronchitis.**

Acute bronchitis is most serious in small children, the chronically ill, and the elderly. The tiny **bronchioles** of children can become easily obstructed. An obstructed bronchus is illustrated in Figure 12–5. The elderly or chronically ill are likely to have a secondary infection develop, such as pneumonia. Acute bronchitis often follows an upper respiratory infection. The patient experiences chest pains, **dyspnea,** a cough, fever, and sometimes chills. The sputum coughed up may contain pus. Depending on the organism causing the bronchitis, antibiotics may be administered. Viruses do not respond to antibiotics, but vapors, sprays, and cough medicines may give relief.

Chronic bronchitis is indicated by repeated attacks of acute bronchitis, coughing, with sputum production, lasting for several months for 2 consecutive years. The symptoms are the same as in acute bronchitis, but they persist. Chronic bronchitis may be a complication of another respiratory infection. Chronic bronchitis can result from long-term exposure to air pollutants or cigarette smoking. It is more common in men than women.

In chronic bronchitis there is an excessive secretion of **mucus** from the mucous glands of the bronchial **mucosa.** The mucous glands hypertrophy, and the mucosa itself is thickened and inflamed. The interference in the air passageway due to the swelling and mucus reduces the patient's oxygen level. **Hypoxia,** an in-

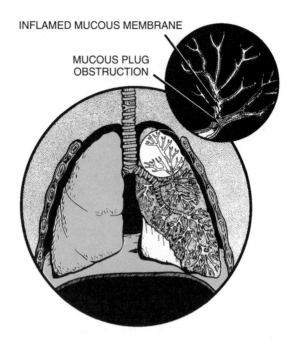

INFLAMED MUCOUS MEMBRANE

MUCOUS PLUG
OBSTRUCTION

Figure 12–5. Obstructed bronchus.

sufficient oxygenation of the tissues, results. Poor drainage of the mucus sets the stage for bacterial infection. Parts of the respiratory tract can become necrotic, and fibrous scarring follows. Chronic bronchitis is aggravated by other respiratory diseases such as the flu or a cold.

No cure for chronic bronchitis exists. The symptoms can be treated with antibiotics and moist vapors to ease the breathing. A cigarette smoker should quit smoking. Pneumonia, emphysema, and bronchiectasis, diseases yet to be described, are frequent complications.

Bronchial Asthma. A very common disease that can have serious consequences is bronchial asthma. Not only is the patient restricted in activities and likely to miss school or work, but the family also experiences a tension and anxiety when attacks are frequent or severe.

Bronchial asthma is not inherited, but there is a hereditary factor involved. A predisposition for hypersensitivity to various **allergens** is inborn. Common allergens are house dust, molds, pollens, animal dander, and various foods. Certain fabrics and cosmetics can also be highly allergenic.

What actually happens in an asthma attack that causes the characteristic wheezing and difficulty in breathing? It is a blockage of the airways, the bronchi. The smooth muscle in the walls of the bronchi suddenly contracts, narrowing the lumen of the tubes. The spasm is a sustained contraction of the musculature, making breathing, particularly expiration, very difficult. Figure 12–6 shows the narrowed bronchi resulting from muscular contraction.

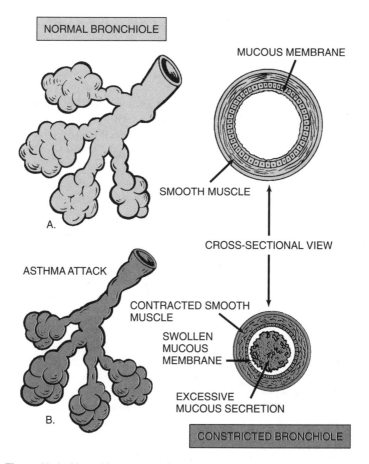

Figure 12–6. Normal bronchiole **(A)** and one constricted **(B)** in asthma attack.

The mucous membrane becomes swollen with fluid, also narrowing the lumen. Excessive secretion of mucus adds to the obstruction. Stale air becomes trapped, which decreases the amount of fresh air that can enter the lungs. The **wheezing** sound results from air passing through the narrowed tubes. The sound can be heard clearly by placing your ear on the patient's chest.

But another question must be asked. What causes the muscular spasm and abnormal reaction of the mucous membrane? This question brings us back to the concept of allergies or hypersensitivity developed in Chapter 2. Some asthmatic people have an excess of an allergic antibody, an immunoglobulin called reagin, or IgE. These reagenic antibodies have an affinity for, or are attracted to, the smooth muscle and mucous membrane of the bronchi. They attach themselves, and when corresponding antigens such as dust, pollen, or mold are introduced, complexes are formed. These antigen–antibody combinations cause certain cells—called **mast cells**—to release histamine and other chemicals. Histamine stimulates the mucous secretion and muscular contraction.

Psychogenic factors are frequently associated with an asthma attack. A tense situation or an emotional experience can trigger one. Other nonallergic causes are overexertion, infection, or inflammation of the bronchi, bronchitis. Exposure of the bronchial mucosa to irritants such as cigarette smoke, aerosol sprays, or perfume may also trigger an attack.

There is no cure for asthma, but attacks may become less severe with age. It is important to identify the offending antigens and avoid contact with them as much as possible. Skin tests, in which minute quantities of allergen are introduced into a scratch, can show various sensitivities. Development of a red hivelike lesion at the site of injection indicates an allergy.

Medication and allergy shots can reduce the incidence or severity of asthma attacks. To counteract an ongoing attack, substances that dilate the bronchi are effective. Ephedrine sprays and **epinephrine (adrenalin)** injections are often effective. Cortisonelike drugs are sometimes used, but these always carry a threat of side effects. All medications used in the treatment of asthma must be carefully controlled and under close supervision of the physician. Antihistamines, although somewhat effective for hay fever, should not be used for asthma.

The most severe form of an asthma attack is called **status asthmaticus,** in which the patient fails to respond to the usual treatment. A procedure as drastic as a **tracheotomy**—opening of the trachea surgically—may be required. Status asthmaticus may end in respiratory failure and death if not treated.

Great strides in asthma research have been made by the National Asthma Center at Denver. A reader with a particular interest in coping with this disease may wish to contact the organization for more detailed information. The following are suggestions offered by the National Asthma Center for reducing the frequency or severity of asthma attacks. These are listed in the Center's publication entitled *Asthma.*

Eliminate house dust as much as possible. Dust catchers such as wool carpeting, heavy draperies, and stuffed furniture should not be used in an asthmatic's bedroom. Dacron, rather than foam rubber pillows, should be used, as the latter can harbor mold spores. Pillows and animals stuffed with feathers or hair should be avoided. Animals should not be kept in the house and cigarette smoking should be avoided, at least in the presence of the asthmatic. Low humidity is desirable to reduce the growth of molds. When common allergens are high outside, the patient should stay in the house with windows closed. The patient should also avoid allergenic substances in food.

■ Bronchiectasis

Many respiratory diseases result from an already-existing disease. **Bronchiectasis** is an example of this. The word element *ectasis* means **dilation** or distention. In bronchiectasis, the smaller bronchi and bronchioles become chronically dilated, as seen in Figure 12–7. If you envision this as a ballooning of these walls, you can understand how they are weakened.

This dilation of the bronchi results from obstruction or infection in the respiratory tract. Obstructions tend to cause infection, as was previously explained.

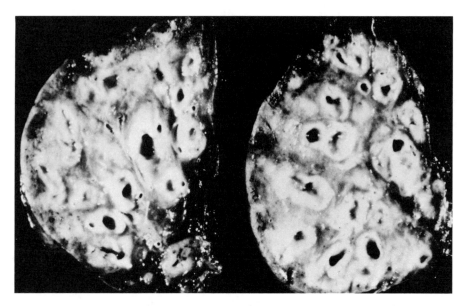

Figure 12–7. Bronchiectasis. Light areas are thickened walls of the dilated bronchi. (*Courtesy of Dr. David R. Duffell.*)

Bronchitis can lead to bronchiectasis because of the mucous plugs that develop. Bronchiectasis is sometimes a complication of influenza, pneumonia, or a chronic sinus infection. Children can develop bronchiectasis after measles or whooping cough.

As the bronchi dilate, pockets are formed where infectious material collects. **Abscesses** develop, which cause pus to be coughed up in the sputum. The weakened walls of the bronchi become necrotic and are destroyed. With the destruction of the smooth muscle in the walls, the ability to cough up mucus is reduced. Stages of bronchiectasis development are shown in Figure 12–8.

The necrotic tissue causes foul-smelling, pus-containing material to be brought up. The patient's breath also has a very bad odor. This infection may spread to the **pleural membrane** on the lung, causing pleurisy. If the infection invades the pleural cavity, empyema results.

Bronchiectasis can be arrested in the early stages but not after the tissue destruction is advanced. Penicillin or other antibiotics prevent secondary bacterial infection. Conditions that promote general good health—fresh air, good diet, and rest—are important.

■ Emphysema

Emphysema is a crippling and **debilitating** (weakening) disease. It is neither a contagious nor an infectious disease, but one of chronic lung obstruction and destruction. The cause of emphysema is not known, but it is most frequently associated with heavy cigarette smoking. Air pollution and long-term exposure to irri-

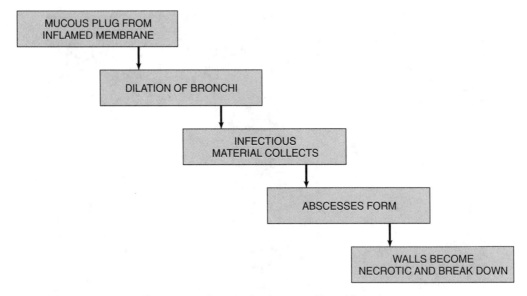

Figure 12–8. Steps in development of bronchiectasis.

tants of the respiratory tract also seem to be factors of its etiology. Emphysema is a frequent complication of chronic bronchitis.

The word *emphysema* means inflation. The lungs become filled with stale air high in carbon dioxide. This air cannot be adequately exhaled to allow oxygen to enter. The patient experiences a suffocating feeling and great distress from the inability to breathe. Severe pain accompanies the difficult breathing.

The emphysema patient shows an increased rate of breathing and a greater than normal expansion of the chest. The chest wall becomes permanently expanded, producing a characteristic "barrel chest." A stethoscope placed on the chest detects abnormal respiratory sounds called **rales.**

Let us go back one step and see what causes this inflation of the lungs with trapped air. The irritants mentioned—smoke, fumes, and pollutants—have their first effect on the cilia of the respiratory mucosa. When their sweeping, cleansing action fails, the mucosa becomes inflamed from the accumulation of foreign particles. In response, the mucosa secretes an excess of mucus that clogs the air passageways. Inadequate oxygen and excess carbon dioxide in the **alveoli,** the tiny air sacs of the lung, cause their thin walls to break down. Deterioration of the walls between alveoli results in a fusion of these tiny air sacs into larger spaces called **bullae.** Fewer alveoli are left to function. Elasticity of the lungs is lost with alveolar deterioration. An emphysematous lung is shown in Figure 12–9.

Emphysema patients are sometimes classified as "pink puffers" or "blue bloaters." The "pink puffers" maintain relatively normal blood gas volumes. They experience progressive dyspnea but no **cyanosis.** It seems that "pink puffers" are able to hyperventilate and they show an increase in lung capacity. The "blue

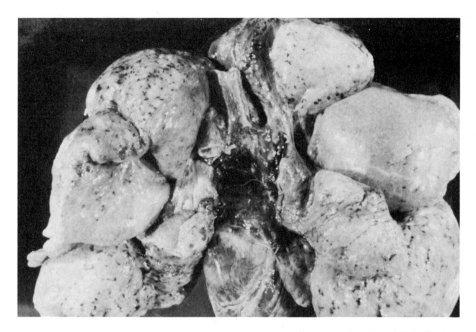

Figure 12–9. Emphysematous lungs viewed posteriorly. (*Courtesy of Dr. David R. Duffell.*)

bloaters," by contrast, show marked cyanosis. They have repeated episodes of right-sided heart failure and hypoxemia.

The loss of elasticity plus the narrowed airways explain the difficulty in exhaling the stale air. As the lungs become less efficient in moving air in and out, a strain is placed on the heart, as the circulatory and respiratory systems work together. The heart tries to pump more blood to meet the body's oxygen needs. This overworking of the heart causes it to enlarge.

Emphysema can last for many years, during which time the damage to the lungs is irreversible. As in any serious disease, complications often develop. With the breakdown of alveolar walls, the surrounding blood capillaries are damaged. This interference with circulation in the lungs can lead to an obstruction of the pulmonary artery.

The large air sacs formed by the fusion of the alveoli, tend to rupture. This allows air into the pleural cavity, the space between the lungs and the chest wall. Air in this space causes the lung to collapse. A ruptured **bulla** is shown in Figure 12–10.

Early detection of emphysema can slow its further development. Symptoms such as a chronic cough (often called smoker's cough), shortness of breath, and abnormally rapid breathing indicate a respiratory disease, and a physician should be consulted. The respiratory rate is increased in emphysema as the body attempts to get more oxygen. The patient tires easily and feels great distress after the slightest exertion, due to the lack of oxygen.

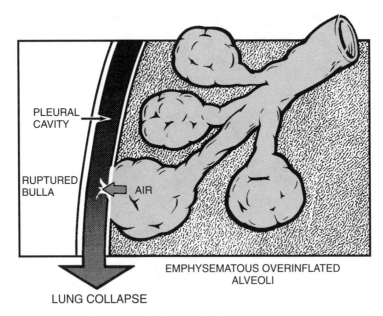

Figure 12–10. Ruptured bulla in emphysema.

The most significant diagnostic test for emphysema is an evaluation of the patient's lung capacity. A simple instrument, a **spirometer,** measures the ability to move air in and out of the lungs. X-rays do not show emphysema in the early stages. Treatment involves stopping the source of the irritation if possible. A smoker will be told to quit smoking and to avoid polluted air, air filled with smoke, fumes, and irritating dust. The patient should observe ozone warnings and limit outdoor activity when the ozone level is high.

Medications can be administered to clear mucus from the lungs. This prevents infection due to stagnation. Some medications give relief from the feeling of not being able to breathe. Physical therapy is sometimes helpful in teaching the patients to use all possible muscles of respiration in the abdomen and chest wall.

■ Pneumothorax

The lungs are surrounded by an airtight space. This is the pleural cavity between the two layers of pleural membrane. An air pressure in the cavity less than that within the lungs keeps the lungs expanded (see Fig. 12–3). If air or gas enters this pleural cavity on either side, the lung will collapse. Admission of air or gas into the pleural cavity is known as a **pneumothorax.**

A pneumothorax can occur in one of two ways. A weakened area of the lung can rupture, letting air into the space. Rupture of a bulla formed in emphysema is a common cause of a pneumothorax. Sometimes ruptures occur spontaneously in young adults. Air can also be admitted into the pleural cavity from outside the body. A chest wound, a stabbing, gunshot, or fractured rib can cause a pneumothorax. The increased air in the pleural cavity puts pressure on the lung and causes it to collapse. The patient experiences sudden, severe chest pain. Breathing becomes difficult and the pulse is rapid and weak.

Treatment depends on the cause of the pneumothorax. If it occurred spontaneously from within it will probably heal itself and the lung will reinflate. In the meantime, the patient must be rested. Drawing out the air from the pleural space, **pleurocentesis,** is sometimes required.

A pneumothorax can be used as a surgical procedure to rest a lung. A measured amount of air is admitted into the pleural cavity. This is sometimes done in the treatment of tuberculosis to give a tuberculous lesion time to heal. Collapse of a lung by this method may follow lung surgery to temporarily immobilize it.

■ Atelectasis

In the discussion of emphysema it was noted that bulging, weakened walls of the alveoli can rupture, admitting air into the pleural cavity. Entrance of air into the pleural cavity is the condition of pneumothorax. The increased pressure in the pleural cavity causes the lung to collapse. Collapse of the lung is called **atelectasis.**

Atelectasis can occur in one of two ways. A lung can collapse when it is compressed. The compression can be due to increased air pressure as in a pneumothorax. Increased fluid secreted by the pleural membranes also compresses the lungs. An accumulation of pus in the pleural cavity resulting from a ruptured lung abscess or malignant tumor can also cause atelectasis.

A lung will also collapse if the air passageway is obstructed. Air is unable to enter and inflate the lung. Severe chronic bronchitis can cause obstruction of a bronchi, because of the excessive secretion of mucus. This occurs if the mucus cannot be coughed up. A malignant tumor growing into the lumen of a bronchi also blocks the airway. Atelectasis can result from any of these events. Figures 12–11A and 12–11B show lung collapse due to compression and obstruction.

■ Pneumonia

There are many different kinds of pneumonia caused by several factors: bacteria, viruses, fungi, chemical/physical agents, and inactivity. Pneumonia is an acute inflammation of the lung. It can affect one lung or both. If both lungs are affected, it is called *double pneumonia*. Primary pneumonia is usually caused by pneumococci, streptococci, or staphylococci. Pneumonia can develop as a secondary disease after influenza, bronchiectasis, bronchitis, or congestive heart failure. One of the difficulties in treating pneumonia is recognizing the causative agent. This is necessary to prescribe the most effective antibiotics. More than one kind of pneumonia may be present at the same time, which makes treatment more difficult.

Lobar pneumonia is generally acquired by pneumococci. The bacteria may come from a person with the disease or from one who carries the organisms in his or her throat.

A person with low resistance is more likely to develop pneumonia. It often de-

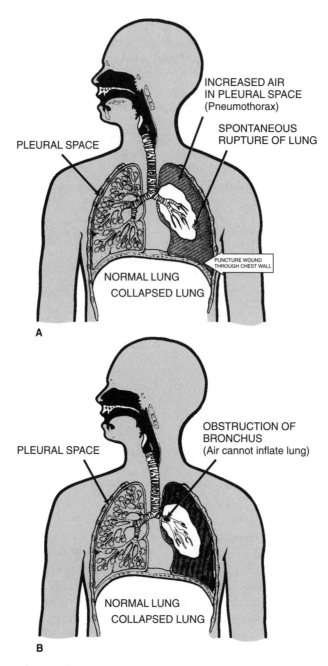

Figure 12–11. Causes of atelectasis due to **(A)** compression of lung and **(B)** obstruction of air passageway.

velops after surgery or immobilization resulting from a severe fracture. Chronic alcoholism is also a predisposing factor to pneumonia.

Lobar pneumonia has a sudden onset. The patient experiences a severe chill possibly accompanied by shaking. A fever develops and both heart rate and respiration rate are increased. Chest pains on breathing may be very severe.

The inflammatory response that produces **inflammatory exudate** was described in Chapter 2. In lobar pneumonia a great amount of exudate containing plasma, leukocytes, and fibrin seeps out of the capillaries into the air spaces, the alveoli. **Fibrin,** a plasma protein essential to blood clotting, becomes stringy when activated. This causes the exudate to solidify. The affected part of the lung becomes solid or **consolidated.** Capillaries can break down, causing the release of red blood cells into the exudate. The exudate takes the place of air in the alveoli. The inflammation spreads rapidly through the lung tissue and may affect an entire lobe. That is the reason for the name lobar pneumonia. It may affect the entire lung.

The severe pain is due to the pleurisy that generally accompanies lobar pneumonia. The pleural membranes, normally very smooth, become covered with exudate. This exudate is described as shaggy because of the consistency produced by the fibrin. A creaking sound is heard with the stethoscope as the two pleural membranes rub on each other.

Lobar pneumonia can be very severe at the onset, but it is relatively short lived, lasting about a week. Antibiotics are effective treatment. The crisis is passed when sweating occurs and the temperature drops; the causative organisms are killed and the exudate softens. Much of the exudate is removed by coughing it up in the sputum. Phagocytic white blood cells digest some of it. The return of the lung to a normal condition is called **resolution.** There is usually no permanent lung damage after lobar pneumonia and the lung returns to normal. As there is no destruction of lung tissue, abscesses do not form.

The symptoms of lobar pneumonia can be related to their causes. The patient's face is flushed because of the fever. Fever develops in response to toxins, the poisonous substances produced by the pneumococci. Fever is considered to be a protective body mechanism, as the elevated temperature kills some microorganisms. Cellular activity, or metabolism, is increased. More antibodies against the invaders are produced with this increase in activity. The respiratory rate is increased, but breathing is shallow. The poor uptake of oxygen by the consolidated lungs stimulates the rapid breathing. Breathing is painful because of the pleurisy that accompanies lobar pneumonia.

Coughing is a reflex, protective mechanism to rid the respiratory tract of an irritant. The sputum that is coughed up is sticky owing to the fibrin in the exudate. The sputum may contain red blood cells, as well as white blood cells and the pneumococci.

Bronchopneumonia (bronchial pneumonia) is primarily an inflammation of the bronchioles, a bronchitis. The infection then spreads into the alveoli at the termination of the bronchioles. The consolidation that develops is spotty. The entire lobe or lung is not consolidated as it is in lobar pneumonia. One or both lungs may be affected.

Bronchopneumonia is more common than lobar. The symptoms are less severe, and it develops more slowly, running a longer course than lobar pneumonia. There is a tendency for bronchopneumonia to recur, and the recurrences can be more serious. Abscesses tend to develop, and the lungs can be scarred with fibrosis.

Predisposing causes to bronchopneumonia are chronic bronchitis and bronchiectasis. It occurs most frequently in children and in the aged. In children, bronchopneumonia sometimes follows measles or whooping cough. In the aged and cancer patients, bronchopneumonia can be the cause of death. Predisposing causes of bronchopneumonia are summarized in Figure 12–12.

Diseases acquired from a hospital environment are called **nosocomial infections.**

The same organisms that cause lobar pneumonia cause bronchopneumonia, namely staphylococci, streptococci, and pneumococci. The infection is spread by coughing. Sometimes antibiotic-resistant staphylococci develop in hospitals and cause serious infections. The weakened patients are very susceptible to pneumonia from this source.

Primary atypical pneumonia is caused by a variety of viruses. Viral pneumonia is the most common pneumonia. It often develops as a complication of a viral disease such as measles or influenza. Primary atypical pneumonia is an acute inflammation of the upper respiratory tract involving the lungs to a lesser degree.

Influenzal pneumonia is a very serious inflammatory disease of the respiratory system. When you hear of great flu epidemics that killed millions of people, it was this disease that was responsible.

The influenza develops when a virus is inhaled and sets up an infection in the nose and throat. The infection spreads into the sinuses and down the trachea and bronchi. The patient becomes very weak, and resistance to bacterial invasion is lessened. Bacteria then attack the susceptible lungs with the development of pneumonia.

Both lungs are always involved. The exudate is not thick as it is in lobar pneumonia, so the lungs are not consolidated. Instead, the exudate is watery and contains blood. The bleeding is from ruptured capillaries, and abscesses form

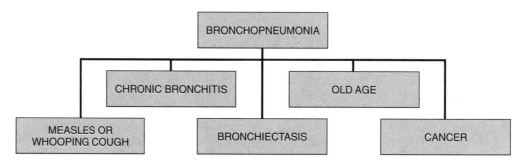

Figure 12–12. Predisposing causes of bronchopneumonia.

throughout the lung. These often rupture into the pleural cavity, spreading the pus and causing empyema, a disease yet to be described.

The patient is totally debilitated, has no strength, and experiences dyspnea. The fluid in the alveoli prevents the normal exchange of carbon dioxide for oxygen. The patient becomes cyanotic owing to the absence of oxygenated hemoglobin. A cough persists from the irritation within the respiratory tract, while the sputum is watery and contains blood. For a patient with lowered resistance, the disease can be fatal. Figure 12–13 summarizes the condition of alveoli in the diseased states described.

■ Pleurisy (Pleuritis)

Reference has been made to **pleurisy,** inflammation of the pleural membranes, as a complication of various lung diseases. Pleurisy may result from infection, pneumonia, or tuberculosis. It may follow an injury or tumor formation. Pleurisy is extremely painful; a sharp, stabbing pain accompanies each inspiration. It is treated with antibiotics, heat applications, and bed rest.

There are two kinds of pleurisy: dry pleurisy, the more painful form, and pleurisy with effusion. Dry pleurisy is a complication of lobar pneumonia. Each layer of pleura is congested, swollen, and covered with a shaggy exudate. Friction results as the pleura rub on each other, and they may stick together, forming adhesions.

Pleurisy with effusion results from an excessive amount of exudate in the pleural cavity. It can interfere with breathing by compressing the lung. Enough fluid may collect to cause the lung to collapse. This type of pleurisy is associated with lung cancer and tuberculosis. Pleural fluid can be drawn out with a needle for diagnostic purposes. Figure 12–14 illustrates the two kinds of pleurisy.

■ Empyema

If the exudate in the pleural cavity contains pus, the condition is known as **empyema.** (The word element, *py*, refers to pus.) Empyema has become rare ever since the development of antibiotics. Pus can enter the pleural cavity from a ruptured lung abscess or from an ulcerated malignant tumor that grows into the pleu-

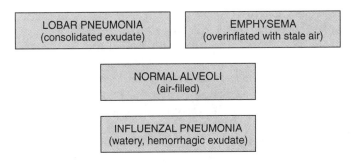

Figure 12–13. Comparison of alveoli in diseased states.

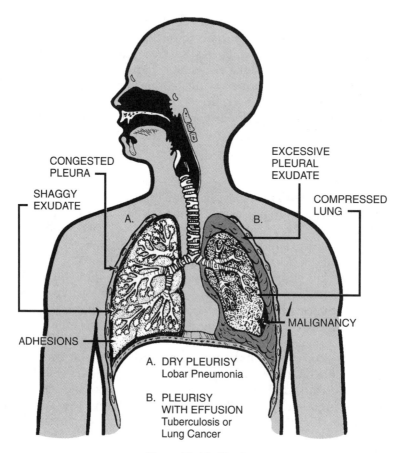

CONGESTED PLEURA

SHAGGY EXUDATE

EXCESSIVE PLEURAL EXUDATE

COMPRESSED LUNG

A.

B.

MALIGNANCY

ADHESIONS

A. DRY PLEURISY
   Lobar Pneumonia

B. PLEURISY
   WITH EFFUSION
   Tuberculosis or
   Lung Cancer

Figure 12–14. Pleurisy.

ral space. Empyema also results from the spread of infection into the pleural cavity in bronchiectasis. Atelectasis, or collapse of the lung, can follow the filling of the pleural cavity with pus.

■ Tuberculosis

The incidence of tuberculosis was greatly reduced several decades ago with early detection and treatment with new antibiotics. Unfortunately it is now making a serious comeback in the United States due to illegal immigrants from tuberculosis infected countries, AIDS patients with poor resistance to infection, homelessness, and the development of drug-resistant bacteria (Fig. 12–15). Tuberculosis is primarily a disease of the lungs, but it can spread to other organs such as the kidney, brain, or bone (see Chapter 16).

Tuberculosis is contracted by the inhalation of infectious material and is spread by coughs and sneezes. The organism that causes tuberculosis, *Mycobacterium tuberculosis,* has a protective waxy coat, enabling it to live outside the body

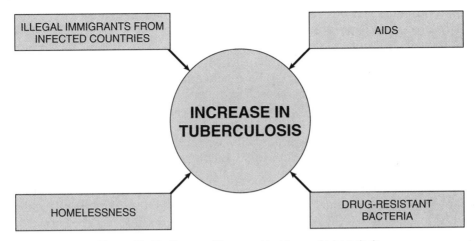

Figure 12–15. Causes of increased incidence of tuberculosis.

for a long time. Infected droplets of sputum dry up and the microorganisms remain as dust. They are killed only by direct sunlight.

Several reasons account for the decrease in the number of tuberculosis cases. Better living conditions, less crowding, and more available fresh air and sunshine are among them. Chest x-rays are required for admission to hospitals, for certain jobs, and are often part of complete physical examinations. If tuberculosis is detected in the early stages, it is easier to treat. Tuberculous patients are taught good hygiene in the management of their infectious sputum.

The symptoms are fever (particularly in the afternoon), night sweats, weight loss, and weakness. A productive cough accompanies the more advanced stages. The outcome of tuberculosis depends on the dosage of the bacilli received and the resistance of the patient. A healthy person fights off the disease, often not even aware of the infection. In the early stages, tuberculosis can be **asymptomatic,** that is, produce no symptoms. A person living in crowded conditions, poorly nourished, overworked, or suffering from chronic alcoholism is susceptible to serious tubercular infection.

The first infection with tuberculosis is called a primary infection. The lung lesion is a small spot, called a Ghon lesion, that drains to a nearby lymph node. The **tubercle bacilli** are surrounded by blood cells, macrophages, lymphocytes, and multinucleated giant cells. Antibodies are produced against the tubercle bacillus and its toxin. The disease can be overcome at this stage. A small scar of fibrous tissue, which limits the spread of the infection, may result. With the production of antibodies, the cells become hypersensitive to the tubercle bacillus, or allergic, so that a reinfection takes a different course.

It is this hypersensitivity to the organism that is the basis for the **tuberculin test.** Injection of the tuberculin protein into the skin triggers an immune response if the antibodies are present. A positive test result, development of a red, raised area within 48 to 72 hours at the site of injection, indicates sensitivity to the organism or previous exposure.

A secondary lesion occurs when there is reactivation of organisms from previously dormant tubercles. The tuberculosis bacillus can lie dormant for many years before a secondary lesion occurs. The reactivation may occur because of a decrease in the body's immune defense. The tubercle bacilli may also be carried to the kidneys or bone, causing a secondary infection (see discussion below and Chapter 16).

Most often the tuberculous lesion will heal with only a fibrous scar remaining. The scar may contain calcium deposits, which can be seen on x-ray. A minimum of lung tissue is actually destroyed.

The standard lesion of chronic tuberculosis is called a **tubercle.** It consists of a clump of bacilli surrounded by inflammatory cells. Within the tubercle, cells are killed by the bacilli—so the core becomes necrotic. It resembles a cheesy mass that is referred to as **caseous** material. Formation of this cheesy mass is called **caseation.**

The mass becomes liquefied and is coughed up in the sputum, leaving a cavity in the lung. Formation of cavities is the way lung tissue is destroyed in advanced tuberculosis. Numerous tubercles form and fuse, and caseation occurs. The result is the formation of large cavities. Blood vessels spanning a cavity can rupture, with a hemorrhage following. Blood is then coughed up, which is known as **hemoptysis.** This advanced form of the disease is called *chronic fibrocaseous tuberculosis.* The name refers to the fibrous scarring and caseation or destruction. Pleurisy is always a complication of chronic tuberculosis.

You have probably heard the term "galloping consumption" used to describe a killing disease. This lethal course of the disease is acute tuberculous pneumonia. The resistance of the patient is totally overwhelmed by the infecting organisms, and no defense is made against them. Frequently, because of the low resistance, secondary bacterial invaders enter, causing the severe pneumonia. If the tuberculosis spreads by means of the bloodstream, setting up minute tubercles in other organs, the condition is called *acute miliary tuberculosis.* Numerous bacilli enter the bloodstream, as blood vessels are destroyed by the disease.

Antituberculous drugs control the progression of the disease in many people. Surgery is sometimes performed to remove the diseased parts of the lung.

Tuberculosis of the Kidney.   Tuberculosis can develop in the kidney as a secondary site of infection. It usually begins in the lung, but the organism that causes tuberculosis, the tubercle bacillus, can be carried to the kidney in the bloodstream.

The lesion is similar to that of tuberculosis in the lungs. Tissue is broken down and cavities form, destroying the kidney. The necrotic tissue enters the ureter and is discharged in the urine. The tuberculous infection can then spread along the urinary tract.

Due to the breakdown of tissue, pus and blood are present in the urine. The tubercle bacilli are also found. If tuberculous lesions form in the bladder wall, urination becomes painful. The bladder is a muscular sac and contractions irritate the lesion. Uremia is the end result if both kidneys are affected.

■ Bronchogenic Carcinoma

Bronchogenic carcinoma, the most common type of lung cancer, arises from the bronchial tree. It can be observed with a **bronchoscope,** a lighted tube that can be placed down the trachea. A biopsy can be made using this instrument. Although bronchogenic cancer is easily diagnosed in this way, it is a most lethal form of cancer and the prognosis is poor.

Lung cancer is more common in men than in women. Although the cause is not known, it is linked to smoking and the inhalation of carcinogens, or cancer-causing agents. This can be an occupational hazard among workers who are constantly exposed to air pollution, exhaust gases, and industrial fumes.

The great danger in bronchogenic carcinoma is blockage of the airway by the malignant tumor as it grows into the lumen of the bronchus. The affected part of the lung collapses for lack of air. A malignant lung tumor is shown in Figure 12–16.

Blockage of any secretions leads to infection. Abscesses form in the obstructed bronchus, and walls become weakened and dilated, resulting in bronchiectasis. Bronchopneumonia is likely to develop and may be the cause of death.

The symptoms of lung cancer are a persistent cough and hemoptysis. The blood in the sputum results from the erosion of blood vessels by the growing malignancy. Anorexia, weight loss, and weakness accompany the disease. The poor oxygenation of the blood explains the generalized weakness. The patient experiences difficulty in breathing due to the obstructed airway.

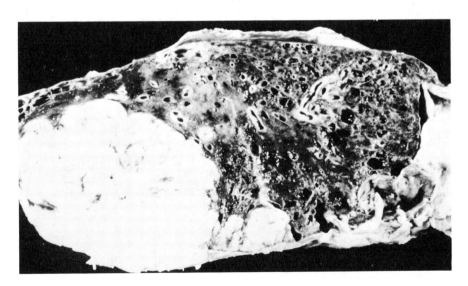

Figure 12–16. Carcinoma of the lung (large white area). (*Courtesy of Dr. David R. Duffell.*)

Diagnosis of lung cancer is made from a biopsy of the tumor, detecting cancer cells in the sputum, or washings from the bronchoscopy examination. Treatment may be surgery, radiation, or chemotherapy, depending on the particular tumor. In addition to primary carcinoma of the lungs, the lungs are a frequent site of metastases from the breast, GI tract, female reproductive system, and kidneys.

■ Cystic Fibrosis

Cystic fibrosis is a disease that affects all the **exocrine glands** of the body, the glands of external secretion. Exocrine glands secrete mucus, perspiration, and digestive enzymes. The abnormality in cystic fibrosis is excessively viscous mucus secretion. Cystic fibrosis is a hereditary disease affecting young children. It is transmitted through a recessive gene carried by each parent (see Chapter 4). Before the disease was understood, the mortality rate of afflicted children was extremely high. The most serious manifestation of cystic fibrosis is in the respiratory system. The trachea and bronchi secrete this thick mucus, and as it accumulates the air passageway is blocked.

Symptoms of cystic fibrosis are wheezing, persistent cough, and thick sputum. The child experiences difficulty in breathing because of the blocked airways. The child is particularly susceptible to respiratory infections due to the abnormal mucosal lining of the respiratory tract. Normally, bacteria are carried away by mucosal secretions, but in cystic fibrosis the bacteria adhere to the sticky mucus. The unmoved secretions serve as a breeding ground for bacteria. **Bronchiectasis** is a common complication of cystic fibrosis. Lung collapse can result from the inability to inflate them, and most deaths occur as a result of respiratory failure.

Not only are the mucous-secreting glands affected, but also the sweat glands. The child perspires excessively and loses large amounts of salt. Susceptibility to heat exhaustion is a result. This abnormal excretion of salt is the basis for the "sweat test" that confirms cystic fibrosis. Complications of cystic fibrosis are summarized in Figure 12–17.

Now that the disease is better understood, the lives of many more children are being saved. Antibiotic treatment reduces the incidence of respiratory tract infection, and respiratory therapy can relieve congestion in the respiratory tract.

This excessive mucus also blocks the ducts of the pancreas, preventing the release of digestive enzymes, and the absence of these enzymes impairs digestion. The child cannot benefit from the food eaten and is underweight. Lack of fat digestion results in large, bulky, foul-smelling stools. In the pancreas the glands become dilated and are converted into cysts that contain the thick mucus. Fibrous tissue then develops, which is how cystic fibrosis gets its name. Supplements for the lacking pancreatic enzymes can be given with food.

■ Sudden Infant Death Syndrome

Sudden Infant Death Syndrome (SIDS), commonly called "crib death," is the major cause of death for infants between one month and one year old. At present there are no adequate medical explanations for these unexpected deaths. Autop-

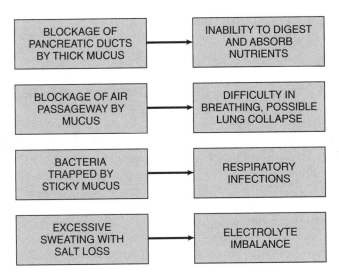

Figure 12–17. Complications of cystic fibrosis.

sies, examinations of the scene of death, and a review of the infant's medical history have failed to reveal the cause of death.

Extensive research is being done on various theories of possible causes of SIDS. Areas of study include the brain, particularly the brain stem, which contains the respiratory control center, the heart, and body chemical balances.

Researchers believe that eventually there will be a combination of factors involved and therefore they continue to study body positions, breathing and sleeping patterns, and environmental conditions. At present SIDS is neither predictable nor preventable.

SIDS occurs in all social, economic, racial, and ethnic groups. There seems to be a slightly higher risk in premature and low birth weight babies, among twins and triplets, and in infants born to teenagers. Risk factors were found by a National Institute of Child Health and Development study to include smoking during pregnancy, poor prenatal care, sexually transmitted diseases, and urinary tract infections which can affect the uterine environment.

■ Hiccoughs

Most everyone has experienced the annoyance of hiccoughs. What causes this phenomenon? Hiccoughs result from a spasm of the muscles of inspiration, particularly the diaphragm. Air is inhaled and the air passageway then closes abruptly, producing the characteristic sound. Hiccoughs can occur in normal people after eating or drinking, and they can usually be stopped by holding the breath, drinking water, or rebreathing from a paper bag.

Hiccoughs can accompany certain diseases and are then more difficult to stop. Persistent hiccoughs are sometimes treated with medication. If this fails, one of the nerves that stimulates the diaphragm—one of the phrenic nerves—can be blocked with local anesthesia.

DIAGNOSTIC PROCEDURES FOR RESPIRATORY DISEASES

Diagnostic procedures include bronchoscopy, chest x-rays, and, when warranted, **fluoroscopy,** which permits visualization of the lungs and diaphragm during respiration. Computerized tomography, or CT scans, augment chest x-rays. A series of exposed x-ray films visualize lung tissue at different depths.

Arterial blood gas analysis evaluates gas exchange, oxygen for carbon dioxide, and blood pH, thus indicating respiratory function. Sputum examination is helpful in the evaluation of pneumonias and suspected malignancies. Gram-stained smears and cultures are useful in identifying causative organisms and determining proper antibiotic treatment. Tuberculosis and fungal lung infections can be similarly diagnosed. **Spirometry** measures and records changes in gas volume in the lungs and thus ventilation capacity and flow rate. Figure 12–18 shows a spirogram and explains lung volumes and capacities.

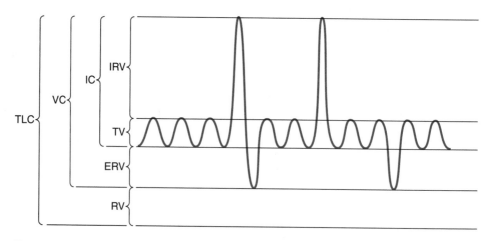

Total lung capacity (TLC)—includes vital capacity plus residual volume.
Vital capacity (VC)—the inspiratory reserve volume plus tidal volume plus expiratory reserve volume. This is the maximum amount of air that can be expelled from the lungs after maximal inspiration. Volume varies with age, sex, body position, and body build.
Inspiratory capacity (IC)—tidal volume plus inspiratory reserve volume (about 3500 mL).
Inspiratory reserve volume (IRV)—the maximal volume of air that can still be inspired after the end of a normal tidal volume (about 3000 mL).
Tidal volume (TV)—the volume of air moved with each normal breath (about 500 mL).
Expiratory reserve (ERV)—the maximal amount of air that can be expired, by forceful expiration, after the end of normal tidal expiration (about 1100 mL).
Residual volume (RV)—the volume of air that remains in the lung after a forced maximal expiration (about 1200 mL).

Figure 12–18. Spirogram explaining lung volumes and capacities.

CHAPTER SUMMARY

Reviewing the respiratory structure and function laid the foundation for understanding diseases of the system. The interaction of the respiratory and circulatory systems in providing the entire body with oxygen was explained.

Diseases of the upper respiratory system can be caused by both viruses and bacteria. Many viral infections, such as the common cold and influenza, are followed by bacterial infections. Pyogenic bacteria—streptococci, staphylococci, and pneumococci—cause the formation of pus. This is added to the excessive mucous secretion resulting from inflammation of the mucous membranes.

In allergic diseases—hay fever and asthma—the cause is hypersensitivity to foreign proteins. The allergy sufferer has abnormal antibodies, or reagins, also called immunoglobulins or IgE, that sensitize parts of the respiratory tract. The sensitization is in the nasal passages with hay fever and in the bronchi with asthma.

Certain respiratory diseases are related as a result of obstruction in the airways. Blockage of secretions sets the stage for bacterial infections. Chronic bronchitis can lead to pneumonia, bronchiectasis, and emphysema. Influenza and pneumonia can also cause bronchiectasis.

Pneumonia is caused by both viruses and bacteria. The elderly and chronically ill are very susceptible to pneumonia, which may even prove fatal. Predisposing causes of bronchopneumonia are chronic bronchitis and bronchiectasis. Again, the relationship between one respiratory disease and another is seen.

The severity of tuberculosis depends on the dosage of tubercle bacilli received and the resistance of the patient. The incidence of tuberculosis had decreased with better living conditions and effective antibiotic treatment after early detection. It is now, however, making a serious comeback in the United States due to illegal immigrants from infected countries. AIDS patients with poor resistance to infection, homelessness, and the development of drug-resistant bacteria are factors in the increase.

Lung cancer, although easily diagnosed, has a poor prognosis. The greatest danger is that the malignancy will obstruct the air passageway and the affected part of the lung will collapse.

Cystic fibrosis is a serious hereditary disease with the most serious manifestation in the respiratory system.

Sudden Infant Death Syndrome (SIDS) is a major cause of death for infants between one month and one year old. At present it is neither predictable nor preventable.

■ Self-Study

True or False

_____ 1. Abscess formation may accompany bronchogenic carcinoma.

_____ 2. A lung may collapse with bronchogenic carcinoma.

_____ 3. Pneumothorax can cause atelectasis.

_____ 4. Empyema is a degenerative condition of the alveoli.

_____ 5. Lobar pneumonia is caused by a virus.

_____ 6. A watery exudate fills the alveoli in lobar pneumonia.

_____ 7. Bronchiectasis is a predisposing cause of bronchopneumonia.

_____ 8. Sputum examination is important in diagnosing tuberculosis and fungal lung infections.

_____ 9. The lumen fills with pus in bronchial asthma.

_____ 10. The alveolar walls degenerate in bronchiectasis.

_____ 11. Rapid, deep breathing is a symptom of lobar pneumonia.

_____ 12. Suppuration can develop with the common cold.

_____ 13. Hypertrophy of the bronchial mucous glands develops in chronic bronchitis.

_____ 14. Dilatation of small bronchi causes bronchial asthma.

_____ 15. Lungs are shrunken in emphysema.

Match

_____ 16. bronchodilators   a) atelectasis

_____ 17. lung collapse   b) pneumothorax

_____ 18. shaggy exudate   c) pleurisy

_____ 19. air in pleural cavity   d) tuberculosis

_____ 20. caseous matter   e) asthma

Multiple Choice

_____ 21. _____ may result from bronchogenic carcinoma.
    a. Atelectasis
    b. Abscess formation
    c. Bronchiectasis
    d. all of the above

_____ 22. Barrel chest appearance develops in _____.
    a. empyema
    b. chronic bronchitis
    c. asthma
    d. emphysema

_____ 23. Changes in gas volume in the lungs can be measured by _____.
    a. sputum examination
    b. arterial blood gas analysis
    c. spirometry

_____ 24. Inflammatory exudate containing polymorphonuclear leukocytes and fibrin is characteristic of _____.
    a. influenzal pneumonia
    b. lobar pneumonia
    c. emphysema
    d. bronchial asthma
    e. tracheobronchitis

_____ 25. Foul-smelling, purulent expectoration is associated with _____.
    a. viral pneumonia
    b. tracheobronchitis
    c. bronchiectasis
    d. emphysema
    e. empyema

(Answers on page 450)

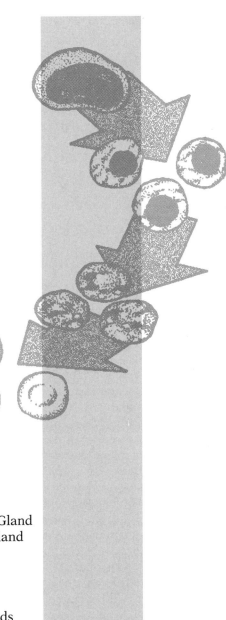

Chapter 13

Diseases of
the Endocrine
System

Chapter Outline

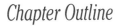

- Functions of the Endocrine
  Glands
- Structure and Function of the
  Pituitary Gland
- Diseases of the Anterior Pituitary Gland
- Function of the Posterior Pituitary Gland
- Hyposecretion of the Posterior Pituitary Gland
- Structure and Function of the Thyroid Gland
- Diseases of the Thyroid Gland
- Structure and Function of the
  Adrenal Glands
- Diseases of the Adrenal Cortex
- Structure and Function of the Parathyroids
- Diseases of the Parathyroid Gland
- Endocrine Function of the Pancreas
- Hyposecretion of the Pancreas
- Abnormalities in Secretion of Sex Hormones
- Diagnostic Procedures for Endocrine
  Diseases
- Chapter Summary
- Self-Study

The functions of the endocrine system cover a broad range of action. Endocrine activity affects the entire body: growth and development, metabolism, sexual activity, and even mental ability and emotions. The endocrine system is a means of communication between one body part and another.

FUNCTIONS OF THE ENDOCRINE GLANDS

All the glands of internal secretions are included in this system. These glands secrete directly into the bloodstream or lymph and possess no ducts. The pituitary gland, the thyroid, the adrenals, and the parathyroids are all part of the endocrine system. A certain area of the pancreas is endocrine in function, as are the sex glands. The sex glands—the ovaries and testes—will be studied with the Reproductive System in Chapter 14. Figure 13–1 shows the location of the endocrine glands.

The secretions of endocrine glands are **hormones**—the chemical messengers that circulate in the blood. Some of these hormones affect the whole body, whereas others act only on a distant organ, a target organ. Hormones may be steroids, proteins, or modified amino acids.

Most glandular activity is controlled by the pituitary, which is sometimes called the *master gland*. The pituitary itself is controlled by an area of the brain called the *hypothalamus*.

The body is conservative and secretes hormones only as needed. For example, **insulin** is secreted when the blood sugar level rises. Another hormone, **glucagon,** works antagonistically to insulin and is released when the blood sugar level falls below normal. Hormones are potent chemicals, so their circulating levels must be carefully controlled. When the level of a hormone is adequate, its further release is stopped. This type of control is called a **negative feedback mechanism.** Its importance will become clearer as specific diseases of the endocrine system are considered.

Overactivity or underactivity of a gland is the malfunction that most commonly causes endocrine diseases. If a gland secretes an excessive amount of its hormone, it is **hyperactive.** This condition is sometimes caused by a hypertrophied gland or by a glandular tumor.

A gland that fails to secrete its hormone or secretes an inadequate amount is **hypoactive.** The gland may be diseased, tumorous, or it may have been adversely affected by trauma, surgery, or radiation. A gland that has decreased in size and consequently is secreting inadequately is said to be atrophied. Each endocrine gland will be discussed with an emphasis on normal function and importance. The

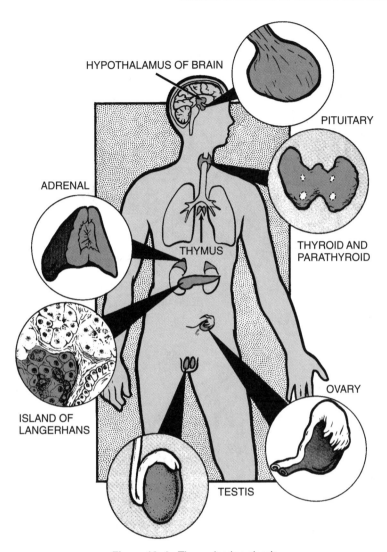

Figure 13–1. The endocrine glands.

diseases caused by hypoactivity and hyperactivity of each gland will then be explained.

STRUCTURE AND FUNCTION OF THE PITUITARY GLAND

The wonder of the pituitary gland is its tiny size and yet its tremendous functions. It is only the size of a pea suspended from the base of the brain by a small stalk. The pituitary gland fits into a bony depression in one of the skull bones that carefully protects it from injury. The pituitary gland is illustrated in Figure 13–2.

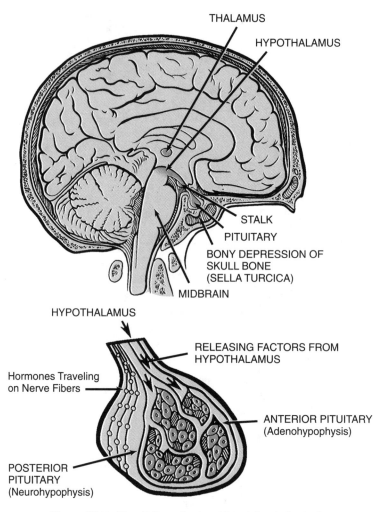

Figure 13–2. The pituitary gland and its relation to the brain.

Another name for the pituitary gland is the **hypophysis.** The hypophysis has two parts to it, each of which acts as a separate gland. Each part is stimulated differently to secrete, and each secretes entirely different hormones.

The anterior and larger portion of the hypophysis is the **adenohypophysis.** *Adeno* means gland, and this part is truly glandular. It is in direct communication with the **hypothalamus** of the brain. Portal blood vessels extending through the stalk connect the two. The hypothalamus is an extremely important coordinating center for the brain. It directs which hormones the anterior pituitary gland should secrete at a particular time. It does this by sending substances called **releasing factors** to the anterior pituitary through the connecting blood vessels. The pituitary then secretes the proper hormone.

The posterior pituitary, or **neurohypophysis** works differently. It receives hormones secreted by the hypothalamus and stores them for subsequent release. These hormones travel over nerve fibers from the hypothalamus to the neurohypophysis. It is because of the neural connection with the hypothalamus, that the posterior portion of the pituitary gland is called the neurohypophysis.

What can this little pea-sized structure control that makes it the master gland? The anterior pituitary, the adenohypophysis, secretes six hormones called *tropic hormones*. The word element *tropic* means going toward. That is what these six hormones do. They go toward a particular target organ.

■ Hormones of the Anterior Pituitary Gland

Growth hormone (GH; also called **somatotropin**) affects all parts of the body by promoting growth and development of the tissues. Before puberty, it stimulates

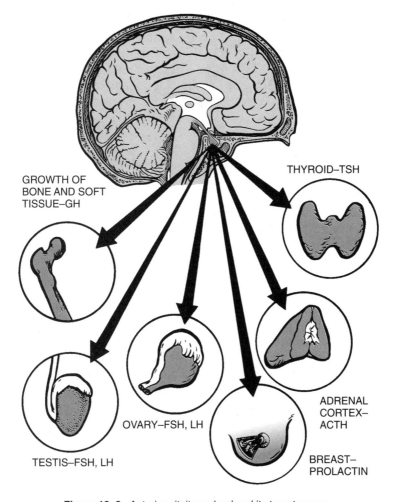

Figure 13–3. Anterior pituitary gland and its target organs.

the growth of long bones, increasing the child's height. Soft tissues—organs such as the liver, heart, and kidneys—also increase in size and develop under the influence of growth hormone. After adolescence, growth hormone is secreted in lesser amounts but continues to function in promoting tissue replacement and repair.

The thyroid gland regulates metabolism, the rate at which the body produces and uses energy. Secretion of thyroid hormone is controlled by the anterior pituitary. The pituitary hormone that stimulates the thyroid gland is *thyroid stimulating hormone* (TSH; also called **thyrotropin**). In the absence of TSH, the thyroid gland stops functioning.

The adrenal glands, essential to life, are also regulated by the anterior pituitary. The adrenal glands have an inner part, the medulla, and an outer portion, the cortex. It is the cortex that is controlled by the anterior pituitary. The tropic hormone affecting the adrenal cortex is **adrenocorticotropic hormone (ACTH).**

The anterior pituitary regulates sexual development and function by means of hormones known as the **gonadotropins.** These are not sex hormones, but they affect the sex organs, the gonads. They are follicle-stimulating hormone (FSH) and luteinizing hormone (LH) and prolactin. These gonadotropic hormones regulate the menstrual cycle and secretion of male and female hormones. The relationship between the anterior pituitary and its target organs is seen in Figure 13–3.

DISEASES OF THE ANTERIOR PITUITARY GLAND

■ Hyperpituitarism

The most noticeable result of **hyperpituitarism** is the effect of excessive growth hormone. The condition produces a giant if the hypersecretion of growth hormone occurs before puberty. Normally at puberty the ends of the long bones seal with the shafts and no further height is attained. Excessive growth hormone retards this normal closure of the bones. Sexual development is usually decreased and mental development may be normal or retarded. **Gigantism** is usually the result of a tumor, an **adenoma,** of the anterior pituitary. Removal of the tumor or radiation treatment to reduce its size decreases the secretion of growth hormone.

If the excessive production of growth hormone occurs after puberty, when full stature is attained, the result is different. This is the condition of **acromegaly;** the word element *megaly* means enlargement. The long bones can no longer grow in length, but the bones of the hands, feet, and face enlarge. There is also excessive growth of soft tissues. The features of the face become coarsened; the nose and lips enlarge, and the lower jaw protrudes, producing an overbite that interferes with chewing. The skin and tongue thicken, the latter causing slurred speech. A curvature of the spine often develops, giving the patient a bent appearance. The curvature is due to an overgrowth of the vertebrae. This hyperactivity of the pituitary gland is generally due to a tumor. A patient with acromegaly is illustrated in Figure 13–4.

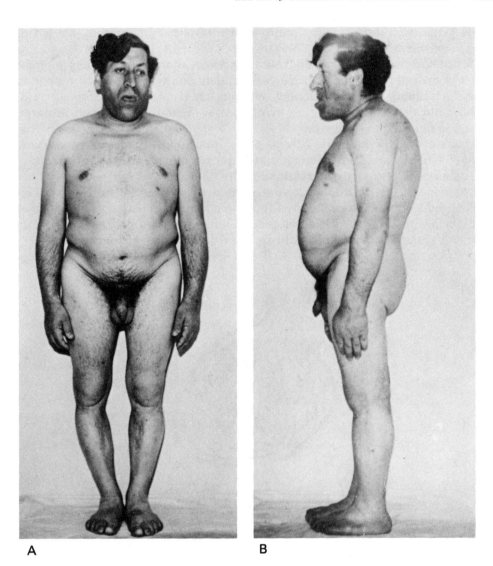

A   B

Figure 13–4. A. A 43-year-old patient with acromegaly. Note heavy, stocky build; broad chest; large head; and heavy hands and feet. **B.** Curvature of the spine causes the arms to appear excessively large. Thickening of the fingers interferes with manual dexterity.

■ Hypopituitarism

Hypopituitarism can result from damage to the anterior lobe of the pituitary gland or from an inadequate secretion of hormones. A fracture at the base of the skull, a tumor, or ischemia (lack of blood flow) can cause pituitary destruction. Lack of blood flow causes an infarction, and the tissue becomes necrotic. Hypopituitarism can be mild or severe. If the entire anterior lobe of the pituitary is destroyed, the condition is called **panhypopituitarism,** *pan* meaning all. No pituitary hormones are secreted.

The abnormalities that result from the absence of tropic hormones are numerous. The thyroid gland, for example, is dependent on thyroid-stimulating hormone from the pituitary for its functioning. Without that tropic hormone, the thyroid atrophies and the functions of the thyroid cease. Mental dullness and **lethargy,** a condition of drowsiness, develop.

Lack of ACTH causes the adrenal cortex to atrophy. Inadequate cortical hormones result in a salt imbalance and improper metabolism of nutrients. The adrenal cortical hormones are essential to life.

Absence of the gonadotropic hormones depresses sexual functions. The gonads atrophy without stimulation of the tropic hormones. If the lack of hormones exists before puberty, sexual development is impaired. In an adult woman menstruation ceases; an adult male will lack sex drive or have **aspermia,** that is, no

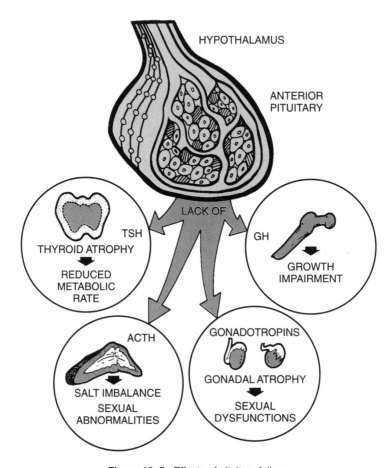

Figure 13–5. Effects of pituitary failure.

OPTIC NERVE

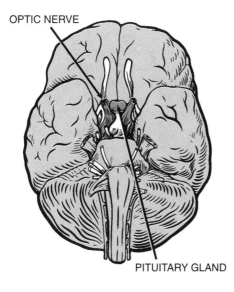

PITUITARY GLAND

Figure 13–6. Base of brain showing proximity of pituitary gland to optic nerves.

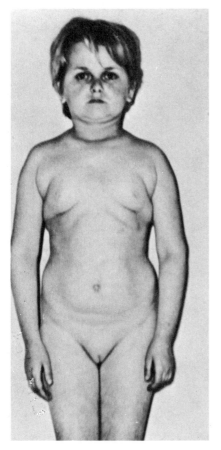

Figure 13–7. This 28-year-old pituitary dwarf is 45 inches tall, with the characteristic round face and fat deposits in breasts and abdomen. No sexual development is observed.

formation or emission of sperm. Figure 13–5 illustrates the glandular failure caused by severe hypopituitarism.

Hypopituitarism caused by a tumor may show additional symptoms. Pressure of the tumor may cause pain, a headache, or a peculiar form of blindness. Figure 13–6 shows the closeness of the pituitary gland to the optic nerves. As the tumor enlarges, it interferes with these nerves.

The patient suffering from hypopituitarism must be treated with hormonal supplements. Administration of **thyroxine, cortisone,** growth hormone, and sex hormones can compensate for the dysfunctional glands. It is significant that all these failures result from hypoactivity of the anterior pituitary. For this reason the anterior pituitary is called the master gland.

A different form of hypopituitarism sometimes occurs in children. Inadequate growth hormone can cause a pituitary dwarf. This patient is mentally bright but small and underdeveloped sexually. All growth processes are retarded; teeth, for example, are late in erupting. A 28-year-old pituitary dwarf is shown in Figure

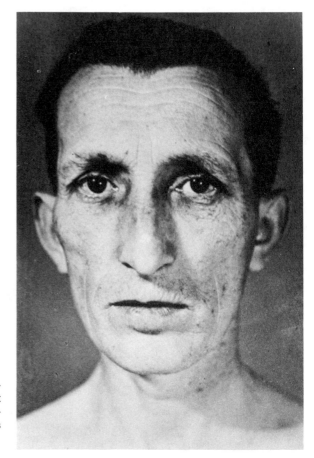

Figure 13–8. Face of a 29-year-old patient with a pituitary tumor and insufficient pituitary hormones. Note premature aging. The skin shows many fine wrinkles and lack of beard growth.

13–7. Growth hormones to prevent this condition are now being synthesized and tested.

Simmond's syndrome, a form of premature senility, is the result of chronic pituitary insufficiency, a case of panhypopituitarism. A child with this disease has the appearance of an old man or woman with pale, wrinkled skin and fine, soft hair. A 29-year-old man with pituitary insufficiency is shown in Figure 13–8.

Simmond's syndrome develops in an adult if the anterior pituitary becomes necrotic. This can follow a serious head injury or pituitary ischemia. Blood vessels to the pituitary occasionally collapse after a hemorrhage from a difficult delivery. A patient affected with this condition is seen in Figure 13–9. The breasts lack normal engorgement after a delivery, and pigmentation around the nipple is decreased. Simmond's syndrome may also be caused by an undifferentiated tumor of the pituitary that secretes no hormones.

Symptoms of this disease include weakness, dry, smooth skin with no sweating, and a loss of pubic and axillary hair. Both blood pressure and the rate of

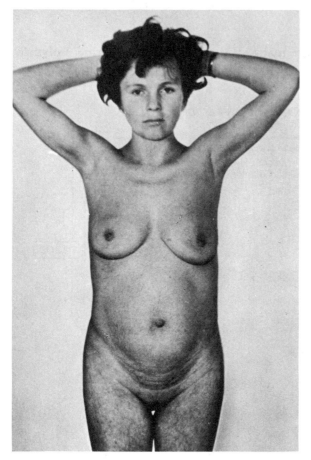

Figure 13–9. A 26-year-old patient with hypopituitarism after childbirth. Her skin is pale, and pubic and axillary hair has ceased to grow. Note lack of breast development.

metabolism are low. Menstruation ceases in a woman, and sex drive is decreased. Since Simmond's syndrome is a form of panhypopituitarism, the symptoms result from widespread glandular failure. The thyroid, adrenal cortex, and glands cease to function because of inadequate stimulation by the anterior pituitary gland.

FUNCTION OF THE POSTERIOR PITUITARY GLAND

The posterior pituitary, or neurohypophysis, secretes two hormones: **oxytocin** and **vasopressin,** also called **antidiuretic hormone** (ADH). Oxytocin causes smooth muscle, particularly that of the uterus, to contract. It strengthens contractions during labor and helps to prevent hemorrhage after delivery. Antidiuretic hormone prevents excessive water loss through the kidneys and makes the collecting ducts permeable to water. Water is then reabsorbed back into the bloodstream by the kidney tubules.

HYPOSECRETION OF THE POSTERIOR PITUITARY GLAND

■ Diabetes Insipidus

In the absence of ADH, water is not reabsorbed and is lost in the urine. **Polyuria,** excessive urination, results. This is the condition of **diabetes insipidus,** a disease

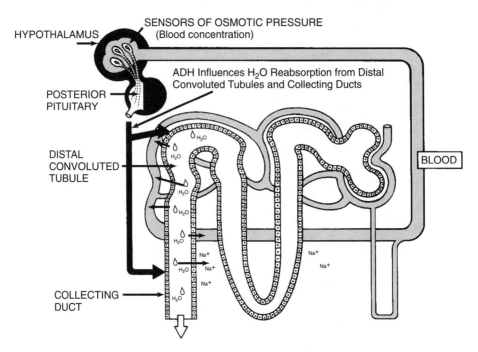

Figure 13–10A. Normal action of antidiuretic hormone (ADH).

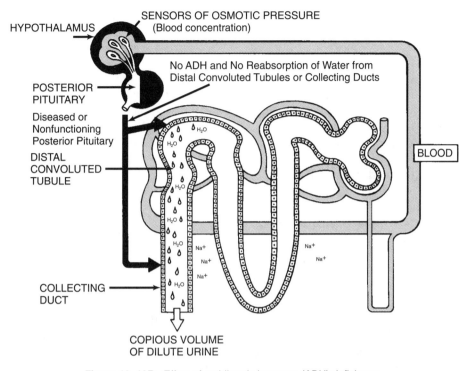

Figure 13–10B. Effect of antidiuretic hormone (ADH) deficiency.

not related to **diabetes mellitus.** The posterior pituitary fails to secrete ADH, and a copious amount of dilute urine is therefore passed. This excessive water loss could quickly lead to dehydration. The body compensates, however, through an insatiable thirst, a condition known as **polydipsia.** Treatment of diabetes insipidus is the administration of ADH. Figure 13–10A shows the normal action of ADH, and Figure 13–10B shows the effects of its absence.

STRUCTURE AND FUNCTION OF THE THYROID GLAND

The activity of the thyroid gland affects the whole body. It regulates the metabolic rate, the rate at which calories are used. The thyroid gland, through its hormone **thyroxine,** governs cellular oxygen consumption and, thus, energy and heat production. The more oxygen that is used, the more calories are metabolized ("burned up"). Thyroxine assures that enough body heat is produced to maintain normal temperature even in a cold environment.

Many people blame obesity on an underactive thyroid, a low rate of metabolism. Although there is a relationship between a person's body weight and metabolic rate, diet is still the critical factor in controlling obesity. A person with a low rate of metabolism requires fewer calories than someone who uses them at a faster rate.

■ Structure of the Thyroid Gland

The thyroid gland is located in the neck region, one lobe on either side of the trachea. A connecting strip, or isthmus, anterior to the trachea connects the two lobes. The thyroid gland lies just below the Adam's apple, the protrusion formed by part of the larynx. Figure 13–11 illustrates the thyroid gland. Internally, the thyroid gland consists of countless follicles, microscopic sacs. Within these protein-containing follicles, the thyroid hormones thyroxine and **triiodothyronine** are made. Thin-walled capillaries run between the follicles in a position ideal to receive the thyroid hormones.

■ Function of the Thyroid Gland

The thyroid gland synthesizes, stores, and releases thyroid hormones, which contain iodine. In fact, most of the iodide ions of the body are taken into the thyroid gland by a mechanism called the iodide trap. Iodine combines with an amino acid; two of these groups join, and the thyroid hormones are formed.

The hormones are stored until needed and then released into the blood capillaries. In the blood the thyroid hormones combine with plasma proteins. Tests to determine the activity of the thyroid gland are based on this combination of triiodothyronine (T_3) and thyroxine (T_4) with plasma proteins. In the T_3 and T_4 tests, a sample of the patient's serum is incubated with radioactive thyroid hormones

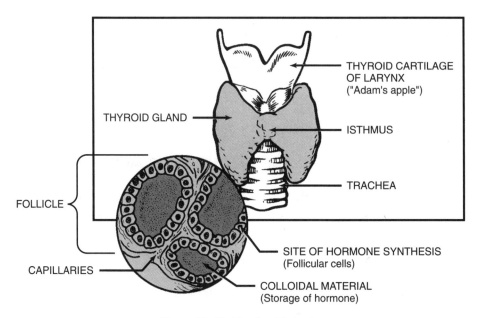

THYROID CARTILAGE
OF LARYNX
("Adam's apple")

THYROID GLAND

ISTHMUS

FOLLICLE

TRACHEA

CAPILLARIES

SITE OF HORMONE SYNTHESIS
(Follicular cells)

COLLOIDAL MATERIAL
(Storage of hormone)

Figure 13–11. The thyroid gland.

and resin. The resin absorbs the hormones that are not bound to the blood proteins. Radioactivity counts of the serum and resin are made and the percentage of thyroid hormones absorbed by the resin is calculated. A low percentage of absorption indicates a poorly functioning thyroid gland. A high percentage of absorption indicates hyperactivity. In the latter case, the patient's own thyroid hormones had saturated the plasma proteins, and the radioactive hormones were absorbed by the resin. This is a more accurate means of measuring thyroid activity than the test used for many years, the BMR, or basal metabolic rate. The term *basal metabolic rate*, however, is still used, and it refers to a person's oxygen consumption while at rest.

■ Effects of Thyroid Hormones

Although there is more than one thyroid hormone, for clarity the thyroid hormones are referred to here as thyroxine, the one that is secreted in the largest quantity. Thyroxine stimulates cellular metabolism by increasing the rate of oxygen use with subsequent energy and heat production.

Keeping in mind that thyroxine stimulates the rate of cellular metabolism, the effect of an increased thyroxine level on heart activity becomes clear. Think of it this way: Faster cellular metabolism increases the cell's demand for oxygen, so more oxygen must be circulated to the cells. Nutrients are converted to energy in the presence of oxygen and the waste products of metabolism, including carbon dioxide, are formed. These must be carried away from the cells. The circulatory system can meet these needs by increasing blood flow to the cells. Increased blood flow is obtained by greater cardiac output, more heart activity.

What about the effect of increased cellular metabolism on respiration? The greater need for oxygen and a corresponding accumulation of carbon dioxide stimulate the respiratory center of the brain. Stimulation of the respiratory center results in a faster rate and greater depth of breathing.

How does thyroxine affect body temperature? Heat is produced through cellular metabolism, and thyroxine stimulates this process. In a cold environment, thyroxine secretion increases to assure adequate body heat. If excessive body heat is produced, it is dissipated in two ways. Blood vessels of the skin dilate, increasing blood flow at the body surface, and giving the body a flushed appearance. As the blood flows through the skin blood vessels, excess heat escapes. The body is also cooled by the perspiration mechanism. Body temperature is controlled by a regulatory center in the brain.

Thyroxine also has a stimulatory effect on the gastrointestinal system. It increases the secretion of digestive juices and the movement of material through the digestive tract. Absorption of carbohydrates from the intestine is also increased under the influence of thyroxine, assuring adequate fuel for cellular metabolism. The effects of thyroxine are illustrated in Figure 13–12.

An understanding of these effects of thyroxine will make the diseases of the thyroid gland meaningful. Basically, the results of inadequate or excessive thyroxine secretion will be considered. The symptoms of each disease will be related to the function of thyroxine.

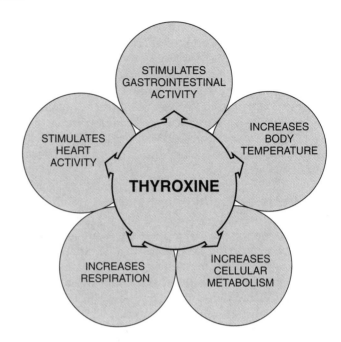

Figure 13–12. Effects of thyroxine.

■ Control of Circulating Thyroxine Level

The anterior pituitary gland stimulates the thyroid by releasing thyroid-stimulating hormone, TSH. The thyroid in turn releases thyroxine, which circulates in the blood to all cells and tissues. When the level of circulating thyroxine is high, the anterior pituitary is inhibited and stops releasing TSH. This is an example of a negative feedback mechanism. An adequate level of thyroxine prevents further synthesis of the hormone. When the level of thyroxine falls, the anterior pituitary is released from the inhibition, and once again sends out TSH. This feedback mechanism is shown in Figure 13–13.

At times this mechanism fails, constituting one basis for a thyroid disease. The thyroid gland may be perfectly healthy, but if the body's iodine supply is inadequate, the gland cannot produce thyroxine. It is possible for the thyroid gland to be overstimulated or understimulated by the anterior pituitary. The thyroid gland itself may be diseased, with a resultant hyperactivity or hypoactivity. These are some of the conditions that will be discussed.

DISEASES OF THE THYROID GLAND

■ Goiter

Goiter is an enlargement of the thyroid gland. The enlargement may be due to hypoactivity or hyperactivity of the thyroid. A goiter develops if the gland is unable

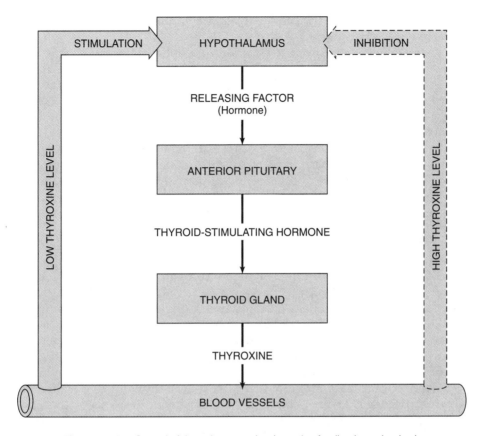

Figure 13–13. Control of thyroxine secretion (negative feedback mechanism).

to produce adequate thyroxine because of an iodine deficiency. The thyroid also enlarges if the gland is hyperactive.

The most common type of goiter is the **diffuse colloidal goiter,** or nontoxic goiter. The follicles of the thyroid gland normally contain colloid, a protein material. In this type of goiter an excessive amount of colloid is secreted into the follicles, increasing the size of the gland. A diffuse colloidal goiter is also called an *endemic goiter* because it is common in a particular geographic region.

The usual cause of an endemic goiter is insufficient iodine in the diet. Inland areas, such as the Great Lakes region, and mountainous regions, like the Alps, have a very low iodine content in the soil and water. As a result, the inhabitants are unable to synthesize thyroxine adequately.

Normally, when the proper level of thyroxine is circulating, the anterior pituitary stops secreting thyroid-stimulating hormone. In the absence of thyroxine there is nothing to inhibit the anterior pituitary. As a result, the continuous secretion of thyroid-stimulating hormone causes the thyroid gland to enlarge as a compensatory mechanism. The thyroid enlarges in an attempt to meet the demand of thyroid-stimulating hormone.

An enlargement of the neck is generally the only symptom. Usually enough thyroxine is produced to prevent the symptoms of **hypothyroidism.** The condition responds well to treatment with iodides, so the use of iodized salt prevents endemic goiter formation. If the goiter is very advanced, surgery may be necessary. A very large goiter puts pressure on the esophagus, causing difficulty in swallowing, or presses on the trachea, causing a cough or choking sensation.

Other factors can cause a simple diffuse colloidal goiter; for example, a defect in the thyroxine-synthesizing mechanism. A young girl entering adolescence may develop this type of goiter because of an increased need for thyroxine at this time.

■ Hyperthyroidism

Another type of goiter is the **adenomatous** or **nodular goiter,** named from adenoma, a glandular tumor. These nodules are secretory and produce an excessive amount of thyroxine, a condition of **hyperthyroidism.** Various goiters are shown in Figure 13–14.

The effects of thyroxine have been discussed, and an excessive amount of this hormone augments these effects. The hyperthyroid patient is very nervous and experiences **tremors,** a shakiness, particularly in the hands. The metabolic rate is high, causing sweating and a rapid pulse. A nodule or adenoma may put pressure on the trachea or esophagus. Surgery is sometimes necessary to remove part of the thyroid gland, but medication is often effective in preventing further enlargement.

Graves' disease is another condition in which goiter develops. In this case the entire gland hypertrophies, and there are no nodules. The patient suffers from severe hyperthyroidism. Graves' disease is far more common in women than in men and usually affects young women.

A patient with Graves' disease has a very characteristic appearance. The facial expression is strained and tense, and there is a stare in the eyes. The eyeballs protrude outward, a condition called **exophthalmos** (Fig. 13–15). This is caused by edema in the tissue behind the eyes. The bulging of the eyes can be so severe that the eyelids do not close, and the swelling sometimes damages the optic nerve. This symptom generally persists even when the hyperthyroidism is corrected.

The patient has a tremendous appetite but loses weight to the point of appearing emaciated, as calories are burned up at a rapid rate. Thyroxine speeds the passage of food through the digestive tract. There is no time for the normal reabsorption of water from the large intestine, so diarrhea frequently accompanies the disease.

Tachycardia, rapid pulse rate, and palpitation are also among the symptoms. The patient is extremely nervous, excitable, and is always tired but has difficulty sleeping because of the hyperactivity of the body. The high metabolic rate causes excessive heat production, which results in profuse perspiration. The skin is always moist, and an insatiable thirst follows the loss of water. The signs of Graves' disease are shown in Figure 13–16.

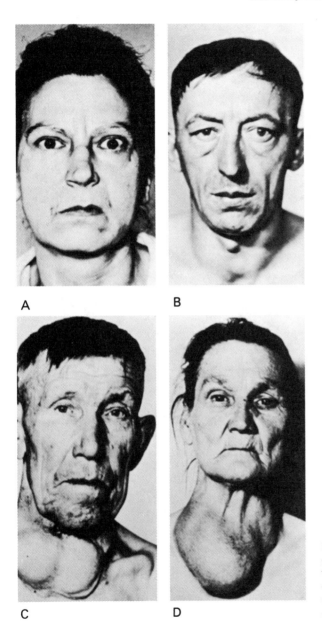

Figure 13–14. A. A nontoxic, nodular goiter. **B.** A 32-year-old man showing diffuse enlargement of the thyroid. **C.** An elderly man with a multinodular and cystic goiter. **D.** A diffuse, multinodular colloid goiter.

Graves' disease is an autoimmune condition in which antibodies to a thyroid antigen stimulate hyperactivity of the thyroid gland. This causes the thyroid to produce too much thyroxine.

Graves' disease can sometimes be treated with medication that inhibits the synthesis of thyroxine, or by administration of radioactive iodine, which destroys the thyroid gland. Removal of the thyroid gland however, may be necessary. If the

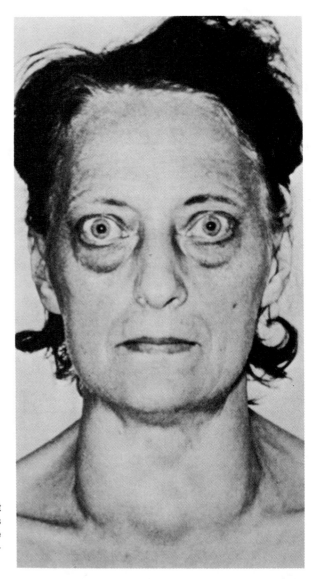

Figure 13–15. A Graves' disease patient with marked exophthalmos. The eyes have a fixed, staring expression. Note marked swelling of neck due to an enlarged thyroid.

gland is removed, hormonal supplements must be given. Partial removal of the thyroid gland allows the remaining portion to secrete hormones.

▪ Hypothyroidism

Myxedema is the condition of severe hypothyroidism, an inadequate level of thyroxine. The symptoms are just the opposite of those in Graves' disease. The patient's face is bloated, the tongue is thick, and the eyelids are puffy. The skin is dry

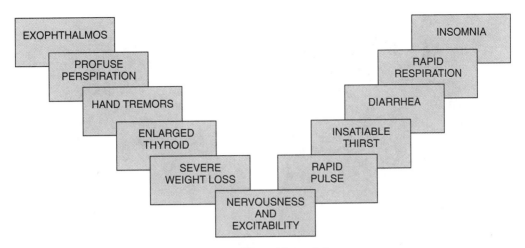

Figure 13–16. Signs of Graves' disease.

and scaly, and there is little perspiration. The patient has no tolerance of a cold environment.

A person with myxedema experiences muscular weakness and **somnolence,** sleeping for 14 to 16 hours a day. The mental and physical processes are sluggish, the speech is slurred, and reflexes are slow. Heart rate is decreased, and the slowed circulation causes edema to develop. Lack of thyroxine increases the amount of circulating lipids, which leads to the development of atherosclerosis (Chapter 8). The digestive system works sluggishly, so the patient suffers from constipation. Weight gain also accompanies the disease.

Myxedema affects women more than men, and usually women of middle age. It can result from radiation damage to the thyroid gland or after thyroid surgery if thyroxine is not administered. Myxedema can be a primary disease of the thyroid gland or secondary to pituitary disease. If the pituitary gland does not secrete thyroid-stimulating hormones, the thyroid gland ceases to function. Patients with myxedema are shown in Figure 13–17. Myxedema is treated by administering thyroxine. The condition generally responds well to treatment and the symptoms disappear.

■ Cretinism

Cretinism is a congenital thyroid deficiency in which thyroxine is not synthesized. Thyroxine is essential to both physical and mental development. Lack of this hormone in an infant or young child causes mental retardation and an abnormal, dwarfed stature. Cretinism can result from an error in fetal development if the thyroid gland fails to form or is nonfunctional. Cretinism sometimes occurs in areas of endemic goiter where the mother suffers from an inadequate iodine supply.

The cretin is a dwarf with a stocky stature and a characteristically protruding abdomen. The sexual organs do not develop, and the face of the cretin is typically misshapen: a broad, sunken nose, small eyes set far apart, puffy eyelids, and a

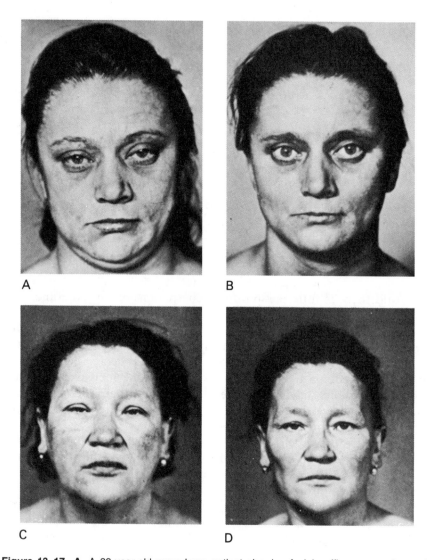

Figure 13–17. A. A 29-year-old myxedema patient showing facial puffiness, muscle weakness, and drooping eyelids, which give a sleepy appearance. **B.** The same patient after 2 months of thyroxine replacement. **C.** A 62-year-old patient with myxedema exhibiting marked edema of the face and a somnolent look. The hair is stiff and without luster. **D.** The same patient after 3 months of treatment with thyroxine.

short forehead. A thick tongue protrudes from a wide-open mouth, and the face is expressionless. Figure 13–18 shows an example of a cretin.

The earlier this condition is diagnosed and treated with thyroxine, the more optimistic is the prognosis. Lifelong hormonal therapy will be required. An untreated 14-year-old patient is shown in Figure 13–19.

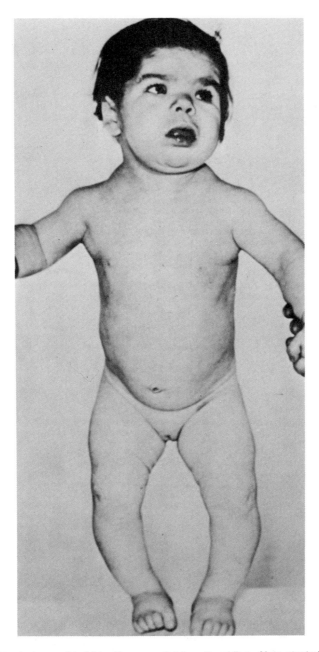

Figure 13–18. A 4-year-old child with congenital hypothyroidism. Note stunted growth (32 inches) and typical facial features: broad, flat nose; open mouth; and protruding tongue. The child cannot stand unsupported or speak.

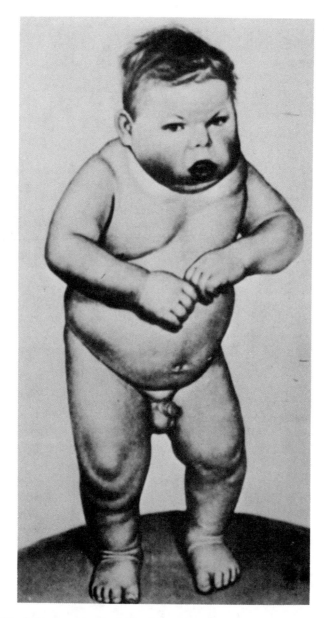

Figure 13–19. A 14-year-old untreated patient with severe, congenital hypothyroidism. The face is greatly swollen, the neck is obscured by fat, and the abdomen protrudes due to lack of muscle tone. The patient has difficulty in standing and walking.

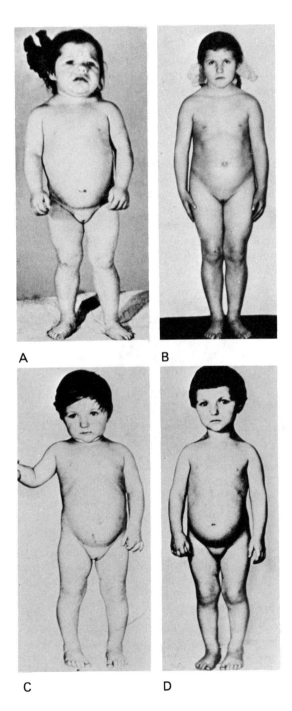

Figure 13–20. A. A 6-year-old child with congenital hypothyroidism, exhibiting marked mental and physical retardation. **B.** The same patient after 3 years of thyroxine therapy, which resulted in a spurt of growth and regression of pathological manifestations. Mental development is delayed. **C.** A 5-year-old patient with congenital hypothyroidism. Mental and physical development are delayed. **D.** The same patient after 3 months of thyroxine treatment. The child began to grow, lost weight, and became more alert.

Even less severe cases of hypothyroidism should be treated in infants. A baby may appear normal at first and only later give indications that the developmental processes are retarded. The baby may be slow in smiling, reaching, sitting, and standing. Valuable treatment time has been lost by then. The American Thyroid Association recommends that all newborn babies be given a simple blood test for hypothyroidism. Some hospitals have already adopted the practice. Figure 13–20 shows the effectiveness of thyroxine replacement therapy.

STRUCTURE AND FUNCTION OF THE ADRENAL GLANDS

The adrenal glands are located at the top of each kidney. Each of the glands consists of two distinct parts: an outer part, the cortex, and an inner section, the medulla. The cortex and the medulla secrete different hormones. The adrenal cortex is stimulated by ACTH, adrenocorticotropic hormone, from the anterior pituitary gland. The adrenal glands are shown in Figure 13–21.

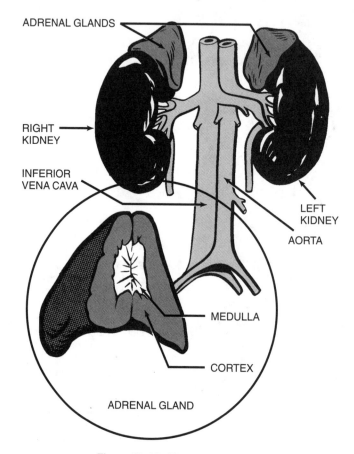

Figure 13–21. The adrenal glands.

On the Practical Side

MUSCLE-BUILDING STEROIDS

Anabolic steroids (muscle-building steroids) were used initially by athletes to increase strength and endurance during athletic competition. Anabolic steroids are closely related to the male hormone, testosterone, and did indeed build muscle. However, it was found that these steroids had serious side effects including kidney damage, increased risk of heart disease, and the development of liver cancer. Increased irritability and aggressive behavior developed, and in women, the growth of facial hair and deepening of the voice. Males were affected by diminished hormone secretion and sperm production. The use of anabolic steroids by athletes is now banned and if they are found to be present, the athlete is severely punished.

The adrenal cortex secretes many steroid hormones, which can be classified into three groups. One group, the **mineralocorticoids,** regulates salt balance. The principal hormone of this group is **aldosterone.** Aldosterone causes sodium retention and potassium secretion by the kidneys. Another group, the **glucocorticoids,** helps to regulate carbohydrate, lipid, and protein metabolism. The principal hormone of this group is **cortisol** or hydrocortisone. The third group of hormones are sex hormones: **androgens,** the male hormones, and **estrogen,** the female hormone.

You may be familiar with one of the hormones of the adrenal cortex called **cortisone.** It is frequently used to treat nonbacterial inflammatory diseases such as rheumatoid arthritis, bursitis, and asthma. It can greatly relieve pain, but it must be understood that it relieves only the symptoms, not the cause of the disease.

There are many side effects to prolonged cortisone use. It can cause high blood pressure, peptic ulcers, and electrolyte imbalance that affects the heart. Cortisone reduces the body's inflammatory response and thus masks the symptoms of a bacterial or viral invasion. An infection therefore can be well established before the patient is aware of it. Cortisone causes a puffiness of the face, referred to as a "moon-face" appearance. This steroid hormone produces a drowsiness that is a danger when driving a car or using power equipment. Research is progressing to reduce the side effects of cortisone while maintaining its valuable actions.

The adrenal medulla secretes **epinephrine,** also called adrenalin. This hormone is secreted in stress situations when additional energy and strength are needed. Epinephrine raises the blood pressure, stimulates heart activity, and causes an increase in blood glucose. Epinephrine, through constriction of some blood vessels and dilation of others, shunts blood to active muscles where oxygen and nutrients are needed. The action of epinephrine is often called the "flight or fight" mechanism.

Hyperactivity of the adrenal cortex is usually caused by hyperplasia (enlargement of the glands), a tumor, or administration of corticosteroids. Hyperactivity may also result from overstimulation by the anterior pituitary gland.

Hypoactivity of the adrenal cortex sometimes results from a destructive disease such as tuberculosis. Some steroid hormones can cause the adrenal glands to atrophy by interfering with the normal control mechanism for corticosteroid release.

DISEASES OF THE ADRENAL CORTEX

■ Hyperadrenalism

Overactivity of the adrenal cortex **(hyperadrenalism)** can take different forms depending on which group of hormones are secreted in excess. **Cushing's syndrome** develops from an excess of glucocorticoid hormones, the hormones that raise the blood sugar level. In excess they cause **hyperglycemia.** Elevation of blood glucose due to hypersecretion by the adrenal cortex is called **adrenal diabetes.** Glucocorticoids mobilize lipids, increasing their level in the blood. A characteristic obesity develops that is confined to the trunk of the body. A fat pad forms behind the shoulders and is referred to as a buffalo hump, but the arms and legs remain normal. The face is round and described as moon-shaped.

The patient with Cushing's syndrome retains salt and water, resulting in hypertension, and atherosclerosis develops as a result of excess circulating lipid. Muscular weakness and fatigue accompany the disease, and the patient finds it difficult even to climb stairs. The skin is thin and tends to bruise easily. Red **striae** (stretch marks) develop on the abdomen, buttocks, and breasts as a result of a loss of elastic tissue and fat accumulation. Figure 13–22 shows a patient with Cushing's syndrome. Wounds heal poorly, and the patient is very susceptible to infection. Bones, particularly the vertebrae and ribs, are likely to fracture. These symptoms result from a decrease in protein synthesis. Surgical removal of the enlarged glands or tumor can correct the condition. Hormonal therapy is then required to replace the hormones normally secreted by the adrenal cortex.

Conn's syndrome is another form of hyperadrenalism. In this disease aldosterone is secreted in excess. This causes retention of sodium and water, and abnormal loss of potassium in the urine. Hypertension develops as a result of the salt imbalance and water retention. Muscles become weak to the point of paralysis. The patient has an excessive thirst (polydipsia) due to the salt retention, and polyuria follows the great intake of water. Conn's syndrome is usually caused by a tumor that can be removed surgically, and the prognosis is usually good.

Adrenogenital syndrome is another form of hyperadrenalism, also called *adrenal virilism.* In this case androgens, male hormones, are secreted in excess. If

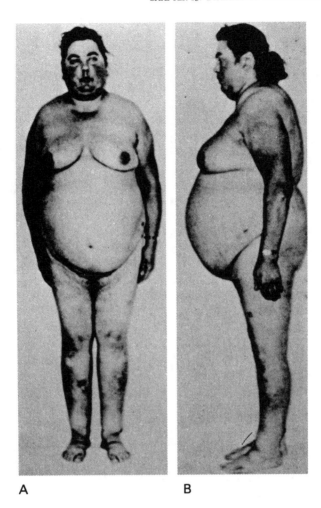

A   B

Figure 13–22. A. Cushing's syndrome patient showing round, red face; stocky neck; and marked obesity of the trunk with protruding abdomen. Note bruises on trunk and legs and also stretch marks. **B.** Note fat pads above the collarbone and on the back of the neck, which produce the "buffalo hump."

this occurs in children, it stimulates premature sexual development. Sex organs of a male child greatly enlarge. In a girl, the clitoris enlarges, a male distribution of hair develops, and the voice deepens. This condition is seen in Figure 13–23A and B.

This excessive production of androgens is usually due to a block in the synthesis of cortisol from cholesterol or from other corticosteroids. Cortisone is generally inactive until it is converted to cortisol. Cortisone is prepared synthetically from animal and plant tissue. Since steroids cannot be converted to cortisol, because of

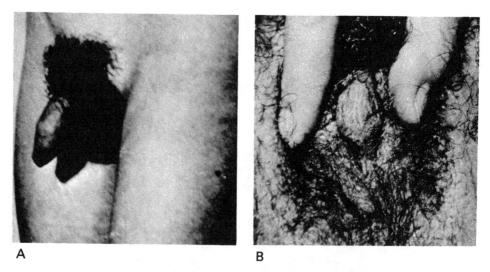

A   B

Figure 13–23. **A.** Genitalia of a 6-year-old boy with adrenogenital syndrome, showing preco-cious sexual development. The penis is enlarged but the testes remain small. **B.** Genitals of an 18-year-old woman with adrenogenital syndrome. The enlarged clitoris resembles a penis, and growth of pubic hair is excessive.

the blockage in the pathway, they are converted to androgens. Cortisol treatment can prevent this overproduction.

Excessive androgen secretion in a woman causes masculinization (adrenal vi-rilism). Hair develops on the face, a condition called **hirsutism,** and the hairline recedes. The breasts diminish in size, the clitoris enlarges, and ovulation and men-struation cease. In an adult the cause is usually an androgen-secreting tumor of the glands. Adrenal virilism is shown in Figure 13–24.

■ Hypoadrenalism

Chronic **hypoadrenalism** is called **Addison's disease.** The indiscriminate use of steroid hormones can cause this disease in which the adrenal glands atrophy. An autoimmune mechanism may also result in destruction of the glands. Surpris-ingly, the adrenal cortex can still function adequately when up to 90 percent of it is destroyed. In Addison's disease the adrenal glands fail to secrete aldosterone, which renders the patient unable to retain salt and water. This causes dehydration and the blood level of potassium rises. Blood pressure is low due to the electrolyte imbalance. There is always a loss of weight, muscle weakness, and fatigue, and gastrointestinal disturbances are common.

A peculiar pigmentation—yellow to deep brown—develops. Normally pig-mented areas such as the areola surrounding the nipples and parts of the genitals become even darker. Areas of the body subjected to friction, the palms and elbows, also darken and pigment develops in scars. This coloration is due to a pituitary hormone normally inhibited by cortisol, but cortisol is not secreted in Addison's

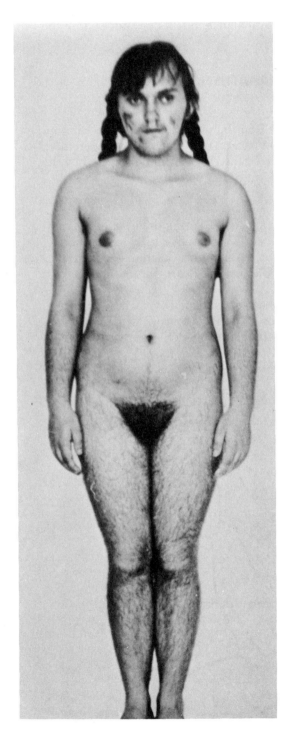

Figure 13–24. A 15-year-old girl with congenital adrenogenital syndrome. Note typical masculine build of broad shoulders and narrow hips. Breast development is poor, and excessive hair has developed on the face, abdomen, and legs.

disease. Steroid therapy can correct the salt imbalance, but it does not restore the adrenal glands.

STRUCTURE AND FUNCTION OF THE PARATHYROIDS

■ Structure of the Parathyroids

The parathyroids are four tiny glands located on the posterior side of the thyroid gland (Fig. 13–25). Before the function of the parathyroid glands was understood, they were sometimes removed with a thyroidectomy. The hormone secreted by the parathyroids is **parathormone,** also called parathyroid hormone.

■ Function of the Parathyroids

The parathyroid glands are extremely important in regulating the level of circulating calcium and phosphate. Ninety-nine percent of the body's calcium is in bone, but the remaining 1 percent has many important functions. Calcium is essential to the blood-clotting mechanism. It increases the tone of heart muscle and plays a significant role in muscle contraction.

Bone is not inert, but rather there is a constant exchange of calcium and phosphate between bone and the blood. Two kinds of cells are at work within bone: **osteoblasts** (which form bone tissue) and **osteoclasts** (which resorb salts out of bone, dissolving it). These salts are then released into the blood. The balance between these two processes, osteoblastic and osteoclastic, is governed by the parathyroid hormone.

When the calcium level falls, parathormone is secreted. The hormone acts at three distinct sites to raise the level of calcium to normal. Parathormone increases

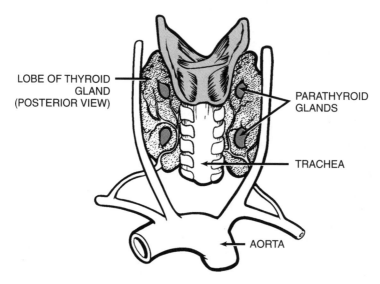

Figure 13–25. Parathyroid glands.

the amount of calcium that is absorbed out of the digestive tract by interaction with ingested vitamin D. It prevents a loss of calcium through the kidneys and releases calcium from bones by stimulating osteoclastic activity. When the proper level of circulating calcium is restored, parathormone is no longer released. An excess or a deficiency of calcium can have disastrous results. These conditions are usually the result of hyperactivity or hypoactivity of the parathyroid glands.

DISEASES OF THE PARATHYROID GLAND

■ Hyperparathyroidism

An overactive parathyroid gland secretes too much parathormone **(hyperparathyroidism).** Excessive parathormone raises the level of circulating calcium above normal, the condition called **hypercalcemia.** Much of the calcium comes from bone resorption mediated by parathormone. As the calcium level rises, the phosphate level falls.

What effect does this have on the bones? With the loss of calcium, the bones are weakened. They tend to bend, become deformed, and fracture spontaneously. Giant cell tumors and cysts of the bone sometimes develop. Excessive calcium causes formation of kidney stones because calcium forms insoluble compounds. Calcium deposited within the walls of the blood vessels makes them hard. It may also be found in the stomach and lungs. Effects of hyperparathyroidism are illustrated in Figure 13–26.

Hyperparathyroidism, with its concurrent excess of calcium, causes generalized symptoms. There may be pain in the bones that is sometimes confused with arthritis. The nervous system is depressed and muscles lose their tone and weaken. Heart muscle is affected and the pulse slows. Gastrointestinal disturbances, abdominal pain, vomiting, and constipation develop. These symptoms result from deposits of calcium in the mucosa of the gastrointestinal tract. Deposits of calcium sometimes form in the eye, causing irritation and excessive tearing. Hyperparathyroidism usually results from a tumor. If the tumor is removed, parathormone se-

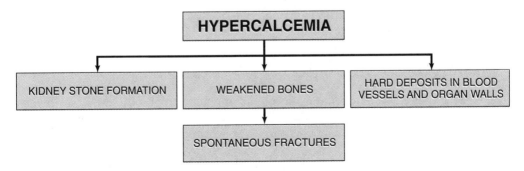

Figure 13–26. Complications of hyperparathyroidism—hypercalcemia.

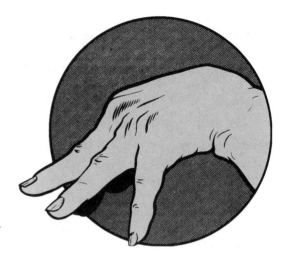

Figure 13–27. Tetany of the hand in hypoparathyroidism.

cretion returns to normal, and the level of circulating calcium is again properly controlled.

Hyperparathyroidism can develop from other conditions that reduce the level of circulating calcium. Any decrease in calcium stimulates the parathyroid glands to hypertrophy and to increase their rate of secretion. During pregnancy and lactation, the mother's supply of calcium is reduced. This reduction will stimulate the parathyroid glands to secrete parathormone.

■ Hypoparathyroidism

The principal manifestation of **hypoparathyroidism** is **tetany,** a sustained muscular contraction. In hypoparathyroidism the muscles of the hands and feet contract in a characteristic fashion. The typical tetanic contraction of the hand is seen in Figure 13–27. Laryngeal muscles are very susceptible to these spasms, which can obstruct the respiratory tract, and death may follow.

The low level of calcium in the blood, **hypocalcemia,** makes the nervous system hyperexcitable. As the nerves discharge spontaneously, the skeletal muscles are overstimulated. Administration of calcium and vitamin D, which assists in the absorption of calcium from the gastrointestinal tract, will correct the condition.

ENDOCRINE FUNCTION OF THE PANCREAS

The structure of the pancreas and its role as an exocrine gland were described in Chapter 11. The pancreas has another critical function: the control of glucose level in the blood. This is accomplished through the secretion of two hormones, **insulin** and **glucagon.**

Insulin is secreted by certain cells of the pancreas called **beta cells,** located in patches of tissue named the islands of Langerhans. Glucagon is secreted by the **al-**

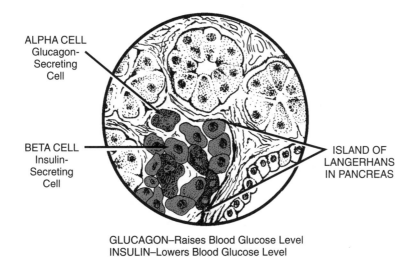

GLUCAGON–Raises Blood Glucose Level
INSULIN–Lowers Blood Glucose Level

Figure 13–28. Islands of Langerhans.

pha cells of the islets. This arrangement is illustrated in Figure 13–28. These hormones work antagonistically to each other. Insulin lowers the level of blood glucose and glucagon elevates it. The combined effect of these hormones maintains the normal level of blood glucose.

Insulin is secreted when the blood glucose level rises. Through a complex mechanism, not completely understood, insulin facilitates the entry of glucose into the cells where it is primarily stored as **glycogen** and metabolized for energy. Glucose enters primarily skeletal muscle cells and fat cells.

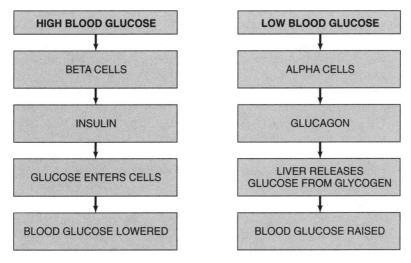

Figure 13–29. Control of blood glucose level.

As glucose enters cells, the level of blood glucose falls. The normal level of glucose in the blood is about 90 milligrams per 100 milliliters (90 mg/100 ml or 90 mg/dl) of blood. This is also expressed as 90 mg percent.

When the level of blood glucose falls below normal, glucagon is released. Glucagon circulates to the liver and stimulates the release of glucose from its stored form, glycogen. This raises the level of blood glucose to normal. The control of glucose is illustrated in Figure 13–29.

HYPOSECRETION OF THE PANCREAS

■ Diabetes Mellitus (Hyperglycemia)

Diabetes mellitus is an endocrine disease in which the beta cells fail to secrete insulin or target cells fail to respond to insulin. In the absence of insulin, glucose cannot enter the cells. The glucose level in the blood increases greatly, resulting in **hyperglycemia.** A diabetic's sugar level can range from 300 to 1200 mg/dl of blood and even higher. The cells are deprived of their principal nutrient, glucose, for the production of energy.

Diabetes that develops in children is called juvenile-onset diabetes or **insulin-dependent diabetes mellitus (IDDM)** also called Type I diabetes. This is the more serious form, and the patient requires daily insulin injections. Diabetes that develops later in life, maturity-onset diabetes, or **non-insulin-dependent diabetes mellitus (NIDDM),** known as Type II diabetes, is less severe and can often be controlled by diet alone. It affects women more often than men, and usually women over 40. Maturity-onset diabetes frequently accompanies obesity. A prolonged, excessively high carbohydrate diet overstimulates the beta cells to secrete insulin. As a result, the beta cells "burn out" and stop functioning. Development of diabetes mellitus may have a genetic basis.

Symptoms of Diabetes Mellitus. One of the principal symptoms of diabetes mellitus is excessive urination, or **polyuria.** This is caused by the great amount of glucose that filters into the kidney tubule and the volume of water required to carry it away. The glucose acts as a diuretic. Normally, glucose that enters the kidney tubules is reabsorbed and does not appear in the urine. In diabetes, however, the amount of glucose that the kidney tubules can reabsorb, the tubular maximum, is surpassed. The excess glucose is excreted in the urine, a condition called **glycosuria.** Glycosuria is a major sign of diabetes mellitus.

The great loss of water with the glucose could result in dehydration, but the diabetic has an excessive thirst, **polydipsia.** By drinking large amounts of water, the diabetic compensates for the fluid loss. An unusual thirst is also one of the symptoms of diabetes.

Cells prefer to metabolize glucose, but in its absence, cells metabolize fats first and proteins last. This is known as the "protein-sparing effect." Because glucose cannot enter the cells without the action of insulin, the diabetic metabolizes a large amount of fat. Fat metabolism produces a large number of fatty acids and

ketone bodies, acetone, and related substances. The presence of ketone bodies in the urine is another sign of diabetes mellitus.

The production of acids lowers the body's pH, and the condition of **acidosis** results. This is one of the most serious consequences of diabetes. The normal pH range is 7.35 to 7.45. If the pH drops below 6.9 to 7.0, the patient goes into a coma and will die if not treated.

Another sign of diabetes mellitus is weight loss, although the diabetic's appetite is good. The patient tires easily and lacks energy. In the absence of glucose to metabolize, the diabetic uses the body's tissue fat and protein, as well as that in the diet, which explains the loss of weight. There is an increased breakdown of tissue protein and a decrease in protein synthesis that results in poor wound healing. Susceptibility to infection also accompanies diabetes.

Complications of Diabetes Mellitus. Lipid is mobilized from fat tissue, and the level of blood lipid, particularly cholesterol, increases. Much of this lipid is deposited within the walls of the blood vessels, causing atherosclerosis. This is one of the greatest dangers in long-term uncontrolled diabetes because blood vessels tend to become occluded. Blockage of a coronary artery causes a myocardial infarction, as explained in Chapter 7. Thromboembolic strokes are also frequent complications of untreated diabetes. Occlusion of a leg artery can result in gangrene. Atherosclerosis generally causes poor circulation, which is another reason for poor wound healing.

Another complication of diabetes is diabetic retinopathy, a vascular disorder of the retina that can result in blindness. The minute retinal blood vessels become sclerotic and rupture. The nervous system is affected by poor circulation, as manifested by pain, tingling sensations, loss of feeling, and paralysis. The kidneys are always affected by long-standing diabetes, and kidney failure is frequently the cause of death in the diabetic. The complications of diabetes are summarized in Figure 13–30.

Treatment of Diabetes Mellitus. The important factors in treating diabetes are diet, insulin, and exercise. The insulin dosage prescribed accompanies a carefully regulated diet that includes some carbohydrates. The diet cannot be altered without creating an insulin excess or deficiency. A person who exercises actively requires less insulin than one who does not. A diabetic's exercise pattern is a factor in prescribing insulin.

Regulation of the proper insulin dosage takes time. Certain factors—illness or emotional stress—can temporarily alter a patient's needs. There are different types of insulin (fast-, intermediate-, and slow-acting), which are effective over various time periods. These are often prescribed in combination. Monitoring of blood-glucose level has had a pivotal breakthrough in the last few years. Self-blood–glucose monitoring (SBGM) enables the diabetic to determine his or her blood glucose level by means of a simple finger-prick blood test.

Insulin must be given by injection because it is a protein and would be digested in the gastrointestinal tract. There are oral compounds that can be used for

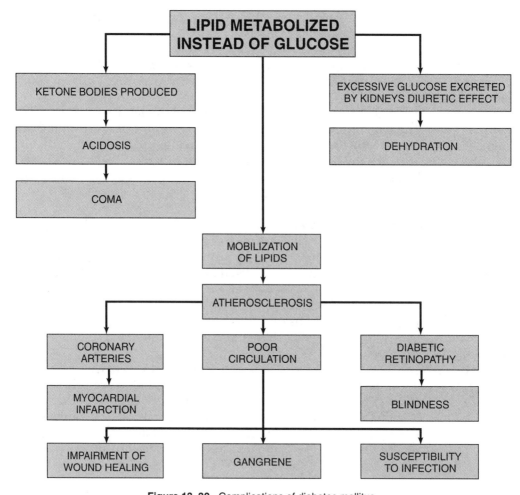

Figure 13–30. Complications of diabetes mellitus.

some Type II diabetes, but they are not insulin. These are oral hypoglycemic agents, which stimulate secretion of insulin from beta cells that still have some capacity or make cells more responsive to insulin. New types of injectors can replace the old needles and are less painful to use. The experimental insulin pump transmits a measured dose of insulin into the body via a tube with its tip embedded under the abdominal skin.

Diabetic Coma and Insulin Shock. Diabetic coma develops when a severe diabetic fails to take enough insulin or deviates markedly from a prescribed diet. Acidosis and dehydration result, and death can follow if proper treatment is not given immediately. One symptom of diabetic coma is deep, labored breathing, which results from the effect of the acidosis on the respiratory center of the brain. The patient's breath has a fruity, acetone smell. The skin is flushed and dry, and the tongue is dry because of the dehydration. A diabetic coma may have a gradual onset, during which time the patient is drowsy and lethargic. If urine and blood samples are taken, a high level of sugar is found.

Treatment of the comatose patient requires a large dosage of insulin, and dehydration must be remedied by administration of fluids. Sodium chloride and sodium bicarbonate, which counteract the acidosis, are administered in the fluid. The patient's level of potassium must be checked, as the entire electrolyte balance is affected by the dehydration.

Insulin shock, also called hypoglycemic shock, results from too much insulin, not enough food, or excessive exercise. The patient feels light-headed and faint, trembles, and begins to perspire. Taking sugar in some form, candy or orange juice for example, may be adequate treatment at this stage. If the glucose level is not raised, the condition becomes more serious. The patient's speech becomes thick and walking becomes unsteady because the low level of glucose affects the brain. Double vision may be experienced, and loss of consciousness may follow.

If the patient becomes comatose, it is difficult for the untrained to determine if the cause is a diabetic coma or insulin shock. A significant difference is that the deep, rapid breathing and acetone breath characteristic of diabetic coma are not present in insulin shock. The patient in shock breathes shallowly. Intravenous injections of glucose must be given immediately for insulin shock. The administration of epinephrine also raises the blood sugar level. Figure 13–31 illustrates the differences between diabetic coma and insulin shock.

Tests for Diabetes Mellitus. A simple test can show the presence or absence of glucose in the urine. If glucose is found, a test of the blood after fasting is made to determine the glucose level. When diabetes is suspected, a glucose tolerance test is performed by having the patient, in a fasting state, drink a standard glucose solution. Blood and urine samples are then analyzed during the next 4 to 5 hours. No food is allowed during the test, but the patient is encouraged to drink water. Smoking and exercise are not permitted during the test period. No glucose should

DIABETIC COMA	INSULIN SHOCK
Deep, labored breathing due to acidosis	Shallow breathing
Skin and tongue dry due to dehydration	Patient perspires
Fruity, acetone smell to breath	Odor of breath normal
Patient drowsy and lethargic before onset	Patient feels light-headed and faint before onset
Comatose	Comatose
Requires large dose of insulin	Requires glucose intravenously
Fluid and salts needed	

Figure 13–31. Differences between diabetic coma and insulin shock.

appear in the urine, and the blood level should not exceed 170 mg/dl of blood if insulin is being produced.

Education of the Diabetic Patient. The American Diabetes Association, physicians, nurses, and dieticians have made a great effort to assist the diabetic patient in leading a normal life. The diabetic who understands the disease knows the importance of insulin dosage, diet, and exercise to lead an active life. A safety precaution advised by the American Diabetes Association is that anyone who takes insulin carry an identification card explaining the emergency treatment required if an insulin reaction occurs.

■ Hypoglycemia

Hypoglycemia is an abnormally low level of glucose in the blood. Symptoms develop when the glucose level falls below 50 mg/dl as compared with the normal of 90 mg/dl. The symptoms of hypoglycemia have been described under hypoglycemic or insulin shock. They include faintness, sweating, nervousness, and mental confusion. A severe condition that is not treated results in coma and possibly convulsions and death. The patient, if conscious, should eat sugar in any form. If the patient is unconscious, glucose must be given by injection.

In addition to hypoglycemic shock in the diabetic resulting from too much insulin, insufficient food, or strenuous exercise, other factors can cause hypoglycemia. A tumor of the beta cells in the pancreas results in a hypersecretion of insulin that lowers blood glucose. A patient with Addison's disease, hypoactivity of the adrenal cortex, secretes an inadequate amount of glucocorticoids to raise the level of blood glucose.

Treatment of hypoglycemia depends on its cause. For the diabetic, precautionary measures can usually prevent its development: exact insulin dosage, careful observance of diet and times for meals, and exercise within the prescribed range. A tumor causing excessive insulin secretion should be removed. The patient with Addison's disease requires hormonal supplements.

ABNORMALITIES IN SECRETION OF SEX HORMONES

The gonads (ovaries and testes) are endocrine glands as well as the source of the ova and sperm (Chapter 14). They secrete the hormones estrogen and testosterone directly into the blood.

■ Hypergonadism (Hypersecretion)

Abnormally increased functional activity of the gonads before puberty produces precocious sexual development in both sexes. In a male child excessive production of testosterone may be due to a tumor in the testes. This causes rapid growth of musculature and bones but premature uniting of the epiphyses and shaft of long bones. Normal height, therefore, is not attained. Hypersecretion of ovarian hormones in the female is rare because of the negative feedback mechanism with gonadotropic hormones.

Hypogonadism in the Male. Several factors can cause **hypogonadism,** that is, the decreased functional activity of the gonads. A person may be born without functional testes, the testes may fail to descend and thus atrophy, or the testes may be lost through castration. Testes fail to develop because of a lack of gonadotropic hormones.

Loss of the male gonads before puberty causes the condition of eunuchism, in which sexual characteristics do not develop. Development of male traits depends on testosterone secretion by the testes. Castration after puberty causes some regression of secondary sexual characteristics, but masculinity is retained. Hormonal therapy, the administration of testosterone, can be effective.

Hypogonadism in the Female. Hyposecretion of hormones by the ovaries may be due to poorly formed or missing ovaries. When ovaries are absent or fail to develop, female eunuchism results. Secondary sexual characteristics do not develop. A characteristic of this condition is excessive growth of long bones because the epiphyses do not seal with the shaft of the bone as normally occurs at adolescence.

DIAGNOSTIC PROCEDURES FOR ENDOCRINE DISEASES

Indications of pituitary hyperactivity or hypoactivity can be confirmed by serum assays (tests). Growth hormone (GH) level can detect hyperpituitarism (gigantism and/or acromegaly) and hypopituitarism (dwarfism). Thyroid-stimulating hormone (TSH) assay is useful in confirming primary hypothyroidism. Activity of the posterior pituitary can be evaluated by the water deprivation and vasopressin injection test. A urine specimen is taken after controlled water deprivation and a blood sample is drawn. Dilute urine and high osmotic pressure in the blood indicates that water is not being absorbed by the kidney tubules. If vasopressin injection corrects the massive polyuria, diabetes insipidus is confirmed.

Diseases of the thyroid gland are diagnosed on the basis of the T_3 and T_4 tests previously described, and by the serum level of thyroid-stimulating hormone (TSH), which can detect hypothyroidism. A thyroid scan provides visualization of the thyroid gland after administration of radioactive iodine. It is usually recommended after discovery of a mass, an enlarged gland, or an asymmetric goiter. Thyroid ultrasonography evaluates characteristics of thyroid nodules and distinguishes between solid or cystic masses in the gland.

Diagnostic tests for parathyroid gland activity measure parathyroid hormone and calcium levels in the blood, and can detect hyperparathyroidism.

Adrenal gland activity can be evaluated by the level of plasma cortisol from the adrenal cortex. Abnormal levels indicate hyperfunction (Cushing's syndrome) or hypofunction (Addison's disease). Urine tests measure steroid level and detect hyperactivity of the gland.

A fasting blood glucose test helps to detect diabetes mellitus and to evaluate the clinical status of diabetic patients. An oral glucose tolerance test, previously described, challenges the ability of the pancreas to secrete insulin in response to large doses of glucose.

CHAPTER SUMMARY

The endocrine system provides a means of chemical communication between body parts. The tiny anterior pituitary gland controls activities of the thyroid, adrenals, and sex glands. It also stimulates growth, development, and tissue repair. The pituitary is called the "master gland" for these reasons. Pituitary activity is governed by the hypothalamus of the brain.

Hyperpituitarism causes an excess of growth hormone. This condition, if present before puberty results in gigantism. In an adult, excessive production of growth hormone leads to abnormal enlargement of facial bones, bones of hands and feet, and soft tissue. This growth in an adult is called acromegaly.

Severe hypopituitarism impedes growth and development in a child, causing the child to be dwarfed in stature. Glands dependent on stimulation by the anterior pituitary—the thyroid, adrenals, and sex glands—cease functioning in hypopituitarism at any age. The posterior pituitary gland secretes vasopressin, also called antidiuretic hormone, and oxytocin. Hypoactivity of this gland causes diabetes insipidus.

The rate of metabolism is controlled by the thyroid gland. An enlargement of this gland is a goiter. Hyperthyroidism, an excess of thyroxine, accelerates heart and respiratory activity, increases metabolic rate, and raises body temperature. Graves' disease is an example of severe hyperthyroidism. A congenital lack of thyroxine results in cretinism, a condition of mental and physical retardation. Myxedema is a disease of severe hypothyroidism in an adult.

Hormones of the adrenal cortex are essential to life. Aldosterone regulates salt balance and cortisol affects the metabolism of nutrients. The sex hormones estrogen and androgen are also produced by this gland. Hypoactivity of the adrenal cortex is called Addison's disease.

Hyperactivity of the adrenal cortex causes different diseases, depending on which hormones are in excess. Cushing's syndrome results from an excess of cortisol, and Conn's syndrome results from excessive aldosterone. Precocious puberty and adrenal virilism develop from too much androgen secretion.

The parathyroid hormone, parathormone, regulates the level of circulating calcium and phosphate. Hyperactivity of the parathyroids causes hypercalcemia. The high level of calcium is primarily from bone resorption that weakens the bones. Hypoparathyroidism reduces the level of calcium in the blood. This causes the nervous system to become hyperexcitable, skeletal muscles are overstimulated, and tetany results. Hormones of the pancreas, insulin and glucagon, control blood sugar level. Lack of insulin causes an increase in blood glucose, the condition of diabetes mellitus.

Hypoglycemia, abnormally low blood glucose, results from insulin excess. This condition can develop in the diabetic from an overdosage of insulin. A tumor of the insulin-producing cells of the pancreas can also cause hypoglycemia. The absence of glucocorticoids in an Addison's disease patient results in low blood glucose.

■ Self-Study

True or False

_____ 1. Blood pressure is very low in Addison's disease.

_____ 2. Kidney stones are likely to form in hypoparathyroidism.

_____ 3. Hypercalcemia causes tetany.

_____ 4. Glucagon prevents hyperglycemia.

_____ 5. Steroids which suppress the inflammatory response, as in arthritis, are produced by the thyroid.

_____ 6. Hypertension accompanies Addison's disease.

_____ 7. Masculinization in women occurs in hyperactivity of the adrenal cortex.

_____ 8. Insulin is sometimes administered orally.

_____ 9. Polyuria is a principal symptom of diabetes mellitus.

_____ 10. Cretinism results from a congenital thyroid deficiency.

_____ 11. A strained, tense expression is characteristic of myxedema.

_____ 12. A person with Graves' disease is very sensitive to cold.

_____ 13. Destruction or removal of the anterior pituitary causes hypertrophy of the thyroid gland.

_____ 14. Diabetics taking insulin must avoid all carbohydrates.

_____ 15. Dehydration can develop in diabetes mellitus.

Match

_____ 16. congenital lack of thyroid gland   a) atrophy of the thyroid

_____ 17. diabetes insipidus   b) masculinization in females

_____ 18. anterior pituitary hyperactivity   c) copious urine excretion

_____ 19. hyperactive adrenal glands   d) gigantism

_____ 20. myxedema   e) cretinism

Multiple Choice

_____ 21. Acromegaly results from the anterior pituitary _____.
   a. hypoactivity
   b. hyperactivity

_____ 22. Epinephrine could be administered in _____.
   a. diabetic coma
   b. insulin shock

_____ 23. Hypoglycemia is a sign in _____.
   a. Cushing's disease
   b. Addison's disease
   c. Simmond's syndrome
   d. Graves' disease

_____ 24. The trunk is obese in _____.
   a. Graves' disease
   b. Cushing's disease
   c. Addison's disease

_____ 25. Adrenal diabetes results in _____.
   a. Graves' disease
   b. Cushing's disease
   c. Addison's disease

(Answers on page 450)

Chapter 14

Diseases of the Reproductive Systems and Sexually Transmitted Diseases

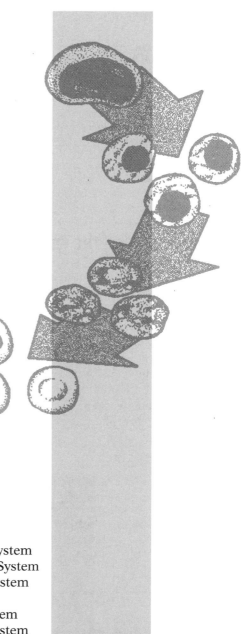

Chapter Outline

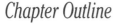

- Anatomy of the Female Reproductive System
- Physiology of the Female Reproductive System
- Diseases of the Female Reproductive System
- Abnormalities of Pregnancy
- Anatomy of the Male Reproductive System
- Physiology of the Male Reproductive System
- Diseases of the Male Reproductive System
- Sexually Transmitted Diseases
- Diagnostic Procedures for Reproductive and Sexually Transmitted Diseases
- Chapter Summary
- Self-Study

*N*ew life is created through the reproductive system. The female body produces ova, nurtures the developing fetus in the uterus, and nourishes the baby at the breast. The male body produces sperm and transmits it to the female. The fertilization that ensues combines characteristics of each parent, and an embryo begins to develop.

ANATOMY OF THE FEMALE REPRODUCTIVE SYSTEM

The female reproductive system consists of the **vagina,** the **uterus,** the **fallopian tubes,** and the **ovaries.** The vagina is a tubular structure extending backward and upward to the **cervix,** the lowest part of the uterus. The expanded, upper portion of the uterus tapers down to form the narrow cervix, giving the organ a pear-shaped appearance. The uterine wall is very strong, comprised of smooth muscle and lined with a mucosal membrane, the endometrium. It is responsive to hormonal changes. Figure 14–1 shows the female reproductive system.

The fallopian tubes extend laterally from each side of the uterus supported by the broad ligament. The outer ends of the tube are open to receive a released ovum. Fringelike projections at the outer ends, the **fimbriae,** propel the ova into the tube.

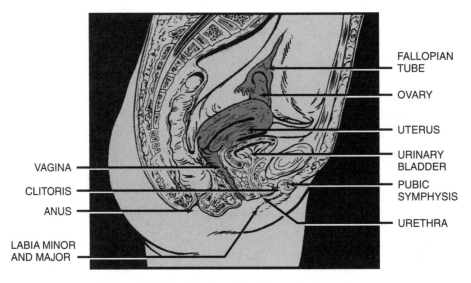

Figure 14–1. Sagittal view of female reproductive organs.

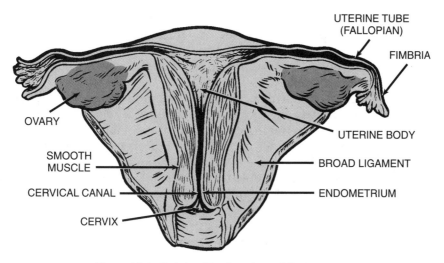

Figure 14–2. Relationship of ovaries to fallopian tubes.

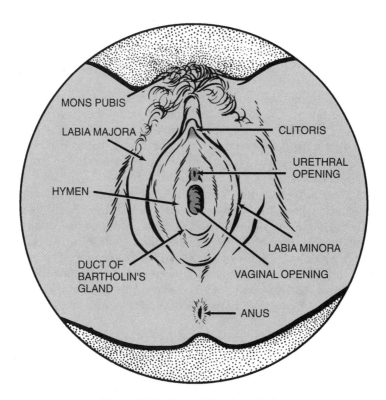

Figure 14–3. External female genitalia.

The ovaries, small oval-shaped glands, are anchored near the open end of the fallopian tubes by ligaments. The ovaries contain hundreds of thousands of ova, which are present at birth. Each ovum is surrounded by a single layer of cells comprising a **primary follicle.** The relationship between the ovaries and the fallopian tubes is shown in Figure 14–2.

The external genitalia, the **vulva,** consists of the **mons pubis,** the labia majora and labia minora, the **clitoris,** and the **vaginal opening.** The urinary meatus is between the clitoris and the vaginal opening. The mons pubis, a pad of fat tissue over the pubic symphysis, becomes covered with hair at puberty. Extending back from the mons pubis to the anus are two pairs of folds, the labia majora and the labia minora. The clitoris, a tuft of erectile tissue, similar to that of the penis, is located at the anterior junction of the minor lips. A membranous fold, the **hymen,** partly or completely closes the vaginal opening. Occasionally this membrane is imperforate or abnormally closed and requires a minor surgical procedure to open it. The external female genitalia are shown in Figure 14–3. A pair of mucus-secreting glands, Bartholin's glands, are situated at the vaginal entrance. These glands produce a lubricating secretion during sexual intercourse.

The breasts, accessory organs of reproduction, consist of milk glands supported by connective tissue covered with fatty tissue and skin. Ducts of the milk glands converge at the nipple, which is surrounded by a darkly pigmented area, the **areola.** The breasts overlie the pectoral muscles of the chest.

PHYSIOLOGY OF THE FEMALE REPRODUCTIVE SYSTEM

The cyclic hormonal changes in the life of a woman prepare the uterus monthly for a possible pregnancy. The secretion of female hormones, estrogen and progesterone, is governed by the gonadotropic hormones of the anterior pituitary gland, which is controlled by the hypothalamus of the brain. Failure of the ovary to secrete sex hormones or to ovulate may result from pituitary disease or disturbances in the central nervous system.

A woman's reproductive life begins with the onset of menstruation, the **menarche,** occurring generally between ages 10 and 15. The reproductive years terminate with the cessation of menstrual periods, **menopause,** which usually begins in the late 40s or early 50s. At the beginning of each monthly cycle a pituitary gonadotropic hormone stimulates ovarian follicles to develop. The particular follicles that are stimulated begin to grow and develop into **Graafian follicles** (see Fig. 14–4). One of these matures first and is released at the midpoint of the cycle, which is the process of ovulation. Ovulation is also controlled by a gonadotropic hormone.

As the follicles are growing, during the first half of the cycle, the ovary secretes estrogen, which is carried by the blood to the uterus. Estrogen stimulates the endometrium of the uterus to thicken and become more vascular. This is the first preparation for pregnancy and is called the proliferative stage.

Once the ovum has been released from the ovary, the empty follicle is converted into the **corpus luteum,** which begins to secrete progesterone. Progesterone continues the stimulation of endometrial growth and promotes the storage of nutrients for nourishing a fertilized ovum. This is the secretory phase of the uterus. Figure 14–4 shows the effect of gonadotropic hormones on the ovary, and the response of the endometrium of the female hormones.

If no fertilization occurs, the corpus luteum ceases to secrete hormones about 8 to 12 days after ovulation. At the end of the monthly cycle the level of estrogen and progesterone drops, and menstruation, the sloughing of the endometrial lining, occurs. If pregnancy occurs, the corpus luteum greatly enlarges and continues to secrete high levels of progesterone. The **placenta** gradually assumes the role of the corpus luteum in secreting these hormones.

The placenta is formed from both maternal and embryonic tissue. Near the site of implantation in the uterus the endometrium greatly thickens, becomes highly vascular, and develops large blood sinuses. An embryonic membrane, the chorion, develops fingerlike projections called villi, which dip into the maternal

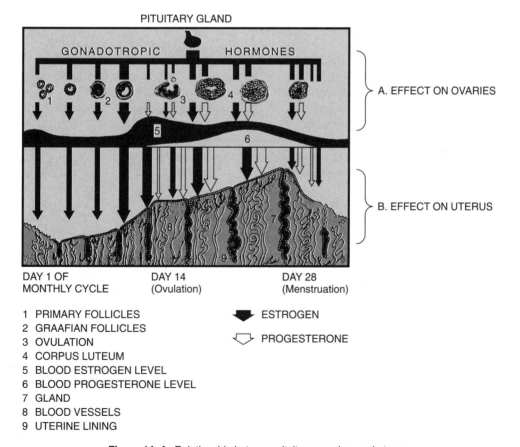

Figure 14–4. Relationship between pituitary, ovaries, and uterus.

blood sinuses. This interdigitation of embryonic and maternal tissue constitutes the placenta.

The umbilical arteries extend into the chorionic villi, where the exchange of carbon dioxide for oxygen and waste material for nutrients occurs. Maternal and fetal blood do not mix; the exchange of these substances is by diffusion across the blood vessel walls. Oxygen and nutrients return to the fetus through the umbilical vein. The fetal–maternal relationship is shown in Figure 6–3 (see Chapter 6, Diseases of the Blood).

DISEASES OF THE FEMALE REPRODUCTIVE SYSTEM

The female reproductive organs are affected by disease in numerous ways. Microorganisms can invade the structures, thus setting up infections. Tumors, both malignant and benign, and cysts develop in the reproductive organs and in the breasts. Abnormalities of the menstrual cycle and of pregnancy also occur.

■ Pelvic Inflammatory Disease (PID)

The pelvic reproductive organs become inflamed as a result of bacterial, viral, fungal, or parasitic invasion. The subsequent infection can ascend to the cervix, the endometrium, the fallopian tubes, and even to the ovaries. **Gonococcus** transmitted by a male with gonorrhea is one of the most common causes of pelvic inflammatory disease. Chlamydia and other sexually transmitted diseases also cause PID. Streptococcal and staphylococcal organisms can enter the female reproductive tract after an abortion or delivery in which sterile procedures were not carefully followed. The symptoms of pelvic inflammatory disease are lower abdominal pain, fever resulting from the infection, and a vaginal discharge of pus. If the infection is not treated, abscesses form. Antibiotics are prescribed to counteract the invading organisms, and aspirin is used to reduce the fever. The patient requires bed rest and fluids.

■ Salpingitis

Salpingitis is an inflammation of the fallopian tubes; the term *salpinx* refers to a tube. Untreated sexually transmitted diseases can cause this inflammation, as can a streptococcal or staphylococcal invasion. These pyogenic organisms cause a purulent, pus-producing infection.

The fallopian tubes become red and swollen, and if the outer ends remain open the infection spreads out into the pelvic cavity to cause pelvic peritonitis. The outer ends of the tubes usually close and the tubes fill with pus, which is then called a **pyosalpinx.** When the inflammation subsides after treatment with antibiotics, the tube is filled with a watery fluid and is referred to as a **hydrosalpinx.** Both tubes are usually affected as the inflammation ascends through the uterus. Sterility results from salpingitis if the ends of both tubes close. Adhesions may form that affect the tubes and cause sterility. The effect of adhesion formation on

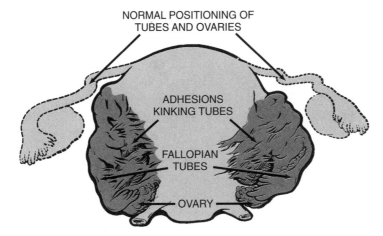

Figure 14–5. The effect of adhesions on the fallopian tubes.

the fallopian tubes is seen in Figure 14–5. Menstrual disturbances generally accompany salpingitis, as do ectopic pregnancies.

■ Vaginitis

Vaginitis, inflammation of the vagina, is a common disease caused by several organisms. A parasite, **trichomonas,** that can be transmitted by sexual intercourse is one causative agent. Trichomonas is sometimes admitted from fecal material. *Candida albicans,* a fungus, is another cause of vaginitis, a yeast infection. An overgrowth of fungus can develop from antibiotic treatment that destroys the normal flora. The normal flora consists of nonpathogenic microorganisms that are generally present and help keep down the number of harmful microbes. If the normal flora is wiped out by antibiotics, fungi, and viruses, antibiotic-resistant organisms thrive. A foul-smelling vaginal discharge is the principal sign of vaginitis. The discharge causes itching, burning, and soreness of the surrounding tissues. Any vaginal discharge other than blood is referred to as **leukorrhea.** Atrophic vaginitis can be a postmenopausal condition. The vaginal lining changes with the loss of estrogen secretion when the ovaries atrophy, and the mucosa becomes more susceptible to infection. Hormonal therapy, antibiotic ointments, or steroid creams may be prescribed.

■ Inflammation of Bartholin's Glands

Bartholin's glands (see Fig. 14–3) are susceptible to infections caused by gonococcal, streptococcal, and staphylococcal organisms. If the duct of the gland becomes occluded from the inflammation, pus collects in the gland and abscesses form. Such abscesses require surgical lancing to allow drainage of the pus.

■ Puerperal Sepsis

Puerperal sepsis is an infection of the endometrium after childbirth or an abortion. Danger of an infection is greater after an abortion. The **puerperium** is the

period after childbirth, when the endometrium is open and particularly susceptible to infection. The trauma and blood loss encountered during delivery provide a
portal of entry for invading microorganisms through the birth canal. The lesions
of the endometrium favor bacterial growth. Streptococci are the principal causative organisms, but staphylococci and *E. coli* enter the uterus through a lack of
aseptic technique. Necrosis of the endometrium develops from the infection.

Infected blood clots can break loose and travel as septic emboli. A systemic infection of the blood, **septicemia,** is often the result. The deep veins of the leg are
frequently affected, resulting in thrombophlebitis, a condition previously described in Chapter 8. The symptoms of puerperal sepsis are fever, chills, and profuse bleeding. A foul-smelling vaginal discharge indicates infection. Pain is experienced in the lower abdomen and pelvis. Puerperal sepsis responds well to
antibiotic treatment.

■ Neoplasms of the Female Organs

Early detection, diagnosis, and treatment of any abnormal mass or lump is extremely important in preventing the growth and spread of cancer. Many tumors
and cysts are harmless, but tests are required to differentiate between malignant
and benign growths.

Carcinoma of the Cervix. Carcinoma of the cervix is one of the cancers most easily
diagnosed in the early stages. Incidence of this malignancy has decreased significantly since the development of the Pap smear. The Pap smear, explained in Chapter 3, enables physicians to obtain scrapings from the cervix. These scrapings are
examined microscopically; cell abnormalities indicate precursors of cancer and
various stages in its development, and biopsies of suspected lesions are also taken.
Carcinoma in situ, a premalignant lesion, is the earliest stage of cancer; the underlying tissue has not been invaded. Progression from a carcinoma in situ to
an invasive malignancy may be slow. Ulceration then occurs, causing vaginal discharge and bleeding. The cancer spreads to surrounding organs: the vagina, bladder, rectum, and pelvic wall. Widespread cancer becomes inoperable, and radiation therapy is the usual treatment. Carcinoma of the cervix appears to follow
chronic irritation, infection, and poor hygiene. Promiscuity, beginning at an early
age and involving many partners, is somehow related to this cancer.

Carcinoma of the Endometrium. Carcinoma of the endometrium, the lining of the
uterus, occurs most often in postmenopausal women who have had no children.
The malignant tumor may grow into the cavity of the uterus or invade the wall itself. Ulcerations develop, and erosion of blood vessels causes vaginal bleeding.
Surgery and radiation are the usual treatments.

Fibroid Tumors. Benign tumors of the smooth muscle of the uterus, **leiomyomas**
or fibroid tumors, are very common and frequently cause no symptoms. Fibroids
are often multiple and vary greatly in size. Fibroid tumors, some of which are
stalked or pedunculated, are shown in Figure 14–6. Fibroid tumor growth is stim-

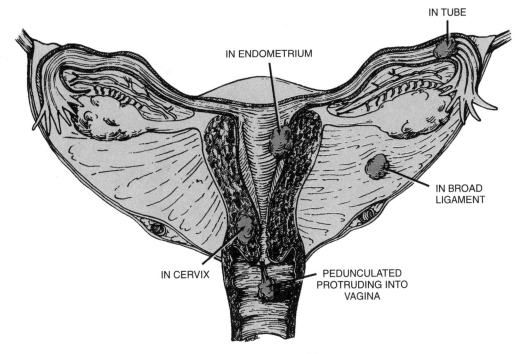

IN TUBE

IN ENDOMETRIUM

IN BROAD
LIGAMENT

IN CERVIX

PEDUNCULATED
PROTRUDING INTO
VAGINA

Figure 14–6. Fibroid tumors of the uterus.

ulated by estrogen because the tumors develop only during the reproductive years. Large tumors putting pressure on surrounding organs and nerve endings cause pelvic pain. Fibroid tumors can also interfere during delivery. Abnormal bleeding between periods or excessively heavy menstrual flow is a common symptom of fibroid tumors. A hysterectomy is generally required if bleeding continues.

Ovarian Neoplasms. The most common ovarian neoplasm is the cyst, a fluid-filled sac. Many cysts have no symptoms but are discovered during a pelvic examination. Large cysts that can interfere with blood flow are removed surgically.

Primary malignant tumors of the ovary are relatively common. Primary tumors tend to be asymptomatic and therefore are discovered only when the disease is advanced. A malignant tumor can be removed surgically before metastases or treated with chemotherapy once it has spread.

A peculiar benign tumor of the ovary is the **dermoid cyst,** or **teratoma,** described in Chapter 3. The dermoid cyst contains all kinds of tissues: skin with its oil glands and hair follicles, teeth, and bone. The cyst is filled with oily material from the glands, and hair grows into the cavity. The tumor is harmless unless its size or other symptoms necessitate surgery. A teratoma is seen in Figure 14–7.

Hydatidiform Mole. The **hydatidiform mole** is a benign tumor of the placenta. It can develop after a pregnancy or in association with an abnormal one. The tumor

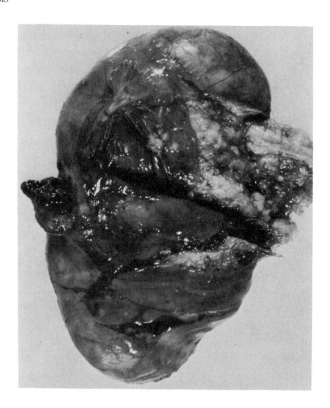

Figure 14–7. Dermoid cyst of ovary. (*Courtesy of Dr. David R. Duffell.*)

consists of multiple cysts and resembles a bunch of grapes. The tumor secretes **chorionic gonadotropic hormone (CGH),** the hormone that indicates a positive pregnancy test. The uterus enlarges greatly, although no fetus develops. Bleeding usually occurs, and the mole is expelled. Scraping of the uterus, the procedure of **dilation** of the cervix and **curettage (D&C),** removes any fragments of the tumor or placenta.

Choriocarcinoma. **Choriocarcinoma** is a highly malignant tumor of the placenta. A part of the placenta is formed by the embryonic membrane called the chorion. This tumor may develop after a hydatidiform mole, a normal delivery, or an abortion. A choriocarcinoma, like the hydatidiform mole, secretes large amounts of CGH. Presence of this hormone in the urine in the absence of pregnancy is significant diagnostically. The tumor is highly invasive and metastasizes rapidly. Chemotherapy rather than surgery is the usual treatment.

Adenocarcinoma of the Vagina. Adenocarcinoma of the vagina has been linked to the synthetic hormone **diethylstilbestrol (DES)** used to prevent spontaneous abortion. This rather rare cancer has developed in some young girls whose mothers were given DES during pregnancy.

Daughters of women who received DES therapy should be checked for possible cancer development, but the incidence is low. DES appears to have only slight effects in sons born to these women. Testes have been found to be smaller than normal in some cases, and some cyst formation has been found in the **epididymis.**

Neoplasms of the Breast. Adenocarcinoma, cancer of the breast ducts, is the most common breast malignancy. It occurs more often in single women, in women who have had no children, and in women with a family history of breast cancer. Adenocarcinoma of the breast usually develops around the time of the menopause, and development of this cancer seems to be related to estrogen activity. Women are strongly urged to examine their breasts monthly for a possible lump. The American Cancer Society and the National Cancer Institute have done a great deal to encourage this practice, and they provide valuable information on the procedure.

The signs that indicate a malignant tumor are presented by an advanced cancer. A hard, fixed lump in the upper, outer quadrant is one such sign. Benign tumors, because they are encapsulated (Chapter 3), are not fixed to underlying structures. The nipple often retracts and the skin dimples due to contraction of dense fibrous connective tissue that extends to the chest muscles and skin.

The lymph nodes of the axillary region may be swollen. Carcinoma spreads principally through the lymph system. Metastases are frequent to the lungs, liver, brain, and bone. **Mammography** can detect small, early cancers and should be performed on the recommended schedule according to age. A biopsy of the suspected malignancy confirms the diagnosis or shows the tumor to be benign.

Treatment of breast cancer varies. In a simple mastectomy, only the breast is removed. The breast, chest muscles, and axillary lymph nodes are removed in a **radical mastectomy.** Some studies indicate that prognosis after a radical mastectomy is not necessarily better than that after a less mutilating procedure. Less mutilating procedures involve removal of the tumor only, a **lumpectomy,** and radiation therapy. The ovaries are often removed to prevent the stimulating effect of estrogen on tumor growth when disease is metastatic.

Paget's disease of the nipple is a rare cancer involving inflammatory changes that affect the nipple and the areola. The nipple becomes granular and crusted with lesions resembling eczema. In advanced Paget's disease, ulceration develops and there is a discharge from the nipple. The breast becomes edematous and is characterized as having a "pigskin" appearance. Treatment depends on the extent of the disease. A significant feature in Paget's disease is that it is accompanied by an underlying infiltrating duct cancer.

Benign Tumors of the Breast. The most common benign tumor of the breast is a fibroadenoma (Fig. 14–8). It is a firm, movable mass easily removed by surgery. The fibroadenoma does not become malignant.

Cystic hyperplasia or **fibrocystic disease** is very common and not serious. Development occurs at any age with the formation of numerous lumps in the breast. The lumps are fluid-filled cysts, not tumors. They tend to be painful at the time of the menstrual period as the breasts themselves respond to hormonal

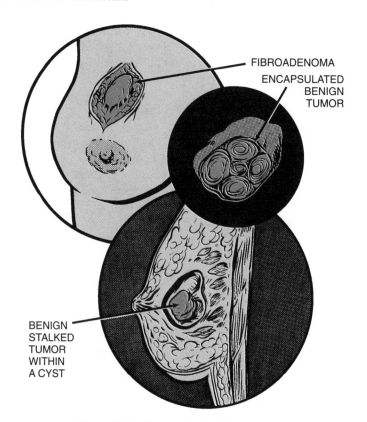

Figure 14–8. Common benign breast tumors.

changes, enlarging and regressing. These cysts are often **aspirated:** A needle is inserted to remove fluid. The withdrawal of fluid confirms that the lump is a cyst and not a solid tumor. There may be a higher incidence of breast cancer development in women who have cystic hyperplasia. These women should be examined regularly to prevent mistaking a tumor for a cyst.

■ Menstrual Abnormalities

Amenorrhea is the absence of menstrual periods and is known as primary amenorrhea if menstruation fails to begin. Lack of gonadotropic hormones from the pituitary gland or a diseased ovary can cause the abnormality and administration of hormones may be effective treatment. The cessation of menstrual periods for more than a year is termed secondary amenorrhea. This can result from an ovarian or uterine disease, as well as hormonal imbalance; pituitary failure and thyroid disease can cause amenorrhea. The absence of menstruation is a sign of a disease that must be diagnosed and treated.

Certain mental disturbances—extreme depression, worry, and continuous stress—can cause cessation of menstruation. The hypothalamus of the brain governs the release of pituitary hormones, including the gonadotropins. The condition of amenorrhea will right itself if the stressful conditions can be eliminated, or if the patient receives counseling on adjustment to the problem.

Menorrhagia is excessive or prolonged bleeding during menstruation. It can result from tumors of the uterus, pelvic inflammatory disease, or endocrine imbalance. Failure to ovulate can also cause menorrhagia. If a corpus luteum is not formed, progesterone is not secreted and estrogen continues to stimulate endometrial thickening. Treatment varies according to the cause of the disease. Tumors should be removed surgically, pelvic inflammatory disease treated with antibiotics, and hormonal therapy administered for endocrine insufficiency.

Metrorrhagia is bleeding between menstrual periods or extreme irregularity of the cycle. It results from an abnormal buildup and sloughing of endometrial tissue. Hormonal imbalance may be the cause of metrorrhagia, or the endometrial response to the hormones may be incorrect. Dilation and curettage, a D&C, is often performed, and the endometrium returns to normal.

■ Toxic Shock Syndrome

Toxic shock syndrome (TSS) is not merely a disease of menstruating women who use tampons but an infection of *Staphylococcus aureus*. The signs include high fever, rash, skin peeling, and decreased blood pressure. Other systemic involvements may include gastrointestinal complaints, elevated liver enzymes, and neuromuscular disturbances. Treatment includes fluid replacement to counteract shock and administration of selected antibiotics.

The relationship between particular tampons and development of TSS is thought to be an increase in staphylococcal toxin production in the environment of certain synthetic fibers. These fibers were found to be the ones used in "super" tampons to increase absorbency. The fibers apparently remove magnesium from the vagina, and this produces an ideal environment for bacteria to make the toxins; these fibers are no longer used. It was found that some surgical dressings also contained the same fibers, a finding that may explain some cases of TSS in nontampon users.

Recommendations for women who use tampons include avoidance of the superabsorptive type, daytime use only, and frequent changes of tampons.

■ Premenstrual Syndrome

Most women experience some mild premenstrual symptoms during their reproductive years but when symptoms become temporarily disabling, disrupt family, business, and social relationships, **premenstrual syndrome (PMS)** is indicated.

PMS consists of a group of severe symptoms, emotional, physical, and behavioral, that are associated with the menstrual cycle. They usually begin at the midpoint of the cycle and worsen until the onset of bleeding.

Physical symptoms include lower abdominal bloating, breast swelling and soreness, headache, and constipation. Episodes of depression, anxiety, irritability, and hostility are characteristics of emotional changes. Typical behavioral symptoms include crying, binge eating, and clumsiness. No tests or physical examinations confirm the presence of PMS. A daily diary which shows the relationship of the monthly cycle and the symptoms can assist in the diagnosis.

The cause of **PMS** is unknown but researchers suspect that the production of cyclic ovarian hormones affect the production of other hormones and chemicals, specifically neurotransmitters. These chemicals may cause the symptoms, but it is not understood why some women are affected and others are not. Whereas in the past it was thought that **PMS** was emotional in origin or caused by stress, it is now known to have a real physical cause.

Treatment has to be very individually prescribed as patients respond differently to various suggestions. For some women dietary changes during the week before the onset of menstruation are helpful. These changes might include the avoidance of salt, sugar, caffeine, and alcohol. Aerobic exercise, brisk walking, or swimming is helpful for others. Support groups and stress management techniques can be positive means of coping with the condition.

■ Endometriosis

Endometriosis is a disease condition in which endometrial tissue from the uterus becomes embedded elsewhere. The tissue may have been pushed backward through the fallopian tubes during menstruation or carried by blood or lymph. It then takes hold on some structure in the peritoneal cavity such as the ovary. The endometrial tissue by nature responds to hormonal changes even when outside the uterus. This tissue goes through a proliferative and secretory phase, along with the sloughing-off phase with subsequent bleeding. Endometriosis causes pelvic pain, abnormal bleeding, and painful menstruation **(dysmenorrhea).** Sterility and pain during sexual intercourse **(dyspareunia)** can result. Treatment of endometriosis varies according to the extent of the abnormal growth and the age of the patient. The only certain means of diagnosing endometriosis is by seeing it. Direct visualization is possible through **laparoscopy** in which an illuminated tube is inserted through a small abdominal incision. A tissue biopsy can be taken and examined. Hormonal therapy is generally used for the young patient. Pregnancy, with the ab-

On the Practical Side

HOT FLASHES

One of the most common complaints of menopausal women is the discomfort of hot flashes. The range in severity is broad but generally involves vasodilation, redness, heat, and sweating. The extensive dilation of superficial blood vessels and increased blood flow accounts for the rapid temperature fluctuations. The cause of hot flashes is attributed to decreased levels of estrogen and progesterone in response to gonadotropic hormone stimulation from the anterior pituitary gland.

sence of menstruation, tends to hold the condition in check. Extensive proliferation of endometrial tissue requires surgery, and cysts filled with blood are usually found at this time.

ABNORMALITIES OF PREGNANCY

A most important factor during pregnancy is good prenatal care. The pregnant woman should be checked regularly for weight gain, blood pressure, and urine abnormalities. She should be instructed on the importance of proper diet and exercise. Most pregnancies progress normally, but occasionally some problems do arise.

■ Ectopic Pregnancy

An **ectopic pregnancy** is a pregnancy in which the fertilized ovum implants in a tissue other than the uterus. The most common site of an ectopic pregnancy is in the fallopian tubes. The fertilized ovum becomes trapped because of a stricture or obstruction such as a tumor. Salpingitis is a predisposing condition for a tubal pregnancy due to the inflammatory effect on the mucosal lining. Embryonic development proceeds for about 2 months, at which time the pregnancy terminates. The tube often ruptures, as seen in Figure 14–9, causing severe internal hemorrhage into the abdominal cavity. Intense pain and bleeding from the uterus result, and the embryo is usually destroyed by the trauma. Once the diagnosis has been made, the ruptured tube and embryo have to be removed surgically.

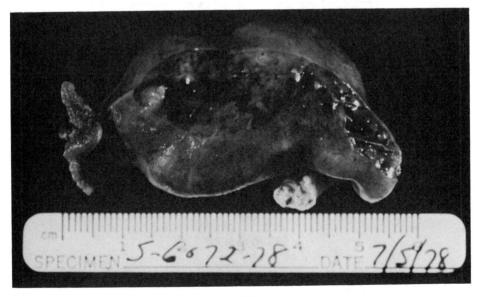

Figure 14–9. Fallopian tube ruptured from an ectopic pregnancy. (*Courtesy of Dr. David R. Duffell.*)

■ Spontaneous Abortion

A spontaneous abortion, commonly called a *miscarriage*, usually results from a genetic abnormality. The fetus is expelled before it is able to live outside of the uterus, and this usually occurs in the second or third month of pregnancy. The first sign is vaginal bleeding with cramping. The woman who has aborted should receive medical attention at once to reduce the hazards of hemorrhage and infection. Dilation and curettage, a D&C, is usually performed to remove any tissue that remains in the uterus.

A woman who has repeated spontaneous abortions should be examined comprehensively to determine the cause. Hormonal imbalances are sometimes responsible and can be corrected by replacement hormones. Emotional and psychological factors may be involved, and professional counseling is advised.

■ Toxemia of Pregnancy

Toxemia of pregnancy sometimes develops during the last trimester. The condition is poorly named because no toxin appears to cause the disease and the cause is not known. The principal signs are hypertension, albuminuria, edema (particu-

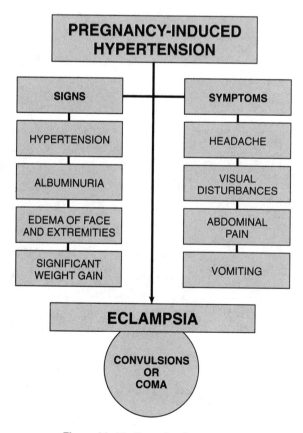

Figure 14–10. Toxemia of pregnancy.

larly in the face and arms), and a significant weight gain. These signs are presented in Figure 14–10. In the first phase of toxemia, pregnancy-induced hypertension (PIH), the patient experiences headache, visual disturbances, abdominal pain, and vomiting. A spasm of blood vessels apparently causes the headache and visual disturbances. If this condition is not treated, **eclampsia** develops and the patient goes into convulsions and coma.

Preventive treatment for toxemia consists of early prenatal care, in which blood pressure is regularly checked, urine is analyzed for albumin, and weight gain is controlled. **Preeclampsia,** diagnosed early and treated, responds well. Restriction of salt (which tends to increase blood pressure), a nutritious low-calorie diet, and diuretics may be prescribed. This must be done with great care to prevent injury to the fetus. If the patient does not respond and eclampsia with convulsions develops, anticonvulsant medications are prescribed with caution.

ANATOMY OF THE MALE REPRODUCTIVE SYSTEM

The male reproductive system consists of a pair of testes in which the sperm develop and hormones are produced, a system of tubules that convey sperm to the outside, and the penis, which transmits the sperm into the female tract. Accessory glands contribute to the formation of semen.

The testes are suspended in the **scrotum,** a saclike structure outside the body wall. The testes contain highly coiled tubules called the **seminiferous tubules,** which are the site of sperm development (Fig. 14–11). When the sperm reach a certain maturity they enter the **epididymis,** a coiled tube that lies along the outer wall of the testis. The epididymis leads into another duct, the **vas deferens,** that passes through the inguinal canal into the abdominal cavity.

Near the base of the urinary bladder the vas deferens joins a duct of the **seminal vesicle,** an accessory gland, to form the **ejaculatory duct.** The ejaculatory ducts from each side penetrate the **prostate gland** to enter the urethra. Ducts of the prostate open into the first part of the male urethra. Another pair of glands, the **bulbourethral glands,** secrete into the urethra as it enters the penis. The male reproductive system is illustrated in Figure 14–12.

The penis consists of three cylindrical bodies of cavernous tissue also known as erectile tissue. This tissue is filled with spaces, or sinuses, that become engorged with blood. The urethra passes through one of these cylindrical bodies as it extends to the outside and connective tissue supports the erectile structures. The distal, expanded end of the penis is the glans penis. A flap of loosely attached skin covering the glans, the **prepuce** or foreskin, is often removed shortly after birth, which is the procedure called circumcision.

PHYSIOLOGY OF THE MALE REPRODUCTIVE SYSTEM

Spermatogenesis, the formation of sperm, begins in the male at about age 13 and continues through life. The development of sperm and the secretion of the male

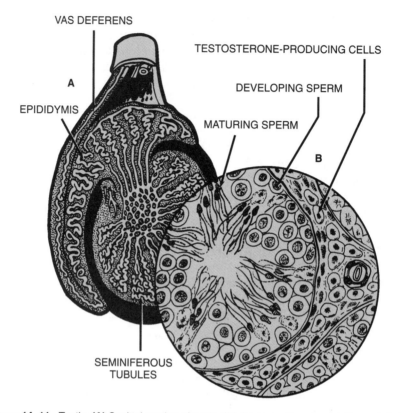

Figure 14–11. Testis: **(A)** Sagittal section of testis. **(B)** Cross-section of seminiferous tubule.

hormone, testosterone, are processes stimulated by gonadotropic hormones of the anterior pituitary gland. Full maturation of the sperm occurs in the epididymis, where they become motile and capable of fertilizing an ovum. Sperm are stored in both the epididymis and vas deferens and can live for several weeks in the male genital ducts. Once they are ejaculated, they live for only 24 to 72 hours.

The accessory glands contribute to the nourishment and protection of the sperm, and mucoid secretions from these glands form the semen. The seminal vesicles provide fructose, other nutrients, and prostaglandin, which increases uterine contractions. This helps to propel the sperm toward the fallopian tubes. The seminal vesicles release their secretions into the ejaculatory ducts at the same time the vas deferens empty the sperm. The muscular prostate gland, which surrounds the first part of the urethra, contracts during ejaculation, releasing its secretions. The secretion is alkaline, which is important to the motility of the sperm, since the highly acidic vaginal secretions would inhibit sperm motility.

Sexual stimulation of the male transmits impulses into the central nervous system, which initiates the male response. Erection of the penis is the first effect. Nerve impulses cause the dilation of penile arteries, allowing blood to flow under

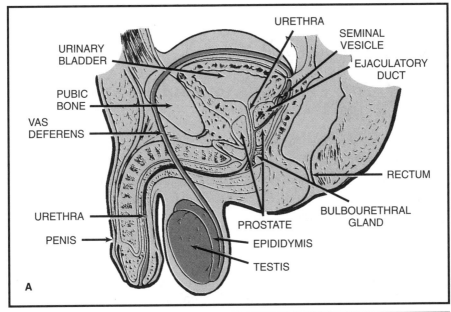

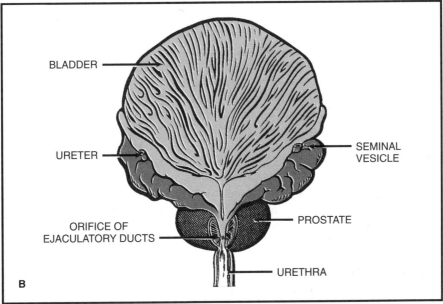

Figure 14–12. Sagittal section **(A)** and posterior view **(B)** of male reproductive system.

On the Practical Side

SEMEN ANALYSIS IN EVALUATING STERILITY

Several factors are analyzed in evaluating possible sterility. Sperm counts below 20 million/ml of semen and/or a high percentage of abnormally shaped sperm are indicators of sterility. Motility of the sperm is essential and a factor which is analyzed. The semen and sugar content, specifically fructose, are also evaluated to determine possible obstruction or absence of accessory glands and ducts.

high pressure into the erectile tissue. The high pressure temporarily impedes the emptying of the penile veins, and causes the penis to become hard, elongated, and erect.

Intense sexual stimulation causes peristaltic contractions in the walls of the epididymis and vas deferens, propelling sperm into the urethra. The seminal vesicles and prostate gland simultaneously release their secretions, which mix with the mucous secretion of the bulbourethral glands forming the semen, the process of emission. Ejaculation of the semen—the culmination of the sexual act—occurs when contraction of this musculature increases pressure on the erectile tissue, and the semen is expressed through the urethral opening.

DISEASES OF THE MALE REPRODUCTIVE SYSTEM

The most common diseases of the male reproductive system are those affecting the prostate gland. This gland can become inflamed or enlarged as a result of bacterial invasion and cause urinary problems. Cancer sometimes develops in the prostate as well as in the testes.

■ Diseases of the Prostate Gland

Inflammation of the prostate can result from urinary tract infections or sexually transmitted diseases. Conversely, an enlarged prostate can cause urinary tract infections by obstructing the outflow of urine from the bladder.

Prostatitis. The cause of **prostatitis,** inflammation of the prostate, is not always known. Infection frequently develops from gonococci in a male with gonorrhea or from *E. coli* that has caused a urinary tract infection. The patient experiences pain and a burning sensation during urination. The prostate may be tender, and pus from the tip of the penis is sometimes noted. Penicillin is the usual treatment unless hypersensitivity to the drug necessitates the use of other antibiotics.

Benign Prostatic Hyperplasia. Enlargement of the prostate gland, benign **prostatic hyperplasia,** is a common occurrence in men over 50. The incidence increases with age, and the enlargement can be felt through rectal examination.

The symptoms resemble urinary tract disturbances (see Chapter 9) as the enlarged prostate partially blocks the flow of urine from the bladder. If the bladder cannot be fully emptied, residual urine provides a medium for bacterial infection and cystitis develops. Figure 14–13 shows an obstruction of the urethra caused by prostatic enlargement.

The blockage of urine outflow places back pressure on the ureters, which causes them to become congested with urine, a condition called *hydroureters*. This back pressure can extend to the kidneys; they swell with fluid, and hydronephrosis results. An imbalance of sex hormones frequently causes prostatic enlargement. The level of testosterone generally decreases with age, but estrogen from the adrenal cortex continues to be secreted, changing the ratio of the two. Treatment for benign prostatic hyperplasia, which is highly symptomatic, is surgical removal.

Carcinoma of the Prostate Gland. Carcinoma of the prostate is common in old age, but the tumor may be small and asymptomatic. Rectal examination may reveal an enlarged prostate that is very hard, harder than a benign enlargement.

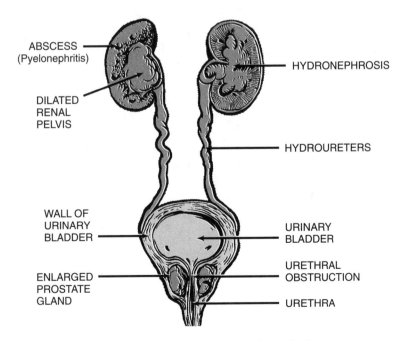

Figure 14–13. Urethral obstruction and complications.

Signs of prostatic cancer are urinary tract obstruction, urinary infections, the need to urinate during the night, or **nocturia,** and at times urinary incontinence.

Prognosis for this carcinoma is poor, as the malignancy spreads rapidly to nearby organs like the bladder and rectum. The cancer invades the lymph and blood vessels and metastasizes to the bone and other organs. Figure 14–14 shows common sites of metastases from cancer of the prostate.

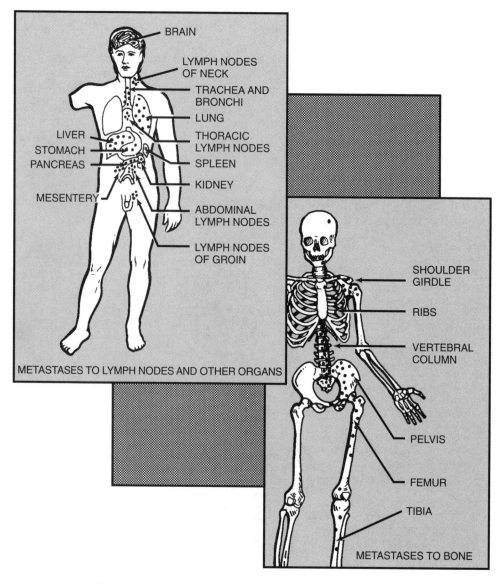

Figure 14–14. Common sites of metastases from prostatic cancer.

Treatment depends on the extent of the cancer, which may be inoperable, and hormonal therapy is generally prescribed. Since testosterone stimulates growth of the tumor, removal of the testes—the source of the hormone—may reduce its size. Estrogen, which has an inhibitory effect on the tumor's growth, is administered.

■ Diseases of the Testes and Epididymis

The testes and epididymis can become inflamed from injury, infection, or some rare tumors that develop in the testes.

Epididymitis. Inflammation of the epididymis **(epididymitis)** is frequently caused by gonococcus, but a urinary tract infection or prostatitis can also be the source of epididymitis. Abscesses sometimes form, and scar tissue develops that can cause sterility if both sides are affected. Symptoms include severe pain in the testes, swelling, and tenderness in the scrotum. Antibiotic treatment is effective when combined with rest and the avoidance of irritants such as alcohol and spicy food.

Orchitis. **Orchitis,** inflammation of the testes, can follow an injury or viral infection such as mumps, with the development of inflammatory edema and pain. The most common cause of orchitis is mumps in an adult man. Swelling of the testes and severe pain usually develop about a week after mumps, an inflammation of the parotid salivary gland. In severe cases, atrophy of the testes can occur, and if both sides are affected, sterility results.

Testicular Tumors. Tumors of the testes are rare, but when they occur it is usually in young men, and these tumors are highly malignant. One such tumor is the **seminoma,** a cancer of the seminiferous tubules. The seminoma is quite radiosensitive, so the prescribed treatment is irradiation.

Another tumor of the testes is the **teratoma,** similar in form to the dermoid cyst of the ovary described previously. The teratoma evidently arises from a primitive germ cell, and the tumor contains a variety of tissues. Whereas the dermoid cyst in the ovary is benign, the teratoma of the testes is highly malignant and spreads through the lymphatics and blood vessels. Chemotherapy and radiotherapy are the usual means of treatment.

Impotence. **Impotence,** the inability of the male to achieve and maintain an erection sufficient for sexual intercourse, is often caused by emotional disturbances. Stress decreases the output of gonadotropic hormones, and, consequently, testosterone production and spermatogenesis are diminished. The dilation of penile arteries that leads to engorgement of the erectile tissue of the penis and then erection is under the control of the autonomic nervous system. Anxiety, fear, and worry are emotions that affect the nervous system. The onset of impotence may be due to fatigue, a form of stress, or distraction.

Impotence may also be physiologic in nature. Arteriosclerosis, diabetes mellitus, surgical complications, urologic disorders, and premature ejaculation are all possible causes. The onset of impotence may be due to certain medications, drug abuse, or alcoholism; changes in these areas may correct the impotence.

Impotence is said to be primary if the man has never been able to complete intercourse successfully. The inability to maintain an adequate erection may stem from worry about satisfactory sexual performance or from psychological concerns about events in adolescence. Impotence is secondary if intercourse has been achieved successfully at least once. The onset of impotence may be due to fatigue, a form of stress, or distraction. Premature ejaculation and alcoholism are also possible causes of impotence. This condition is not generally the result of a physical disorder, but it may be.

Treatment should be directed toward the source of the problem which requires openness on the part of the patient with the physician or therapist. The man must be helped to overcome his personal insecurity and frustration, and his partner should also be supported and instructed about the problem. With good counseling, impotence can usually be overcome.

Cryptorchidism. **Cryptorchidism** is not a disease but a failure of the testes to descend from the abdominal cavity, where they develop during fetal life, to the scrotum. Undescended testes are shown in Figure 14–15. This condition should be corrected through surgery or hormonal therapy. Sterility results if this condition is not rectified. Maturation of the sperm cannot occur in the abdominal cavity, where the temperature is slightly higher than that of the scrotum. If the testes are not brought down into the scrotum, they should be removed. Undescended testes atrophy and may become the potential site of cancer.

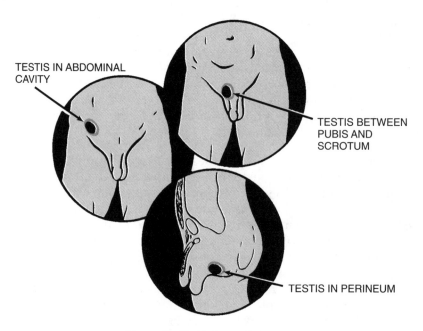

Figure 14–15. Undescended testes.

SEXUALLY TRANSMITTED DISEASES (STDs)

The incidence of diseases transmitted by sexual intercourse has increased dramatically in recent years, especially among women and teenagers. If untreated, serious conditions may develop that can gravely affect a person's life. An estimated 1 million women contract pelvic infections each year as a result of undetected STDs. Infected women are often asymptomatic and spread the diseases to other sexual partners and to their offspring during pregnancy. Sterility and life-threatening ectopic pregnancies are common complications of sexually transmitted diseases.

◼ AIDS (Acquired Immune Deficiency Syndrome)
AIDS, the most dreaded disease in today's society is not only transmitted sexually, but can also be acquired as a blood-borne infection. Because the immune system is destroyed by AIDS, the disease is discussed in Chapter 2 with Immunity.

◼ Gonorrhea
Gonorrhea is one of the most common and widespread of venereal diseases. It is caused by the organism **gonococcus** and is transmitted through sexual intercourse. Gonococci do not live outside the body, and the organisms are acquired by direct sexual contact with an infected person.

The initial site of infection is the genitals or urethra. Symptoms usually occur within 2 to 8 days of infection. The vaginal glands in the female are frequently affected and fill with pus; the organisms may spread to the cervix. Acute urethritis develops in the male, causing difficulty and pain during urination. A copious discharge of pus ensues and prostatitis frequently develops with abscess formation.

Symptoms of urethritis or cervicitis may be ignored in the female or she may be asymptomatic. The female can be a reservoir for organisms and not be aware that she is infected.

Gonorrhea usually responds rapidly to penicillin but early detection and treatment are extremely important. Diagnosis of gonorrhea is made by examining pus from the urethra or vaginal discharge for the presence of gonococci.

If untreated, a chronic condition develops, and the infection spreads upward. The inflammation causes fibrosis, which can produce a stricture in the male urethra or in the vas deferens. If both vas deferens become stenotic, sterility results.

The fallopian tubes in the female are frequently affected by untreated gonorrhea, and salpingitis results. The pus-filled tubes can empty into the peritoneal cavity, causing peritonitis.

One of the most common causes of pelvic inflammatory disease (PID) is untreated gonorrhea. Chills, fever, and weakness develop with intestinal upset. Chronic pelvic inflammatory disease causes abscesses to develop in the fallopian tubes, with fibrous scarring and sterility resulting. Ectopic pregnancies may also result.

The baby of an infected mother can be born with acute purulent conjunctivitis, inflammation of the conjunctiva. The gonococcal organisms enter the eye during delivery, and if the cornea becomes ulcerated, blindness results. To prevent this infection from developing, a drop of silver nitrate is routinely placed in the eyes of newborn babies.

A new danger exists in treating gonorrhea with penicillin; a superinfection can develop in which the causative organisms become resistant to penicillin and actually use it as a nutrient.

■ Syphilis

Syphilis, commonly called "lues," is a most serious venereal disease. The causative organism is a spirochete, ***Treponema pallidum,*** transmitted by sexual intercourse or intimate contact with an infectious lesion. The baby of an infected mother may be born syphilitic.

A **chancre,** or ulceration, develops on the genitals in the primary stage of infection. This lesion, which may vary from a small erosion to a deep ulcer, appears within a few days to a few weeks after sexual contact. The chancre usually develops on the vulva of the female and on the penis of the male as shown in Figure 14–16. The chancre may develop elsewhere: on the lips, the tongue, or anus. Anal chancres are common in male homosexuals.

The lesion, which sometimes goes unnoticed, heals after a few weeks. If un-

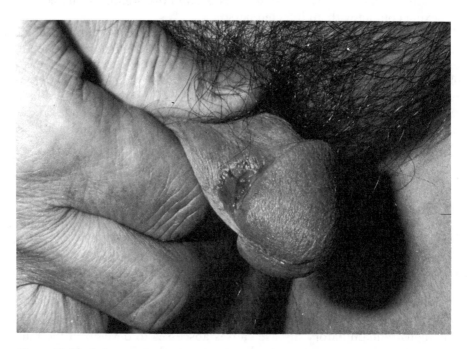

Figure 14–16. A chancre of primary syphilis seen on the penis. (*From Feinstein,* Dermatology, *1975. Courtesy of Robert J. Brady Co.*)

treated with penicillin, the secondary phase of the disease occurs in a matter of weeks. The principal sign of the secondary phase is a nonitching rash that affects any part of the body: the trunk, soles of the feet, palms, mouth, vulva, or rectum. The patient is still infectious at this stage, but he or she can be treated with penicillin.

An untreated case of syphilis may be dormant for many years, but the organisms are in the bloodstream and a systemic spread occurs. The appearance of symptoms, years after the primary infection, marks the tertiary and most serious phase of syphilis.

The cardiovascular system is severely damaged at this stage of infection. The inflammatory response to the spirochetes in the blood causes fibrosis, scarring, and obstruction of blood vessels, particularly of the aorta. Lesions develop on the cerebral cortex, causing mental disorders, deafness, and blindness. Loss of sensation in the legs and feet due to spinal cord damage cause a characteristic gait to develop. **Paresis,** a general paralysis associated with organic loss of brain function, results in death if untreated. The tertiary lesions of the syphilitic infection are irreversible.

Congenital defects are numerous in an infant born to an infectious mother; mental retardation, physical deformities, deafness, and blindness are common. The syphilitic infection can cause death of the fetus and spontaneous abortion.

The severe consequences of syphilis point out the urgent need for early detection and treatment. Diagnostic procedures include screening tests—the **VDRL test** perfected by the Venereal Disease Research Laboratory of the United States Public Health Service, and the **rapid plasma reagin (RPR) test.** The most sensitive and specific test for syphilis is the *Treponema pallidum* **immobilization test (TPI),** which detects specific antibodies against the spirochete. Treatment with penicillin is successful except in reversing tertiary lesions. Development of a superinfection, described under gonorrhea, is a serious threat.

■ Genital Herpes

Genital herpes is an extremely painful, viral disease that tends to recur periodically and for which there is no cure. Herpes virus is transmitted by intimate contact between mucous membrane surfaces, the site of herpes-virus affinity. There are two types of **herpes simplex** virus—type I causing "fever blisters" or "cold sores" and type II involving the mucous membranes of the genital tracts.

Symptoms generally appear within 3 weeks after exposure to the virus. The symptoms intensify from a burning, itching sensation to severe pain. Multiple blisters appear on the genitalia and at times on the buttocks or thigh. As the blisters rupture, they become secondarily infected and ulcerate. Painful urination and vaginal discharge are common.

The active phase subsides as the lesions heal, but the virus remains dormant until reactivated, perhaps at a time of stress or low resistance.

The disease is transmitted by contact with an active sore that is releasing (shedding) the infectious virus. The virus can be spread from a cold sore on the lips to the genitals; the reverse is also true. Great caution should be used to avoid self-infection of the mucous membrane of the eye.

Use of condoms or diaphragms provides partial protection from transmitting the virus during intercourse, but abstention from sexual contact during the active phase is essential.

Diagnosis is most accurate based on a positive viral culture on living tissue. The Tzanck smear test, which involves examination of lesion fluid, is also available.

There is no cure for a herpes infection, but secondary infections can be prevented and healing promoted. The lesions must be kept clean and dry, and ice-cold compresses may be used to relieve the pain.

Active herpes genitalis has very serious consequences during pregnancy, not only causing spontaneous abortion or premature delivery, but also increasing the risk of transmitting the infection to the newborn.

■ Genital Warts

Genital or venereal warts can develop in both men and women and are caused by a virus in the group called HPV (human papilloma virus) which also causes other types of warts. The warts may appear within weeks after sexual relations, vaginal, anal, or oral, with an infected partner or they might not develop for several months. In men the warts occur on the penis or scrotum. In women, the most common site is the perineum, but they may occur on the vulva, vaginal opening, or skin of the thighs. The warts may even develop within the vagina and on the cervix.

Genital warts may cause symptoms such as itching or bleeding, although often they are first detected during a physical exam. An abnormal Pap smear might be an indication of HPV infection. The types of HPV that cause genital warts are being studied as risk factors for cervical cancer when combined with other factors such as multiple sex partners, first intercourse at an early age and other sexually transmitted diseases. Treatment of genital warts depends on their size and number. Some are treated with medication applied by a health care provider but the procedure is very painful. Electrocautery (burning), cryosurgery (freezing), and laser surgery are alternative treatments. Some prescription drugs are now available for home use.

■ Chlamydial Infections

Chlamydial infections are among the most prevalent venereal diseases in the United States. Several strains of the chlamydia organism are responsible for sexually transmitted genitourinary infections in both men and women, as well as in newborns of infected mothers. The disease is a leading cause of pelvic inflammatory disease (PID) in women, with resultant infertility, and severe urethritis in both sexes. Women are often asymptomatic carriers of the infection and continue to infect partners and offspring. Improved tests for the diagnosis of chlamydia infection have recently been developed. The disease responds to certain antibiotics but not to penicillin. The infection often coexists with gonorrhea.

DIAGNOSTIC PROCEDURES FOR REPRODUCTIVE AND SEXUALLY TRANSMITTED DISEASES

In addition to the Pap smear and biopsies of suspicious lesions previously mentioned, pelvic ultrasonography may also be used. It can detect foreign bodies and distinguish between cystic and solid masses or tumors. Ultrasonography is also used in obstetrics. Enlargement of the prostate can be felt by rectal examination.

Specific tests are used to diagnose sexually transmitted diseases. The VDRL test perfected by the Venereal Disease Research Laboratory, the rapid plasma reagin (RPR) test, and the *Treponema pallidum* immobilization test (TPI) are used to diagnose syphilis. The diagnosis of chlamydia is made by direct examination of smears prepared from tissues and scrapings. Microscopic examination of urethral and vaginal discharge reveals the gonococci which cause gonorrhea. Diagnosis of AIDS (discussed in Chapter 2) is made by the clinical picture and blood tests which demonstrate antibodies against the viral antigen. In the very early stages of the disease, before antibodies can be formed, the individual may be infectious and the blood infected.

CHAPTER SUMMARY

Disease can affect the reproductive system in many ways. In the female, tumors and cysts develop in the ovary, uterus, and breast. Infections invade the vagina and vaginal glands, the fallopian tubes, and the endometrium. Menstrual abnormalities result from a diseased organ or from a hormonal imbalance. A pregnancy can develop in the fallopian tubes, a fetus can be spontaneously aborted, and toxemia can occur in pregnancy.

Diseases of the male affect the prostate gland by infection, enlargement, or tumor formation, causing urinary complications. Infections of the testes and epididymis can result in sterility. Inadequate testosterone secretion affects the male secondary characteristics.

Sexually transmitted diseases were discussed. AIDS, the most devastating disease in today's society, sexually transmitted but also a blood-borne infection, was discussed in Chapter 2 as a failure of the immune system. Gonorrhea and syphilis have far-reaching consequences if untreated. Early detection of these diseases and administration of penicillin prevent numerous complications providing that a superinfection does not develop. Chlamydial infections, among the most prevalent venereal diseases, responds to certain antibiotics but not penicillin.

There is no cure for genital herpes which tends to recur periodically. Types of the human papilloma virus (HPV) that causes genital warts are being studied as risk factors for cervical cancer.

Self-Study

True or False

_____ 1. Dermoid cysts secrete large amounts of CGT.

_____ 2. Hydatidiform mole is malignant.

_____ 3. Carcinoma of the prostate is treated with testosterone.

_____ 4. Blood pressure is elevated in toxic shock syndrome.

_____ 5. Orchitis can lead to sterility.

_____ 6. Female vaginal glands can be infected with gonococcal organisms.

_____ 7. In chronic PID, an ectopic pregnancy may develop.

_____ 8. Cancer of the endometrium most commonly occurs following multiple pregnancies.

_____ 9. Chronic cystic mastitis is a malignant condition.

_____ 10. Albuminuria accompanies eclampsia.

Match

_____ 11. salpingitis   a) convulsions

_____ 12. vaginitis   b) spread of infection

_____ 13. septic emboli   c) can cause sterility

_____ 14. eclampsia   d) spontaneous abortion

_____ 15. ectopic pregnancy e) *Candida albicans*

Multiple Choice

_____ 16. _____ is the most common cause of vaginitis.
   a. *Candida albicans*
   b. Staphylococcus

_____ 17. Carcinoma of the _____ is detected through a Pap smear.
   a. endometrium
   b. cervix

_____ 18. Carcinoma of the _____ is linked to promiscuity at an early age.
      a. cervix
      b. endometrium

_____ 19. Adenocarcinoma of the breast occurs more often in women _____.
      a. who have had children
      b. who have not had children

_____ 20. _____ is a sexually transmitted viral disease that tends to recur and for which there is no cure.
      a. Genital herpes
      b. Genital warts

Match

_____ 21. genital warts		a)	degeneration of neurons
_____ 22. chancre		b)	multiple blisters
_____ 23. paresis		c)	penicillin resistance
_____ 24. genital herpes		d)	syphilis lesion
_____ 25. chlamydia		e)	human papilloma virus

(Answers on page 450)

Chapter 15

Diseases of the Nervous System

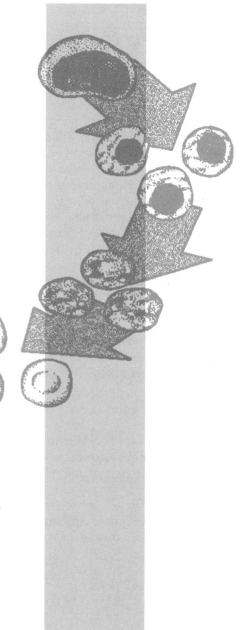

Chapter Outline

- A Highly Organized Communication System
- Structure of the Nervous System
- Function of the Nervous System
- Diseases of the Nervous System
- Convulsions
- Developmental Errors
- Brain Damage
- Cerebrovascular Accident (Stroke) (CVA)
- Traumatic Disorders
- Brain Tumors
- Diagnostic Procedures for the Nervous System
- Chapter Summary
- Self-Study

*T*he body is constantly subjected to changes in its internal and external environment. The body's response is to react appropriately to these changing conditions. How is this accomplished, often with no deliberate thought?

A HIGHLY ORGANIZED COMMUNICATION SYSTEM

The body is equipped to receive all kinds of sensory information: visual, auditory, olfactory, tactile, temperature, pressure, and pain. This input is processed with lightning speed and an action results. It may be an action such as squinting in overly bright light, a turn of the head to detect a faint sound, withdrawal from pain, or shivering to keep warm.

This response to various stimuli is accomplished through the complex nervous system. Certain nerves are specialized to receive sensory information and to convey it to the central nervous system, the brain and spinal cord. Other nerves carry messages from the central nervous system to all parts of the body and initiate action by stimulating a muscle to contract or a gland to secrete. The nervous system is basically a highly organized communication system serving the body.

Disorders of the nervous system may be manifested by such conditions as lack of sensation, paralysis, mental confusion, **seizures,** or the inability to speak. To understand the basis of the various neural disorders, understanding the structure and function of the nervous system is required.

STRUCTURE OF THE NERVOUS SYSTEM

The basic unit of the nervous system is the neuron, or nerve cell. The neuron consists of a cell body and long extensions or fibers—a single axon leading from the cell body and various numbers of dendrites leading toward it. A neuron is shown in Figure 15–1. Some **neurons** are **sensory,** capable of detecting an environmental change and transmitting the message to the brain or spinal cord. Other neurons, the **motor neurons,** convey messages from the central nervous system to a muscle, causing it to contract, or to a gland, triggering its secretion. The response to a stimulus is known as a reflex arc. The fibers of sensory and motor neurons are insulated by a lipid covering called the **myelin** sheath, which increases the rate of transmission of an impulse. Deterioration of this sheath accompanies multiple sclerosis, a disease to be described. The reflex arc pattern is shown in Figure 15–2.

A nerve such as the optic or sciatic nerve consists of a bundle of neuronal fibers. Twelve pairs of nerves—the cranial nerves—enter or exit from the brain. Thirty-one pairs of nerves—the spinal nerves—enter and exit the spinal cord and innervate all parts of the body. The nervous system is illustrated in Figure 15–3.

■ The Spinal Cord

The spinal cord is housed within the vertebral column and is continuous with the brain stem. Numerous tracts of nerve fibers within the cord ascend to the brain, whereas others descend, carrying messages destined for muscles and glands. Three coverings, the **meninges,** protect the delicate nerve tissue. The innermost covering is the pia mater, the next is the arachnoid, and the toughest, outermost covering is the dura mater. Meningitis is an inflammation of these coverings that also surround the brain.

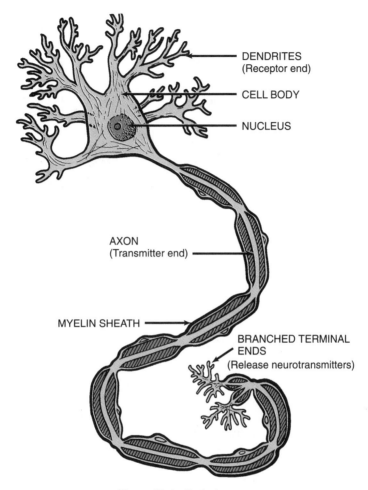

DENDRITES
(Receptor end)

CELL BODY

NUCLEUS

AXON
(Transmitter end)

MYELIN SHEATH

BRANCHED TERMINAL
ENDS
(Release neurotransmitters)

Figure 15–1. Typical neuron.

■ The Brain

The largest portion of the brain is the cerebrum, or cerebral hemispheres. The surface is highly convoluted and has many elevations and depressions. The outer surface of the brain, the cortex, consists of gray matter, where the nerve cell bodies are concentrated. The inner area consists of white matter, the nerve fiber tracts. Deep within the white matter are concentrations of nerve cell bodies known as **basal ganglia,** which help control position and automatic movements. It is the basal ganglia (also gray matter) that are disturbed in Parkinson's disease.

Within the brain are four spaces called **ventricles** that are continuous with the central canal of the spinal cord. **Cerebrospinal fluid** formation takes place in these ventricles. This fluid, derived from plasma, flows out of the ventricles

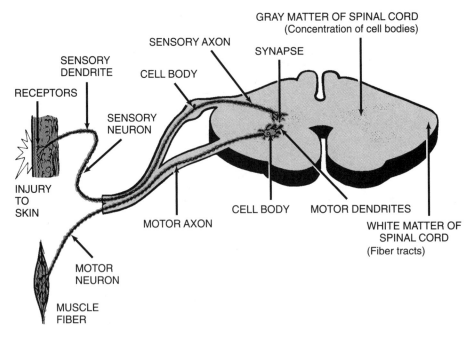

Figure 15–2. Reflex arc pattern.

through small openings and is channeled to circulate over the brain and spinal cord. It flows under the arachnoid covering, acting as a watery, protective cushion. Cerebrospinal fluid is reabsorbed into the venous sinuses of the dura mater, and new fluid is formed. Obstruction of cerebrospinal fluid circulation results in hydrocephalus, which will be described.

■ The Autonomic Nervous System

Another part of the nervous system is the **autonomic nervous system.** This part controls internal functioning of the body. The autonomic nervous system contains the sympathetic and the parasympathetic nervous systems, which often work antagonistically to each other. The hypothalamus, located in the brain, controls activity for a large part of the autonomic nervous system, but it is also affected by other parts of the central nervous system.

The autonomic nervous system controls arterial blood pressure, heart rate, gastrointestinal functions, sweating, temperature regulation, and many other involuntary actions. Whereas the peripheral nerves affect skeletal or voluntary muscle, the autonomic nervous system acts on smooth or involuntary muscle and cardiac muscle. Diseases of the digestive system affected by nerves—ulcers, regional enteritis, and ulcerative colitis (Chapter 10)—are influenced by the autonomic nervous system and the response of the adrenal cortex to stress (Chapter 18).

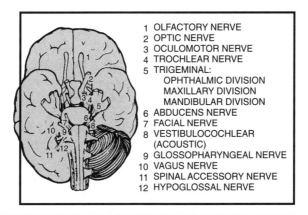

1 OLFACTORY NERVE
2 OPTIC NERVE
3 OCULOMOTOR NERVE
4 TROCHLEAR NERVE
5 TRIGEMINAL:
       OPHTHALMIC DIVISION
       MAXILLARY DIVISION
       MANDIBULAR DIVISION
6 ABDUCENS NERVE
7 FACIAL NERVE
8 VESTIBULOCOCHLEAR
   (ACOUSTIC)
9 GLOSSOPHARYNGEAL NERVE
10 VAGUS NERVE
11 SPINAL ACCESSORY NERVE
12 HYPOGLOSSAL NERVE

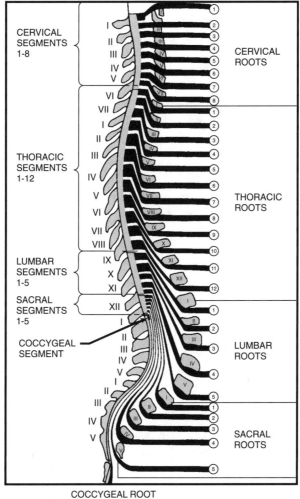

Figure 15–3. The central nervous system. **Top.** Cranial nerves. **Bottom.** Spinal nerves.

FUNCTION OF THE NERVOUS SYSTEM

The transmission of impulses along nerve fibers is an electrical occurrence. For a detailed explanation of the transmission of nerve impulses, you might consult a physiology textbook. Impulses are passed from one neuron to another at a junction called the *synapse*. Transmission at the synapse is a chemical reaction in which the terminal ends of the axon release a transmitter substance that affects the dendrites of the next neuron. One-way transmission of the impulse is assured because only the axons release these chemicals. A similar phenomenon occurs when a motor neuron stimulates a muscle fiber to contract by releasing a transmitter substance, which affects the muscle fiber membrane. This junction is referred to as the neuromuscular or myoneural junction.

■ The Sensory Nervous System

Sensations detected by sensory neurons in the skin, the muscles, tendons, or internal organs are sent into the spinal cord, where they may trigger a simple cord response. A synapse is made with a motor neuron that will bring about an action. More complex actions require that the impulse be sent to various parts of the brain. Impulses reaching the brain stem and cerebellum bring about many automatic actions that are unconscious, but sensory information involving thought processes must reach the highest area of the brain, the cerebral cortex.

The cerebral cortex has specialized areas to receive sensory information from all parts of the body such as the foot, the hand, the abdomen. These areas are just posterior to the central sulcus. Visual impulses are transmitted to the posterior part of the brain, whereas olfactory and auditory impulses are received in the lateral parts. Association areas of the brain interpret deeper meaning of the sensations, and all the sensory messages are integrated in the "knowing area" where

On the Practical Side

PHANTOM PAIN

A patient who has undergone an amputation may perceive pain from the amputated limb. This pain may be similar to that experienced before the surgery. It would seem that pain signals continue in the severed nerve cell fibers and travel to the brain. The brain interprets these signals as pain even though pain receptors at the distal ends of the nerve fibers are no longer present.

they may be stored as memory. Creative thought becomes possible through use of all sensory input.

■ The Motor Nervous System

Just as the cerebral cortex has areas specialized for the reception of sensory information, there are areas that govern motor activity. The primary motor cortex is just anterior to the central sulcus and controls discrete movements of skeletal muscles. Stimulation on one side of the cerebral cortex affects particular muscles on the opposite side of the body because the nerve fibers cross over in the medulla and spinal cord.

Anterior to the primary motor cortex is the premotor cortex, which controls coordinate movements of muscles. This is accomplished by stimulating groups of muscles that work together. The speech area is located here and is usually on the left side in right-handed people. Specialized areas of the brain are shown in Figure 15–4.

Damage to any part of the brain from trauma, hemorrhage, blood clot formation with subsequent ischemia, or infection will have varying effects depending on the degree of injury and the location of the lesion.

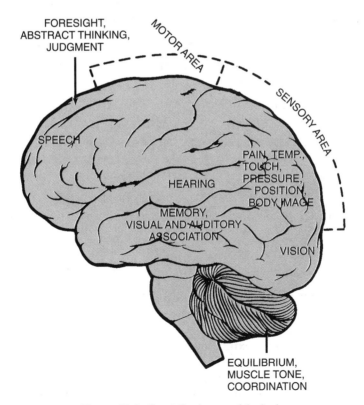

Figure 15–4. Specialized areas of the brain.

DISEASES OF THE NERVOUS SYSTEM

The nervous system is affected by disease in numerous ways. Bacteria and viruses can invade the system and cause infection. Degeneration of nerve tissue is another type of disease. Seizures result from abnormal transmission of neuronal impulses in the brain. Errors in fetal development are responsible for other neural disorders. The brain may be damaged by trauma, cerebral hemorrhages, blood clot formation, and tumors. Many diseases of the nervous system manifest themselves in abnormal muscular activity.

Only neural diseases that have a structural or physiologic basis will be treated in this book. Functional diseases such as schizophrenia, in which there is no apparent brain lesion, are better covered in a psychology text.

On the Practical Side

DRUGS AND THE NERVOUS SYSTEM: "UPPERS" AND "DOWNERS"

Amphetamines known as "uppers," "pep pills," and "speed" are stimulants to the central nervous system. They are subject to abuse as they produce wakefulness and euphoria but they also produce a dangerous dependency. Amphetamines are sometimes used in "diet pills" to suppress appetite, but they are ineffective for weight reduction. Appetite returns when the pills are discontinued, lost weight is regained and it is difficult to get off the pills. Abuse of amphetamines can lead to compulsive behavior, paranoia, hallucinations, and suicidal tendencies.

Barbiturates, or "downers," are sedatives or hypnotics and depress the central nervous system. Blood pressure and body temperature are depressed and the drugs become addictive.

■ Infectious Diseases of the Nervous System

Many diseases are **neurotropic** in that the causative agent, a virus or bacterium, has an affinity for the nervous system. Most viruses in this class affect the nerve tissue directly, although the toxin produced by bacteria is the offending agent in another neural disease.

Infectious neural diseases have numerous causes, such as an infection elsewhere in the body, a contaminated puncture wound, a dog or insect bite, and exposure to chicken pox.

Meningitis. **Meningitis** is an acute inflammation of the first two meninges of the brain and spinal cord, the pia mater and the arachnoid. It is a disease usually affecting children and young adults and may have serious complications if not diagnosed and treated early. There are many forms of meningitis, some being more contagious than others. The most common causative organism is the *Neisseria meningitidis,* but other bacteria, as well as viruses, cause meningitis.

The infecting organisms can reach the meninges from a middle ear, upper respiratory tract, or frontal sinus infection; or they can be carried in the blood from the lungs or other infected site. Healthy children may be carriers of the bacteria and spread the organisms by sneezing or coughing. Viral meningitis may be caused by mumps, polio viruses, and occasionally by herpes simplex.

The symptoms of meningitis are high fever, chills, and a severe headache due to increased intracranial pressure. The patient has a very stiff neck and holds the head rigidly. Any movement of neck muscles stretches the meninges and increases the pain. Nausea, vomiting, and a rash may also be symptomatic. The high fever often causes delirium and convulsions in children, and they may lapse into a coma.

Diagnosis of meningitis is made through a **lumbar puncture,** or spinal tap, in which a hollow needle is inserted into the spinal canal between vertebrae in the lumbar region. This procedure is possible because the spinal cord terminates at the first lumbar vertebra but the sac containing cerebrospinal fluid extends down to the sacrum. Increased pressure of the cerebrospinal fluid with an elevated protein level, numerous polymorphs, and infecting organisms confirms the diagnosis of meningitis. The level of glucose in the cerebrospinal fluid is below normal because the bacteria use the sugar for their own growth.

Treatment with antibiotics is very effective if the meningitis is bacterial. If not treated, permanent brain damage usually results, manifesting itself by sight or hearing loss, paralysis, or mental retardation. The opening in the roof of the fourth ventricle may become blocked by the pyogenic infection. This results in the accumulation of cerebrospinal fluid in the brain, causing a form of **hydrocephalus.**

Encephalitis. **Encephalitis,** an inflammation of the brain and meninges, is caused by a viral infection. The virus may be harbored by wild birds and transmitted to man by mosquitoes. There are many forms of the disease, and they occur in epidemics. Lethargic encephalitis, or "sleeping sickness," is one type of encephalitis in which persistent drowsiness, delirium, and sometimes coma are present. Symptoms of encephalitis range from mild to severe and may include headache, fever, cerebral dysfunction, disordered thought patterns, and, often, seizures. Secondary encephalitis may develop from viral childhood diseases such as chicken pox, measles, and mumps.

Diagnosis of encephalitis is made by lumbar puncture. Treatment is essentially aimed at the symptoms, control of the high fever, maintenance of fluid and electrolyte balance, and careful monitoring of respiratory and kidney function.

In serious cases involving extensive brain damage, convalescence is slow and requires prolonged physical rehabilitation. Nerve damage may cause paralysis. Personality changes occur, as well as emotional disturbances requiring therapy.

Poliomyelitis. **Poliomyelitis,** once a crippling and killing disease that struck primarily children, has nearly been eradicated through the development of the Salk and Sabin vaccines and immunization programs to assure that all children are protected.

Polio is an infectious disease of the brain and spinal cord caused by a virus. Motor neurons of the medulla oblongata and of the spinal cord are primarily affected, and without motor nerve stimulations, muscles become paralyzed. If the respiratory muscles are affected, artificial means of respiration are required.

Symptoms of poliomyelitis are stiff neck, fever, headache, sore throat, and gastrointestinal disturbances. When diagnosed and treated early, severe damage to the nervous system is prevented.

The tremendous value of Dr. Jonas Salk's vaccine to prevent poliomyelitis cannot be measured. Salk used inactivated polio virus, injected intramuscularly, that stimulated production of antibodies against polio. The decrease in the number of polio cases with the institution of immunization programs was immediate. Dr. Albert Sabin developed an oral vaccine against polio that is more convenient to administer, particularly to large groups, and is extremely effective. The Sabin vaccine, because it is taken orally, stimulates the production of antibodies within the digestive system, where the viruses first reside. Destruction of the viruses in the digestive system prevents their transmission and eliminates carriers, which the Salk vaccine does not do.

Tetanus. Most people are familiar with the need for a tetanus shot after a puncture wound or an animal bite. Why are these wounds particularly dangerous?

Tetanus, commonly called "lockjaw," is an infection of nerve tissue caused by the tetanus bacillus that lives in the intestines of animals and human beings. The organisms are excreted in fecal material and persist as spores indefinitely in the soil. The bacilli are prevalent in rural areas and in garden soil fertilized with manure.

The organism that enters the wound with dirt remains in the wound. This organism flourishes in the necrotic tissue of a pus infection and in the absence of oxygen. Deep wounds with ragged, lacerated tissue contaminated with fecal material are the most dangerous type. The bacillus produces a powerful toxin that circulates to the nerves. The toxin becomes anchored to motor nerve cells and stimulates them, which in turn stimulate muscles.

Muscles become rigid, and painful spasms and convulsions develop. The jaw muscles are often the first to be affected, hence the name "lockjaw." These muscles cannot relax, and the mouth is tightly closed. The neck is stiff, and swallowing becomes difficult. If the muscles of respiration are affected, asphyxiation occurs. Death can result from even a minor wound if the condition is not treated.

Tetanus has an incubation period ranging from 1 to a few weeks. The toxin travels slowly, so the distance from the wound to the spinal cord is significant.

Treatment includes a thorough cleansing of the wound, removal of dead tissue and any foreign substance, and immediate immunization to inactivate the toxin before it reaches the spinal cord.

The type of immunization administered depends on the patient's history. If the patient has had no previous immunization, **tetanus antitoxin** is given. If 5 years have elapsed since the previous tetanus injection, the patient receives a booster injection of **tetanus toxoid** to increase the antitoxin level.

Additional treatment includes the administration of antibiotics to prevent secondary infections and the use of sedatives to decrease the frequency of convulsions. Oxygen under high pressure is also used as the bacillus is **anaerobic,** that is, it thrives in the absence of oxygen.

Tetanus may be prevented by adequate immunization. Tetanus toxoid, which stimulates antibody formation, should be given to infants and small children at prescribed times. This should be done in combination with diphtheria toxoid and pertussis vaccine, which prevents whooping cough.

Rabies. **Rabies** is primarily a disease of warm-blooded animals such as dogs, cats, raccoons, skunks, wolves, foxes, and bats; but it can be transmitted to humans through bites or scratches from a rabid animal. Rabies is an infectious disease of the brain and spinal cord caused by a virus that is transmitted by the saliva of an infected animal.

The virus passes from the wound along nerves to the spinal cord and brain where it causes acute encephalomyelitis. The incubation period is long, 40 to 60 days or more, depending on the severity of the wound and the distance of the wound from the brain. Bites on the face, neck, and hands are the most serious. The mode of tetanus and rabies transmission to the central nervous system is illustrated in Figure 15–5.

The symptoms include fever, pain, mental derangement, rage, convulsions, and paralysis. The muscles of the throat go into spasm at the sight of water, and the patient is unable to drink; hydrophobia is an aversion to water related to rabies. A profuse, sticky saliva is secreted because of the inability to swallow.

The disease is fatal in humans once it reaches the central nervous system and the symptoms described have developed. A series of antirabies injections must be administered before the virus reaches the brain.

In the case of an animal bite, it is extremely important to know if the animal is rabid; thus, investigation of the animal must be made whenever possible. If rabies is suspected, immunization injections are started. The patient receives repeated injections of an altered virus to stimulate antibody production and immune serum to provide passive immunity.

The severity of rabies explains the critical need for the vaccination of dogs and cats against the disease. Certain signs indicate that an animal is rabid. The animal goes through several stages, the first of which is an anxiety stage manifested by a change of temperament. As an example, wild animals may act friendly. A furious stage follows in which the animal bites at everything. When paralysis of the throat occurs, the animal cannot swallow and it foams at the mouth. The

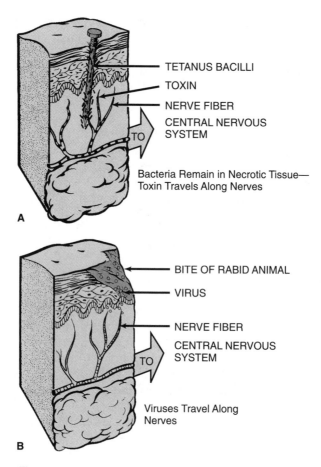

Figure 15–5. Nerve involvement in **(A)** tetanus and **(B)** rabies.

last stage of rabies is called the dumb stage. The animal appears to have something caught in the throat but makes no attempt to remove it and death then follows.

Shingles (Herpes Zoster). **Shingles** is an acute inflammation of nerve cells caused by the chicken pox virus, herpes zoster. It is manifested by pain and a rash consisting of small water blisters surrounded by a red area. The lesions follow a sensory nerve, forming a zone toward the midline of the body trunk, are generally confined to one side of the body, and do not cross the midline. The optic nerve can be affected, causing severe conjunctivitis, and if not treated properly, ulcerations form on the cornea and scarring results. The lesions dry up and become encrusted. They cause severe itching, pain, and heal with scarring.

Shingles can develop from exposure to a patient with shingles in the infectious stage or from exposure to chicken pox within an incubation period of about

2 weeks. It sometimes accompanies another disease such as pneumonia or tuberculosis. Shingles may also result from trauma or a reaction to certain drug injections. If there has been no known exposure to the virus, it is thought that chicken pox virus may have been dormant in the body for a time and been activated.

Treatment of shingles is directed toward alleviating the symptoms and relieving the pain and itchiness. Lotions such as calamine are often applied. Glucocorticoids may be prescribed to suppress the inflammatory reaction.

Reye's Syndrome. Reye's syndrome is a potentially devastating neurologic illness that sometimes develops in young children following a viral infection. Viruses often associated with Reye's syndrome include Epstein-Barr, influenza B, and varicella, which causes chickenpox. There may be a link between the viral infection and the use of aspirin, but the question is controversial. The actual cause of the disease is unknown.

Manifestations of Reye's syndrome include persistent vomiting, often a rash, and lethargy about 1 week after a viral infection. Neurologic dysfunction can progress from confusion to seizures and coma. The encephalopathy includes cerebral swelling with elevated intracranial pressure.

Management is geared toward lowering intracranial pressure. Meticulous monitoring of all vital functions is essential with correction of any imbalance. Blood gases and blood pH must be analyzed.

The outcome is very satisfactory when diagnosed early and proper therapy is given. The cure rate is about 85 to 90 percent.

Abscess of the Brain. Pyogenic organisms such as streptococci, staphylococci, and *E. coli* can travel to the brain from other infected areas and cause a brain abscess. Infections of the middle ear, skull bones, or sinuses, as well as pneumonia and endocarditis are potential sources of a brain abscess. Figure 15–6 shows abscesses of the brain.

The symptoms of brain abscess may be misleading. The patient has a fever and headache due to increased intracranial pressure, which can suggest a tumor. Analysis of the cerebrospinal fluid shows increased pressure and the presence of neutrophils and lymphocytes, indicating infection.

Once the diagnosis of a brain abscess has been made, the abscess must be opened surgically and drained and the patient treated with antibiotics. Brain abscesses are not as common today because the spread of most infections is checked by antibiotics.

■ Degenerative Neural Diseases

Some diseases of the nervous system involve the degeneration of nerves and brain tissue. Abnormalities in muscle function result from neural degeneration.

Multiple Sclerosis. **Multiple sclerosis (MS)** is a major disorder of the central nervous system. It is a chronic, progressive disease of unknown origin. Possible

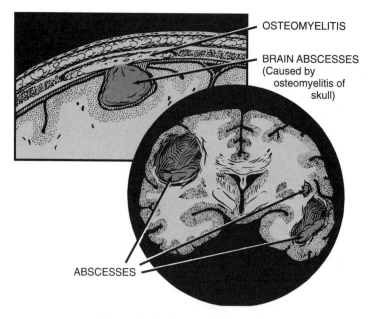

Figure 15–6. Abscesses of the brain.

causes that have been researched are viruses or immunologic reaction to a virus, bacteria, trauma, autoimmunity, and heredity, but the findings have remained inconclusive.

The disease manifests itself at first by muscle impairment. The patient experiences a loss of balance and poor coordination. Tingling and numbing sensations progress to a shaking tremor and muscular weakness. The MS patient has difficulty in speaking clearly and bladder dysfunction frequently develops.

Vision may suddenly be impaired, and double vision frequently occurs. Lesions on the optic nerve can lead to blindness. The patient may have **nystagmus,** an involuntary, rapid movement of the eyeball in all directions. Emotional changes also accompany the disease.

Multiple sclerosis usually affects young adults between the ages of 20 and 40. The disease is difficult to diagnose in the early stages, as many disorders of the nervous system have similar symptoms. It is characterized by periods of remissions and exacerbations and progresses at very different rates.

The degeneration of nerve tissue in MS involves a breaking up of the neuronal myelin sheath, the white matter of the central nervous system. Patchy areas of demyelination appear and become sclerotic. The degeneration of myelin impairs nerve conduction. MRI (magnetic resonance imaging) demonstrates plaques of demyelination of nerve fibers.

There is no effective treatment for MS. Physical therapy enables the patient to use the muscles that are operable. Muscle relaxants help to reduce spasticity, and steroids are often helpful. Psychological counseling is advantageous in dealing with the emotional changes brought about by the disease.

Amyotrophic Lateral Sclerosis (ALS). **Amyotrophic lateral sclerosis**, also known as Lou Gehrig's disease, is a chronic, terminal neurological disease in which there is a progressive loss of motor neurons. Cause of the disease is not known. ALS is characterized by disturbances in motility and atrophy of muscles of the hands, forearms, and legs due to degeneration of neurons in the ventral horns of the spinal cord. Also affected are certain cranial nerves, particularly the hypoglossal, trigeminal, and facial nerves (Fig. 15–3), which impairs muscles of the mouth and throat. Swallowing and tongue movements are affected, and speech becomes difficult or impossible. ALS occurs later in life, most commonly in the 50s and 60s, and is slightly more common in men than in women.

ALS is diagnosed by an **electromyogram (EMG),** which shows reduction in the number of motor units active with muscle contraction. Also observed are fasiculations, spontaneous, uncontrolled discharges of motor neurons seen as irregular twitchings.

Early education of the patient and patient's family is important so that a proper management team can be provided to anticipate and correct certain hazards. Of primary concern is prevention of upper airway obstruction and **pathologic aspiration,** drawing of vomitus or mucus into the respiratory tract. Aspiration can occur from weakened respiratory musculature and an ineffective cough. Death usually occurs within 3 to 4 years after onset of symptoms and generally results from pulmonary failure.

Parkinson's Disease (PD). **Parkinson's disease,** also known as shaking palsy, is a disease of brain degeneration that appears gradually and progresses slowly. It is a chronic disease that usually develops late in life and can be very disabling. Early symptoms include mild tremors of the hands and a nodding movement of the head. The patient is likely to fall frequently, as postural reflexes are lost.

As the disease progresses, muscular movements become slower and more difficult. The stiffness of the muscles affects the facial expressions, making them rigid and masklike. A characteristic tremor develops in the fingers, referred to as a pill-rolling tremor, that disappears with voluntary movement of the hands. The posture is stooped. The forward-leaning position causes a peculiar gait of short, running steps to maintain balance.

Three obvious signs of Parkinson's disease are **bradykinesia** (slowness of movement), tremor, and rigidity. Actions that were once automatic become deliberate. Experts recommend frequent brief rests, moving slowly, and learning how to manage difficult movements such as descending stairs. The most important factor in maintaining flexibility, motility, and mental well-being is prescribed exercise. Relaxation is particularly important for PD patients as stressful situations worsen the condition. Figure 15–7 summarizes possible effects of PD.

The degeneration of nerve cells occurs in the **basal ganglia,** the nerve centers

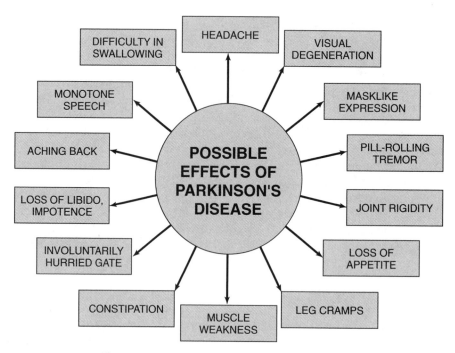

Figure 15–7. Summary of Parkinson's disease effects.

responsible for regulation of certain involuntary body movements. It has been discovered that a neuronal transmitter substance, **dopamine,** is inadequately produced. Treatment includes the administration of L-dopa, a substance that is converted to dopamine in the brain. Although the drug therapy does not stop the neuronal degeneration, the symptoms are relieved. The drug is not recommended for patients with previous mental disorders or cardiovascular disease. Alcohol consumption should be limited because alcohol acts antagonistically to L-dopa.

Physical therapy, including heat and massage, helps to reduce muscle cramps and relieve tension headaches caused by the rigidity of neck muscles. The patient is aided by psychological support while learning to cope with the disability.

The cause of Parkinson's disease is unknown, but a hereditary factor may be involved.

Huntington's Disease (Huntington's Chorea). Huntington's disease is an inherited disease, but symptoms may not appear until middle age. If either parent has the disease, all their children will have a 50 percent chance of inheriting it. (See Chapter 4 for the manner of transmission.) **Huntington's chorea** is a progressive degenerative disease of the brain that results in the loss of muscle control. The word element *chorea* means ceaseless, rapid, jerky movements, which are involuntary—an appropriate description of Huntington's symptoms. Some abnormality of the neurotransmitters causes bizarre transmission of nerve impulses.

The disease affects both the mind and body. Personality changes include care-lessness, poor judgment, and impaired memory, with conditions deteriorating to total mental incompetence, **dementia.** The physical disabilities include speech loss and a difficulty in swallowing coupled with involuntary jerking, twisting, and muscle spasms. There is no cure for Huntington's chorea. In families afflicted with this disease, the risk for the offspring should be clearly understood. Genetic engi-neering has now developed techniques for mapping defective genes on a chromo-some. The gene responsible for Huntington's chorea has been identified, thus mak-ing testing of family members possible to determine if one has the gene.

CONVULSIONS

A **convulsion** is an involuntary contraction, or series of contractions, by voluntary muscles. Numerous factors, often involving a chemical imbalance within the body, can cause convulsions. The accumulation of waste products in the blood resulting from uremia, toxemia of pregnancy, drug poisoning, and withdrawal from alcohol or drugs are all capable of causing convulsions.

Any irritation of the nerve cells can lead to convulsions. Infectious diseases of the brain such as meningitis and encephalitis are frequently accompanied by con-vulsions. They sometimes occur in infants and young children with high fevers.

The bases of convulsions are abnormal electrical discharges that spread over the brain. The excited nerves abnormally stimulate voluntary muscles to contract. Prevention of injury to the patient during a convulsion is the principal treatment.

■ Epilepsy

The seizures associated with **epilepsy** are a form of convulsion. Brain impulses are temporarily disturbed, with resultant involuntary convulsive movements. Epilepsy can be acquired as a result of injury to the brain, birth trauma, a pene-trating wound, or depressed skull fracture. A tumor can irritate the brain, causing abnormal electrical discharges to be released. Alcoholism can also lead to the de-velopment of epilepsy. Most cases of epilepsy are idiopathic, but a predisposition to epilepsy may be inherited.

Epilepsy may manifest itself mildly, particularly in children. Loss of con-sciousness may last only a few seconds, during which time the child appears ab-sent-minded. Some muscular twitching may be noticed around the eyes and mouth and the child's head may sway rhythmically. The child does not fall to the floor. This form of epilepsy is known as **petit mal** and usually disappears by the late teens or early 20s.

Major seizures of epilepsy involve a loss of consciousness during which the person falls to the floor. Generalized convulsions are mild to severe, with violent shaking and thrashing movements. Hypersalivation causes a foaming at the mouth. The patient loses control of urine and sometimes feces. These features are characteristic of **grand mal epilepsy.**

Patients sometimes have a warning of an approaching seizure that gives them time to lie down or reach for support. This warning, known as an **aura,** may come as a ringing sound in the ears, a tingling sensation in the fingers, or spots before the eyes. The signs described are characteristic of grand mal epilepsy. After a seizure the patient is groggy and unaware of what happened. Seizures last for varying lengths of time and appear with varying frequencies.

Epileptic seizures may take different forms. The classification system adopted by the World Health Organization is called the International Classification of Epileptic Seizures. It classifies seizures into four categories.

1. Partial seizures begin locally and may or may not involve a larger area of brain tissue.
2. Generalized seizures are bilaterally symmetrical and without local onset.
3. Unilateral seizures generally involve only one side of the brain.
4. Unclassified epileptic seizures.

Diagnosis of epilepsy has been made on the basis of the **electroencephalogram (EEG),** a recording of brain waves. X-ray films are also used to identify any brain lesions, and family histories of epilepsy are very important in diagnosing the condition. The diagnosis of epilepsy and the seizure type has become more accurate with new techniques for imaging the brain. Computerized tomography (CT) using x-rays and magnetic resonance imaging (MRI) using magnetic fields visualize brain anatomy.

Medication is very effective in controlling epilepsy, particularly the anticonvulsant drugs such as Dilantin. Alcohol must be avoided with these medications. Molecular neurobiology research is providing new information on how nerve cells control electrical activity, thus making possible development of more effective anti-epileptic drugs. It is now known which drugs are best for treating the various kinds of seizures. Finally, treatment during a seizure is directed toward preventing physical injury to the patient.

DEVELOPMENTAL ERRORS

Fetal development is so complex that the relatively small number of errors is miraculous. Some errors are minor and cause no problems, but others that affect a system, such as the nervous system, can cause severe problems.

■ Spina Bifida

Spina bifida is a condition in which one or more vertebrae fail to fuse, leaving an opening in the vertebral canal. The word *bifid* means a cleft or split into two parts, which is the condition of the vertebra in spina bifida. The consequences of spina bifida depend on the extent of the opening and the involvement of the spinal cord.

One form of spina bifida, **spina bifida occulta** (hidden), may not be apparent at birth. Other malformations that tend to accompany this developmental error may point to the disorder. Such malformations are hydrocephalus, cleft palate, cleft lip, club foot, and **strabismus** (crossed eyes). The spinal cord is affected, and muscular abnormalities appearing later—such as incorrect posture, inability to walk, lack of bladder or bowel control—may signal spina bifida occulta. A slight dimpling of the skin and tuft of hair over the vertebral defect indicate the site of the lesion, usually located in the lower part of the vertebral column. The opening can be seen on x-ray films.

One form of spina bifida noticeable at birth is **meningocele.** In this condition, meninges protrude through the opening in the vertebra as a sac filled with cerebrospinal fluid. The spinal cord is not involved in this defect.

Meningomyelocele is a serious anomaly in which the nerve elements protrude into the sac and are trapped and prevented from reaching their destination. The child with this defect may be mentally retarded, fail to develop, lack sensation, or be paralyzed. The consequences of the defect depend on the part of the spinal cord affected. Surgical correction of various forms of spina bifida have been very effective.

The most severe form of spina bifida is **myelocele,** in which the neural tube itself fails to close and the nerve tissue is totally disorganized. This condition is usually fatal. The various forms of spina bifida are shown in Figure 15–8.

■ Hydrocephalus

The name **hydrocephalus** means water or fluid on the brain or head. The formation, circulation, and absorption of cerebrospinal fluid was described in the sec-

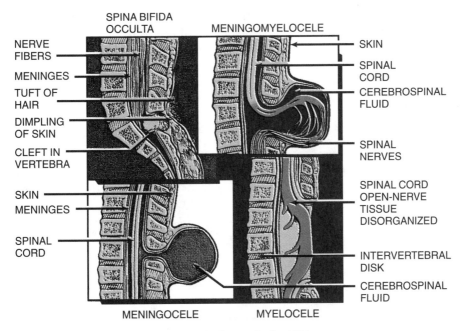

Figure 15–8. Forms of spina bifida.

tion earlier. In hydrocephalus this fluid accumulates abnormally, causing the ventricles to enlarge and push the brain against the skull.

An obstruction in the normal flow of cerebrospinal fluid is the usual cause of hydrocephalus. A congenital defect or an acquired lesion can block the cerebrospinal fluid flow. Meningitis or a tumor may result in acquired hydrocephalus. Trauma at birth is another possible cause. Congenital stenosis of an opening from the ventricles blocks cerebrospinal fluid flow. The error may also be a failure to absorb the fluid into the circulatory system.

There are two types of hydrocephalus, called *communicating* and *noncommunicating*. In the communicating type, the increased cerebrospinal fluid enters the subarachnoid space. In the noncommunicating hydrocephalus, the increased pressure of the cerebrospinal fluid is confined within the ventricles and is not evident in a lumbar puncture.

The head of a child born with hydrocephalus may appear normal at birth, but it will enlarge rapidly in the early months of life as the fluid accumulates. The brain is compressed, the cranial bones are thin, and the sutures of the skull separate under the pressure. The appearance of a hydrocephalic infant is typical; the forehead is prominent and the eyes bulge, giving a frightened expression. The scalp is stretched and the veins of the head are prominent. A hydrocephalic infant is shown in Figure 15–9. The weight of the excessive fluid in the head makes it impossible for the baby to lift its head. The infant fails to grow normally and is mentally retarded.

There have been cases of self-arrested hydrocephalus in which expansion of the head stops. A balance is reached between production and absorption of the fluid. The cranial sutures fill in and the skull bones thicken. The extent of brain damage before the arrest determines the degree of retardation.

Success in relieving the excessive cerebrospinal fluid has been achieved by

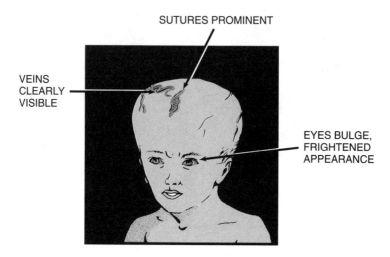

Figure 15–9. Hydrocephalus.

placing a shunt between the blocked ventricle and the veins, the heart, or peritoneal cavity. This allows the fluid to enter the general circulation.

BRAIN DAMAGE

The impact of damage to the brain depends on the location and extent of the injury. Manifestations of brain damage are mental retardation or muscular disorders, such as the lack of coordination and partial paralysis.

■ Cerebral Palsy

Cerebral palsy is a disease of nonprogressive brain damage manifested by motor retardation and sometimes also mental retardation that becomes apparent before age 3. The brain damage may be due to injury at or near the time of birth, an infection in the mother such as rubella (German measles), or infection of the brain even after birth. Lack of oxygen causes brain damage, as can incompatible blood. An Rh⁻ mother produces antibodies against the blood of an Rh⁺ fetus, as previously described. The excessive destruction of fetal blood cells that result causes hyperbilirubinemia, a level of bilirubin that is toxic to the brain. Often no cause is found for the brain damage in a case of cerebral palsy.

There are three forms of cerebral palsy: spastic, athetoid, and atactic. The largest number of cerebral palsy victims have the spastic type of condition; muscles are tense, and the reflexes are exaggerated. In the athetoid form, there are constant, purposeless movements that are uncontrollable. A tremor or shaking of the hands and feet is continuous. Cerebral palsy patients with the atactic form have poor balance and are prone to fall, muscular coordination is poor, and a staggering gait is characteristic.

Depending on the area of the brain affected, there may be seizures or visual or auditory impairment. If the muscles controlling the tongue are affected, speech defects result. Intelligence may be normal, but there is often mental retardation. Treatment depends on the nature of the brain damage. Muscle relaxants can relieve spasms; anticonvulsant drugs reduce seizures; casts or braces may aid walking; and traction or surgery is helpful in some cases. Muscle training is the most important therapy, and the earlier it is started, the more effective it is.

CEREBROVASCULAR ACCIDENT (STROKE) (CVA)

Vascular disturbances are the most frequent causes of brain lesions. The term **stroke** is used broadly to include cerebral hemorrhages and blood-clot formation within cerebral blood vessels. Nerves damaged by the lack of blood flow or hemorrhage do not regenerate and are replaced by scar tissue.

■ Cerebral Hemorrhage

The main cause of cerebral hemorrhage is hypertension. Prolonged hypertension leads to arteriosclerosis, explained in Chapter 8. The combination of high blood pressure and hard, brittle blood vessels is a predisposing condition for cerebral hemorrhage. **Aneurysms,** weakened areas in vascular walls, are also susceptible to rupture. Various aneurysms are shown in Figure 15–10. Subsequent hemorrhage into the brain tissue damages the neurons, and when this occurs there is usually a sudden loss of consciousness. Death can follow, or, if the bleeding stops, varying degrees of brain damage can result.

■ Thrombosis and Embolism

Blood clots that block the cerebral arteries cause infarction of brain tissue. Thromboses develop on walls of atherosclerotic vessels, particularly in the carotid arteries. The clots take time to form, and some warning may precede the occlusion of the vessel. The patient may experience blindness in one eye, difficulty in speaking, or a generalized state of confusion. When the cerebral blood vessel is completely blocked, the patient may lose consciousness.

Because an embolism is a traveling clot, it usually occludes a blood vessel suddenly. The embolism is most fruquently a clot from the heart, but it can travel from another part of the body. Consciousness is generally lost suddenly.

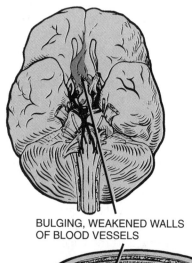

BULGING, WEAKENED WALLS
OF BLOOD VESSELS

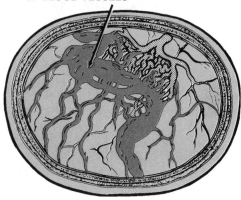

Figure 15–10. Cerebral aneurysms.

The site and extent of the brain damage, regardless of its cause, determines the outcome for the patient. Consciousness is usually regained, but speech is often impaired immediately after the stroke. Loss of speech **(aphasia)** requires therapy, but the ability to speak is often restored.

Damage to the motor nerves where they are about to pass down the spinal cord causes weakness (paresis) or paralysis on the side of the body opposite the brain lesion. This is because of the crossover of nerve fibers in the brain stem. Paralysis on one side of the body is referred to as **hemiplegia.**

Various techniques make it possible to determine the site of blockage in a cerebral blood vessel. Angiography, a process in which radiopaque material is injected into cerebral arteries, allows x-rays to locate the lesion.

A blockage in a carotid artery can be treated surgically. **Endarterectomy,** the more common procedure, removes the thickened area of the inner coat. Carotid bypass surgery removes the blocked segment, and a graft is inserted to allow blood flow to the brain.

■ Transient Ischemic Attack (TIA)

Transient ischemic attacks are caused by brief but critical periods of reduced blood flow in a cerebral artery. The reduced flow may be due to an atherosclerotic narrowing of the blood vessel or to small emboli that temporarily lodge in the vessel. The attacks may last for a minute or two or up to several hours, with the average being 15 minutes. Manifestation can include visual disturbances, transient hemiparesis (muscular weakness on one side), or sensory loss on one side. Lips and tongue may become numb, causing slurred speech. TIAs often precede a complete stroke and often serve as warning of a cerebral vascular disturbance. Further testing such as a cerebral angiogram or CT scan may be indicated.

TRAUMATIC DISORDERS

Physical injury to the head can damage the brain by causing a cerebral hemorrhage, by the increased pressure of resulting edema, or by creating a route for bacterial invasion.

■ Concussion of the Brain

A **concussion** is a transient disorder of the nervous system resulting from a violent blow on the head, as may occur in an automobile accident. The patient loses consciousness and cannot remember the events of the accident. The brain is not actually damaged, but the whole body is affected; the pulse rate is weak, and when consciousness is regained the patient may be nauseous and dizzy. A severe headache follows, and the patient should be watched closely as a coma may ensue.

A person suffering from a concussion should be kept quiet, and drugs that stimulate or depress the nervous system, such as painkillers, should not be administered. The condition will correct itself with rest.

■ Contusion

In a **contusion** there is an injury to brain tissue without a breaking of the skin at the site of the trauma. The brain injury may be on the side of the impact or on the opposite side, where the brain is forced against the skull. Blood from broken blood vessels accumulates in the brain, causing swelling and pain. Blood clots and necrotic tissue form, and the flow of cerebrospinal fluid can be blocked, causing a form of hydrocephalus.

The body attempts to clear the debris through phagocytosis by white blood cells and macrophages. Treatment includes the application of cold compresses to reduce the bleeding, which in turn reduces the swelling. Later, the application of heat facilitates the absorption of blood.

■ Skull Fractures

The most serious danger in a skull fracture is damage to the brain. A fracture at the base of the skull is likely to affect vital centers in the brain stem. The pressure that increases due to accumulation of cerebrospinal fluid must be reduced by medications. Another danger of a skull fracture is that bacteria may be able to reach the brain.

■ Hemorrhages

Hemorrhages can occur in the meninges, causing blood to accumulate between the brain and the skull. A severe injury to the temple can cause an artery just inside the skull to rupture. The blood then flows between the dura mater and the skull: This is called an **extradural** or **epidural hemorrhage.** The increased pressure of the blood causes the patient to lose consciousness, and surgery is required immediately to tie off the bleeding vessel and remove the blood. No blood is found in a lumbar puncture because the blood accumulation is outside the dura mater.

A hemorrhage under the dura mater, a **subdural hemorrhage,** is from the large venous sinuses of the brain rather than an artery. This may occur from a severe blow to the front or back of the brain. The blood clots, and cerebrospinal fluid accumulates in the cystlike clot. Pressure builds up, but the cerebral symptoms may not develop for a time. Subdural hemorrhages are sometimes chronic in alcoholics and abused children.

The surface of the brain may be torn by a skull fracture, causing a **subarachnoid hemorrhage.** Blood flows into the subarachnoid space in which cerebrospinal fluid circulates, and blood is found with a lumbar puncture. Rupture of an aneurysm can also cause a subarachnoid hemorrhage.

BRAIN TUMORS

Tumors of the brain may be malignant or benign. Even the benign tumors are serious, however, since they grow and strangle vital nerve centers. As explained in the chapter on neoplasia (Chapter 3), benign tumors are usually encapsulated and they can be completely removed surgically. Malignant tumors have extensive roots

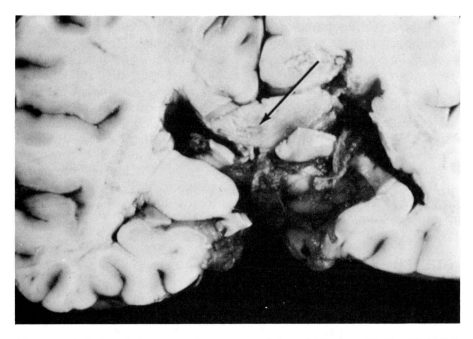

Figure 15–11. A glioma in the corpus callosum of the brain (arrow). (*Courtesy of Dr. David R. Duffell.*)

and are extremely difficult or impossible to remove in their entirety. Most malignant tumors of the brain are metastatic from other organs. Primary malignant tumors of the brain are called **gliomas,** tumors of the glial cells that support nerve tissue rather than of the neurons themselves. Figure 15–11 shows a glioma in the corpus callosum of the brain.

Brain tumors manifest themselves in different ways depending on the site and growth rate of the tumor. **Astrocytomas** are basically benign, slow growing tumors. **Glioblastomas** are highly malignant, rapid growing tumors. Brain function is affected by the increased intracranial pressure. Blood supply to an area of the brain may be reduced by an infiltrating tumor or edema causing the tissue to become necrotic.

Symptoms of brain tumors may include a severe headache due to the increased pressure of the tumor. Personality changes, loss of memory, or poor judgment in a person of normally good judgment can signal a brain tumor. Visual disturbances, double vision, or partial blindness often occur and the ability to speak may be impaired. The patient may be unsteady while standing and have seizures. A drowsy condition can progress to a coma.

DIAGNOSTIC PROCEDURES FOR THE NERVOUS SYSTEM

Neurologic laboratory tests include cerebrospinal fluid (CSF) examination obtained by a lumbar spinal tap as previously described. Angiography allows visualization of the cerebral circulation through the injection of radiopaque material. Computed tomographic (CT) scans are particularly valuable for diagnosing pathologic conditions such as tumors, hemorrhages, hematomas, and hydrocephalus. Electromyelography (EMG) is a radiographic process by which the spinal cord and spinal subarachnoid space are viewed and photographed following injection of contrast medium into the lumbar subarachnoid space. Myelography is used to identify spinal lesions caused by trauma or disease such as amyotrophic lateral sclerosis (ALS). Electroencephalography (EEG) records the electrical activity of the brain (brain waves). It is used to diagnose lesions or tumors, seizures, and impaired consciousness. Magnetic resonance imaging (MRI) utilizes magnetic fields in conjunction with a computer to view and record tissue characteristics at different planes. MRI is excellent for visualizing brain soft tissue, spinal cord, white matter diseases, tumors, and hemorrhages.

CHAPTER SUMMARY

The nervous system enables the human body to respond to changes in the external and internal environment. This system is affected by diseases in numerous ways. Microorganisms that enter the nervous system by various routes cause infectious diseases such as meningitis, encephalitis, polio, tetanus, rabies, Reye's syndrome, and shingles.

A degeneration of nerves and brain tissue results in multiple sclerosis, amyotrophic lateral sclerosis, Parkinson's disease, and Huntington's chorea. A manifestation of these progressively degenerative diseases is abnormal functioning of the muscles.

Convulsions often result from some chemical imbalance that causes irritation to nerve cells. The seizures of epilepsy are a form of convulsions resulting from abnormal electrical discharges in the brain.

Hydrocephalus and the various forms of spina bifida are caused by developmental errors, obstruction to the flow of cerebrospinal fluid, and failure of the vertebral column to close. Damage to the brain during fetal life or at birth can result in cerebral palsy, which is manifested by various forms of muscular abnormalities. Cerebrovascular accidents, cerebral hemorrhages, and blood clots damage brain tissue. The result of the injury depends on the site and extent of the brain lesion.

A severe head injury that causes hemorrhaging within the brain or in the meninges has serious effects on the nerve tissue and may even be fatal. Tumors of the brain, both malignant and benign, strangle nerve fibers and obstruct blood flow. No other tissue of the body depends on a good supply of oxygenated blood as does the brain.

■ Self-Study

True or False

_____ 1. Rabies is a viral infection.

_____ 2. The Sabin vaccine works in the digestive tract.

_____ 3. Oxygen under high pressure would be effective in treating rabies.

_____ 4. Blood is not normally found in cerebrospinal fluid.

_____ 5. Dopamine deficiency causes epilepsy.

_____ 6. Polio is a viral disease of the muscles.

_____ 7. Rabies in man is known as "lock-jaw."

_____ 8. The tetanus bacilli travels along the nerve fiber.

_____ 9. Tetanus is a pyogenic infection.

_____ 10. Cerebral palsy is a hereditary disease.

_____ 11. Reye's syndrome is thought to be caused by a bacterial infection.

_____ 12. Amyotrophic lateral sclerosis occurs most commonly in later life.

_____ 13. Amyotrophic lateral sclerosis is diagnosed by electromyography.

_____ 14. Transient ischemic attacks are characterized by loss of consciousness.

_____ 15. Epilepsy can be acquired through a brain injury.

Match

_____ 16. spina bifida   a) degenerative condition

_____ 17. polio   b) virus

_____ 18. Huntington's disease   c) bacteria

_____ 19. multiple sclerosis   d) heredity

_____ 20. tetanus   e) developmental error

(Answers on page 450)

Chapter 16

Diseases of the Bones, Joints, and Muscles

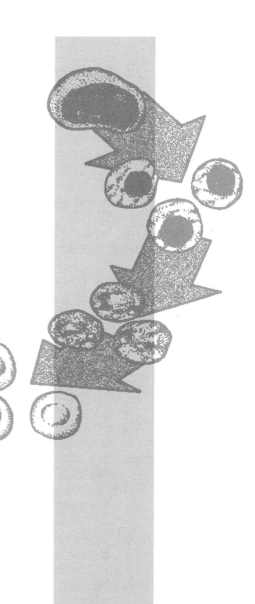

Chapter Outline

- Interaction of Bones, Muscles, and Joints
- The Structure and Function of Bone, Joints, and Muscle
- Diseases of Bone
- Diseases of the Joints
- Diseases of Muscles
- Diagnostic Tests for Bone, Joint, and Muscle Diseases
- Chapter Summary
- Self-Study

*A*ll bodily movements are the result of muscular contractions. These movements range from the wink of an eye to the acrobatic performance of a gymnast. All facial expressions—happiness, sorrow, anger, or surprise—are the result of muscle action.

INTERACTION OF BONES, MUSCLES, AND JOINTS

The attachment of muscles to bones allows contraction, or shortening, of a muscle to move a bone. Muscles that span a joint bring about an action at that joint, and they work antagonistically to muscles on the opposite side of the joint.

Bones cannot move without muscle contractions and muscles cannot contract without nerve stimulation. Diseases of the nervous system, described in the previous chapter, are generally manifested by their effect on the musculature. In this chapter the principal diseases of bone, joints, and muscles will be explained.

THE STRUCTURE AND FUNCTION OF BONE, JOINTS, AND MUSCLE

Bone may appear inert but it is a truly dynamic tissue, with changes constantly occurring within it. The outer surface of bone is hard and smooth due to the arrangement of its constituent protein and minerals. Bone cells, osteoblasts and osteoclasts, are situated within this bony framework and nourished by a highly organized system of blood vessels. These cells constantly remodel bone.

Bones are long, flat, or irregularly shaped, but they are all covered with a layer of compact bone. Spongy bone consisting of a different arrangement of the same material is found inside the bones. This material contains many spaces that are filled with bone marrow. The red bone marrow within flat bones and at the end of long bones is the production site for many blood cells.

The long bones found in the arms and legs contain a hollow cavity, the **medullary cavity,** that is filled with yellow bone marrow primarily consisting of fat. The growth of long bones occurs at the growth plate, an area of cartilage near each expanded end of the bone (Fig. 16–1). At this site new bone is formed, pushing the ends apart from each other until full growth is achieved, at which time the cartilage ossifies. Damage to the growth plate before maturity prevents the bone from reaching its proper length.

The **periosteum** is a highly vascular layer of fibrous connective tissue that covers the surface of the bones. It contains cells that are capable of forming new bone tissue and serves as a site of attachment for tendons or muscles.

Joints are the articulating sites between bones. Various degrees of movement are possible in different kinds of joints. This is referred to as *range of motion.* The shoulder is the most freely movable joint, but it is also the one most easily dislocated.

Articulating bones are held together by **ligaments;** a joint capsule consisting of ligaments and connective tissue surrounds the bone ends. The inner surface of the capsule is lined with a synovial membrane that secretes a lubricating fluid. Sacs of this fluid, the **bursae,** are situated near the joint to reduce friction on movement. The articulating surfaces of the bone ends are covered with a layer of smooth cartilage, which also prevents friction. A typical joint is illustrated in Figure 16–2.

Skeletal or voluntary muscles are firmly attached to bones by **tendons.** Some

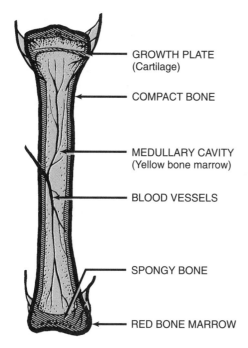

GROWTH PLATE
(Cartilage)

COMPACT BONE

MEDULLARY CAVITY
(Yellow bone marrow)

BLOOD VESSELS

SPONGY BONE

RED BONE MARROW

Figure 16–1. Cut view of long bone.

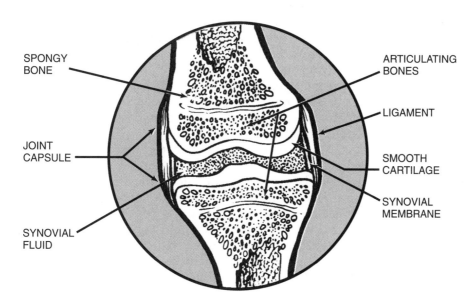

SPONGY
BONE

JOINT
CAPSULE

SYNOVIAL
FLUID

ARTICULATING
BONES

LIGAMENT

SMOOTH
CARTILAGE

SYNOVIAL
MEMBRANE

Figure 16–2. Typical joint.

muscles, the muscles of facial expression, for example, are attached to soft tissue. Muscles consist of bundles of muscle fibers held together by connective tissue. When stimulated by nerves at the myoneural junction, muscle fibers contract, and the shortening of the muscles moves the bones. The diseases of muscle described in this chapter are diseases of voluntary muscle. Smooth muscle, involuntary muscle, is a different type of muscle found in the walls of the internal organs and the walls of blood vessels. Cardiac muscle is present only in the heart.

DISEASES OF BONE

Bone, which is comprised of cells of organic material that gives some flexibility, and of inorganic salts that provide hardness, can be affected by disease in various ways. Infectious agents can enter bone through a compound fracture, transmission in the blood, or extension from an adjacent infection. Mineral and vitamin deficiencies prevent proper formation or maintenance of bone structure. Bones atrophy with disuse and fracture spontaneously in certain diseases. Tumors can also develop in bone.

■ Infectious Diseases of Bone

Bone infections were far more difficult to treat before the availability of antibiotics. These infections still occur and should be properly diagnosed and treated as soon as possible.

Osteomyelitis. **Osteomyelitis** is an inflammation of the bone, particularly of the bone marrow in the medullary cavity and in the spaces of spongy bone. Osteomyelitis affects principally children and adolescents whose bones are still growing. The long bones—the femur, the tibia, and the humerus—are most frequently affected in the area of the growth plate. Pyogenic organisms, such as staphylococci, carried in the bloodstream enter the bone from an infection somewhere in the body or from one adjacent to the bone. Infectious microorganisms can also enter a bone through the open wound of a compound fracture. An injury to the bone can cause small blood vessels to rupture. A clot then forms to stop the bleeding, and microorganisms invade the clot.

An abscess forms within the bone, and pus extends throughout the medullary cavity. A typical inflammatory reaction results in swelling, heat, and pain. Small blood vessels are compressed by the swelling, reducing the blood flow and causing necrosis. The infection spreads to the outer surface of the bone and extends along the bone under the periosteum. Blood supply to the bone is further reduced as the vascular periosteum is lifted from the bone. An area of bone that dies through lack of circulation and becomes separated from sound bone through necrosis is called a **sequestrum.** The periosteum attempts to make new bone around the sequestrum. Blood clots from the necrotic tissue infected with bacteria travel to other sites, initiating new abscesses.

Osteomyelitis is both a local and systemic infection. Not only is there pain at the site of the lesion, but the patient experiences chills, fever, and **leukocytosis.** The infection responds well to antibiotic therapy, particularly if it is started early, and the incidence of osteomyelitis is therefore decreased significantly. Surgery is sometimes required to clean out the dead bone tissue.

Tuberculosis of the Bone. Tuberculosis is primarily a disease of the lungs, but the infection can spread to bone. The ends of long bones, those of the arms and legs, are most frequently affected. The knee is a common site of tuberculosis infection. Similar to tuberculosis of the lung (see Chapter 12), cavity formation leads to destruction of the tissue.

When a joint such as the knee is involved, movement becomes limited. The articular cartilage is destroyed, causing pain due to friction between the articulating bones. In children, the growth plate is destroyed, resulting in the affected limb being shorter than the other.

Pott's disease is a special form of tuberculosis that affects the vertebral column of children. Vertebrae are destroyed and collapse, producing a malformation of the spine such as a humpback. The collapsed vertebrae put pressure on the spinal cord, and this can result in paralysis.

Tuberculosis of the bone responds well to antibiotic treatment. If the condition is advanced and irreversible damage to the vertebral column has already occurred, surgery may be required to correct the deformity.

▪ Bone Diseases of Vitamin and Mineral Deficiencies

Inadequate levels of calcium and phosphorus in the blood prevent proper bone formation and maintenance. These mineral deficiencies cause the bones to become soft and deformed. The absorption of calcium from the digestive tract requires vitamin D.

Rickets. **Rickets** is a disease of infancy and early childhood in which the bones do not properly ossify, or harden. The disease is generally caused by a vitamin D deficiency. Vitamin D is necessary for proper absorption of calcium and phosphorus from the gastrointestinal tract. It is calcium and phosphorus that give hardness to bone. Calcium may be adequate in the diet, but in the absence of vitamin D it cannot be used.

The bones of a child with rickets are soft and tend to bend. The weight-bearing bones of the body become deformed. The legs appear bowed or knock-kneed and the spine is curved. The sternum projects forward and nodules, referred to as "the rickety rosary," form on the rib ends. Nodular swellings also form at the joints—the wrists, ankles, and knees—and the head is often large and square. The pelvic opening in a girl may narrow, causing problems during childbirth later in life.

Other symptoms may also indicate rickets. The child's muscles are flabby because calcium, the deficient mineral, is essential for proper muscle contraction. Teething may be delayed, and the child has a characteristic pot belly.

Rickets can be prevented with vitamin D-fortified milk and sunlight. Sunlight converts a substance in the skin to vitamin D in the body. This need for sunlight explains the higher incidence of rickets in large, smoky cities where buildings are close together and shut out the sun. Children with rickets respond well to sunlight exposure and treatment with vitamin D concentrate or cod liver oil, which is high in vitamin D.

Osteomalacia. **Osteomalacia** is similar to rickets, but it is a softening or decalcification of bone in adults. It is characterized by muscular weakness, weight loss, and pain in the bones. The bones particularly affected are the spine, pelvis, and legs. They are bent, deformed, and tend to fracture with only mild stress.

A vitamin D deficiency and inadequate calcium or phosphorus in the diet causes osteomalacia. As in the case of rickets, a vitamin D deficiency prevents absorption of calcium from the digestive tract. The vitamin D deficiency may result from lack of sunshine, insufficient vitamin D in the diet, or the inability to absorb the vitamin, which is fat-soluble and is not absorbed in a disease such as malabsorption syndrome (Chapter 10). Treatment consists of vitamin D supplements and adequate calcium and phosphorous in the diet.

■ Secondary Bone Diseases

Bone diseases can result from a hormonal imbalance, as in hyperparathyroidism. In the aged, particularly in patients confined to bed, bone disease develops from disuse. Immobilization of a bone in a cast for a long time can have the same effect.

Osteitis Fibrosa Cystica. The name **osteitis fibrosa cystica** may seem threatening, but each word has meaning. The word element *oste(o)* refers to bone, so *osteitis* is an inflammation of the bone. In this disease, fibrous nodules and cysts form in the bones, which become very porous and decalcified. The loss of calcium causes the bones, particularly the long bones and those of the spine, to become deformed and subject to spontaneous fracture.

Osteitis fibrosa cystica generally results from hyperparathyroidism (Chapter 13). The excessive production of parathyroid hormone causes calcium removal from the bone. The blood level of calcium rises, and calcium is deposited in the form of insoluble salts. Kidney stone formation with possible renal obstruction is a complication of the condition.

Treatment involves reducing the parathyroid hormone level. A tumor of the parathyroid can be the cause of the excessive secretion and it should be removed. Orthopedic surgery may be required to correct severe bone deformities.

Osteoporosis. The word **osteoporosis** means increased porosity of the bone, which makes the bone abnormally fragile. The loss or thinning of bone tissue, **osteopenia,** due to increased calcium resorption from the bone is a predisposition to fractures, particularly of the weight-bearing bones of the vertebral column and pelvis. Compression fractures of the vertebra cause a decrease in height and bend-ing or curvature of the spine. The compressed vertebrae cause severe pain by pressing on spinal nerves. Hip and wrist fractures also occur frequently.

Osteoporosis may develop as part of the aging process, or the condition may be related to the estrogen level reduction that occurs after menopause. Certain people seem more susceptible to osteoporosis than others; there is a hereditary tendency to develop the disease. Osteoporosis is most common in patients who are bedridden. Bones that are immobilized, such as an arm or a leg in a cast, show this deterioration. This phenomenon is referred to as **disuse atrophy.** Women with small bone mass develop the condition more frequently than taller, larger women. Dietary inadequacies of calcium and protein, as well as lack of exercise, may contribute to development of osteoporosis. The manner of interaction between estrogen and the loss of bone tissue is unknown. Controversy exists between the value and the risk of estrogen therapy. Improved diet with adequate calcium and exercise are perhaps the most significant measures in preventing osteoporosis.

Paget's Disease. **Paget's disease,** or osteitis deformans, results in overproduction of bone, particularly in the skull, vertebrae, and pelvis. The disease begins with bone softening and is followed by bone overgrowth. The new bone tissue is abnormal and tends to fracture easily. The excessive bony growth causes the skull to enlarge, which often affects the cranial nerves; neurologic complications then follow. Curvatures develop in the spine from the new bone growth and the legs are deformed. The cause of Paget's disease is unknown, but it may have a hereditary basis. A complication of this disease is the development of **osteogenic sarcoma.**

■ Bone Fractures

Excessive stress on a bone will cause it to fracture. There are many types of fractures. A break in the bone that does not penetrate the skin is a simple fracture. A break in which the skin is pierced by the bone, resulting in an open wound, is a **compound fracture.** If the bone is splintered or crushed, it is a **comminuted fracture.** A **greenstick fracture** is one in which the bone is cracked, broken on one side, and bent on the other. These fractures are illustrated in Figure 16–3.

Fractures often occur spontaneously when bones are diseased, and these are called pathologic fractures. They may signal a malignancy that has metastasized from another site in the body or osteoporosis.

Some fractures are particularly dangerous because their location causes them to damage adjacent structures. A skull fracture can cause hemorrhages in the meninges and possible brain damage. A depressed skull fracture, one in which the bone has a caved-in appearance, puts pressure on the brain. The patient may become disoriented or lose consciousness. Shock often develops as a result of the injury.

A fracture of the spine can crush or sever the spinal cord, causing paralysis or death. A patient who has suffered this injury must be moved extremely carefully to prevent damage to the spinal cord by the broken bone ends. Figure 16–4 shows a young man's vertebrae fractured in a motorcycle accident. The 3-D image was reconstructed from 63 CT scans.

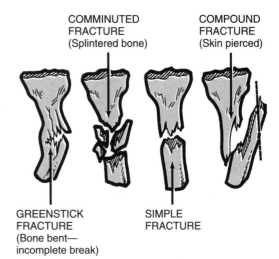

COMMINUTED
FRACTURE
(Splintered bone)

COMPOUND
FRACTURE
(Skin pierced)

GREENSTICK
FRACTURE
(Bone bent—
incomplete break)

SIMPLE
FRACTURE

Figure 16–3. Common bone fractures.

Pelvic bone fractures suffered in the crushing injury of an automobile accident or from the pressure of a heavy weight can cause internal injury to the bladder or rectum. Internal bleeding into surrounding soft tissue results.

Treatment of a fracture involves immediate **reduction,** which means that the broken ends of the bone are brought into proper alignment. Closed reduction is

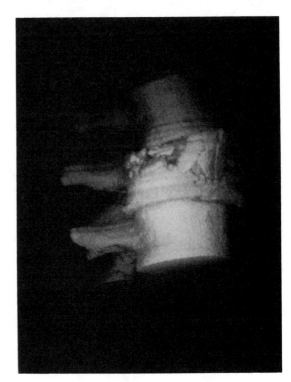

Figure 16–4. Compressed and fractured vertebrae constructed from CT scans. (*From Sochurek,* Medicine's New Vision, *1988. Courtesy of Mack Printing Company.*)

the manipulation of bone from the outside, without surgery. A compound fracture often requires open reduction, opening by exposing the wound to allow cleansing of the damaged tissue or removal of soft tissue lodged between the broken bone ends. The insertion of pins or plates to assure stability of the broken bone requires open reduction. After reduction, the bone is immobilized by a cast, splint, or traction to assure healing.

As the bone heals, new tissue is formed by osteoblasts at the fracture site. Hard material called a **bone callus** develops and unites the bone ends. New blood vessels grow into the tissue, and the fractured ends of the bone die and are resorbed. The length of time required for healing increases with the age of the patient. Bones may fail to heal due to infection or poor blood supply, and excessive motion prevents development of the bony tissue growth necessary for healing.

■ Neoplasia of Bone

Tumors of bone generally cause pain as they progress and make the bone susceptible to fractures. These tumors can be either malignant or benign.

Benign Bone Tumors. The most common benign tumor of the bone is an **osteoma.** This tumor may give no symptoms, or it may appear as a swelling. If a joint is affected, decreased motility is experienced. The tumor consists of hard, bony material, and it usually develops at the end of a long bone. Surgical removal of the osteoma is sometimes required if it causes pain or a pathologic fracture problem.

Giant cell tumors range from benign to malignant. On an x-ray film the tumor appears to consist of large bubbles. Microscopically, numerous multinucleated giant cells are seen. These tumors are usually removed through orthopedic surgery.

Malignant Bone Tumors. A primary malignancy of the bone is an **osteogenic sarcoma** (see Chapter 3). It generally affects the ends of long bones and is more common in young people. The knee is a frequent site, and expansion of the bone end is observed. The newest procedure is to pretreat with chemotherapy over weeks until the tumor stops shrinking. The extent of the surgery that follows is thus minimized, and the amputations previously performed are avoided.

Secondary tumors affecting the bone are carcinomas that have metastasized. They cause bone destruction and are very painful. The bone fractures easily, which is often the signal that carcinoma is present elsewhere. The flat bones that are highly vascular—the ribs, sternum, and skull—are the bones most affected by carcinoma.

DISEASES OF THE JOINTS

Joints are the movable parts of the body subjected to wear and tear. The joints that bear the weight of the body—the lower spine, the hip, and the knee—receive the most stress. Disease of the joints cause pain and limit movement, and muscles, nerves, and bones can all be affected by joint disease.

On the Practical Side

KNUCKLE CRACKING

What causes the sound of cracking knuckles? Contracting the joints quickly can force the synovial fluid of the joint capsule from one side to the other. It does not cause enlarged knuckles as has been proposed.

■ Dislocations, Sprains, and Strains

A dislocated bone is forcibly displaced from its joint. Dislocations are most common in the shoulder and finger joints, but they can occur anywhere. The patient experiences pain and lack of mobility at the involved joint. The bone must be resituated and immobilized to allow healing of torn ligaments and tendons. Congenital dislocations of the hip result from an improperly formed joint, and they are treated in infancy with a cast or surgery.

Sprains result from the wrenching or twisting of a joint such as an ankle that injures the ligaments. Blood vessels and surrounding tissues—muscles, tendons, and nerves—may also be damaged. Swelling and discoloration due to hemorrhaging from the ruptured blood vessels occur. A sprain is very painful, and the joint should not be used while it is severely inflamed. Cold compresses reduce the swelling immediately after the injury, whereas later heat applications reduce the discoloration. A whiplash injury is a sprain in which the cervical (neck) ligaments and tissues are torn.

Strains, also called "pulled muscles," result from a tearing of a muscle and/or its tendon from excessive use or stretching, such as a pulled hamstring. Conditioning and warm-up before exercise prevents strains, which are very painful.

■ Carpal Tunnel Syndrome

An annoying condition of the hand has become quite prevalent in recent years and is known as **carpal tunnel syndrome (CTS).** It is actually one of a larger class of problems known as repetitive strain injuries. It usually begins as numbness or tingling in the hand but progresses to pain which can radiate up the arm to the shoulder; the pain is most severe at night. Simple tasks requiring finger movements become difficult. The condition is much more common in women than in men and usually strikes around middle age. Many women report the symptoms during pregnancy which is attributed to accumulation of fluid within the tissues.

Carpal tunnel syndrome typically develops when the wrists are kept in a bent position for extended periods of time to perform repetitive tasks such as knitting, driving, typing, computer use, and playing the piano.

On the Practical Side

CARPAL TUNNEL SYNDROME: AN OCCUPATIONAL HAZARD

Carpal tunnel syndrome, caused by damage to the median nerve is a common problem of data processors, computer users, typists, beauticians, and dentists who often maintain a flexed wrist position. If surgery is required to relieve pressure on the nerve, a new technique is greatly reducing recovery time and lost work. A tiny video camera enables the surgeon to make two tiny incisions in the wrist and palm, each requiring only one stitch. Recovery is therefore much faster than with the traditional longer incision.

A physician may diagnose carpal tunnel syndrome by requiring certain hand maneuvers. The diagnosis is confirmed by an electrodiagnostic test called **electromyography.** The test measures the velocity of sensory and motor nerve conduction. If electrical impulses are slowed as they travel through the carpal tunnel, compression of the nerve is indicated.

Conservative treatments begin with avoiding the repetitive action where possible, at least temporarily. Splinting the hand and wrist with a lightweight molded plastic splint is often adequate for the inflammation to subside. Injection of a cortisone-like drug into the carpal tunnel is sometimes effective. For some individuals nonsteroidal anti-inflammatory drugs such as aspirin and ibuprofen can reduce symptoms. Surgery may be required to divide the transverse ligament which is compressing the median nerve. The procedure generally provides permanent relief without affecting hand movement or strength.

■ Arthritis

The word element *arthr(o)* refers to a joint. Although arthritis means inflammation of a joint, the disease may be more or less inflammatory depending on the type. The warning signs of arthritis are persistent pain and stiffness, particularly in the morning. One or more joints may be swollen, and pain is often experienced in the neck, lower back, and hip, as well as in the joints of the arms, hands, legs, and feet.

Rheumatoid Arthritis. Rheumatoid arthritis is the most serious and crippling form of arthritis. It is a systemic disease in which more and more joints become affected and the patient feels sick all over. Rheumatoid arthritis is a chronic, inflammatory disease for which there is no cure, but early diagnosis and treatment can prevent severe crippling. Rheumatoid arthritis generally affects young adults, women more often than men. There is also a juvenile form, which can be very serious. The disease may have a sudden onset or begin slowly. Periods of exacerbation and remission are common, so that a patient may experience symptoms that disappear only to recur.

The symptoms of rheumatoid arthritis are pain and stiffness in the joints, particularly on waking. The joints are swollen, red, and warm—the typical signs of inflammation. The same joints are often affected on both sides of the body. As the disease is systemic, the patient experiences fatigue, weakness, and weight loss.

Rheumatoid arthritis begins with an inflammation of the **synovial membrane** that lines the joints, particularly the small joints of the hands and feet. The membrane thickens and extends into the joint cavity, sometimes filling the space. The inflammation affects the articular cartilage of the bone ends by eroding them. Scar tissue that can turn to bone develops between the bone ends, causing the ends to fuse, **ankylosis.** The fusion makes the joint immovable and a characteristic crippling of the hands often develops. Figure 16–5 shows the crippling effect of this disease. Rheumatoid nodules form under the skin, usually near the joints, but they sometimes develop on the white of the eye, too.

The cause of rheumatoid arthritis is not known but it is possibly an autoimmune disease in which a tissue hypersensitivity is involved. Rheumatoid factors, antiglobulin antibodies, combine with immunoglobulin in the synovial fluid to form complexes. Neutrophils are attracted to the joint space and cause destruction. The condition is aggravated by stress. There is a genetic predisposition to develop the disease.

Early diagnosis and a good treatment program can reduce pain and the amount of damage done to the joints. A balance between exercise and rest should be achieved. In an acute phase the joint should be rested to prevent further inflam-

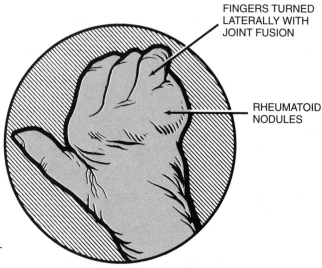

FINGERS TURNED
LATERALLY WITH
JOINT FUSION

RHEUMATOID
NODULES

Figure 16–5. Crippling effect of rheumatoid arthritis.

mation. The prescribed exercises help to maintain joint function. Exercises for good posture are directed toward removing stress on weight-bearing joints. Anti-inflammatory medications are effective when prescribed by a physician, with aspirin and similar drugs being the most commonly used. Steroids are administered with caution, as they mask the symptoms but do not stop the disease process.

Osteoarthritis. **Osteoarthritis** is the most common form of arthritis and is generally a chronic disease that accompanies aging. It results from wear and tear of the joints, chronic irritation, or a joint injury. Unlike rheumatoid arthritis, in which there is a progressive involvement of joints, osteoarthritis may affect only one joint.

The patient experiences aches, pain, and stiffness in the joint. It is pressure on the nerve endings, tense muscles, and muscle fatigue that cause the pain. Arthritis in the lower spine can exert pressure on the spinal cord or pinch a spinal nerve, and pain then radiates down the sciatic nerve of the leg. Range of motion is limited at the affected joint and the nearby muscles become weak from lack of use.

The degenerative process in osteoarthritis begins in the articular cartilage on the bone ends. As it is eroded, the underlying bone is exposed, and it degenerates. New bone forms in and around the joint, causing the bone ends to thicken and limit movement. The spicules of new bone are referred to as bony **spurs.** Small joints such as the knuckles enlarge and appear knobby.

Diagnosis of osteoarthritis is made principally by x-ray films that show the joint damage; a history of the symptoms also aids in the diagnosis.

There is no cure for osteoarthritis, but treatment can greatly relieve the pain. A combination of rest and special exercises, medication, and heat applications is generally prescribed. Steroids such as cortisone are not given orally but are sometimes injected into the joint capsule to relieve pain. Surgical replacement of a damaged joint like the hip has been very effective.

Perfectly functioning joints are least likely to become arthritic, but joints that have been injured or overworked in athletics are most susceptible. Knee and hip

On the Practical Side
HIGH HEELS VS. FLATS

The arches of the foot are designed to facilitate leverage for motion. The heel and the ball of the foot support body weight, the heel normally carrying the greater load. High-heeled shoes shift the greater amount of weight to the ball of the foot and the excessive pressure can cause structural damage. Painful corns and calluses often develop on the ball of the foot and joint pain at the base of the toes can result.

joints are frequently affected in a person who is overweight. Heredity may play a part in the development of osteoarthritis.

■ Gout

Gout, often called "gouty arthritis," affects the joints of the feet, particularly those of the big toe. This is a very painful condition caused by deposits of **uric acid** crystals in the joints. An excessively high uric acid level in the blood results in the precipitation of the crystals. Uric acid crystals are also deposited in the kidneys, stimulating kidney stone formation and irritating the kidney.

The cause of gout is unknown, but a hereditary tendency to the disease is common. It most frequently affects middle-age men. Improper metabolism of purines, a component of nucleic acids, causes the uric acid excess.

The onset of an acute attack of gout is generally sudden. It sometimes follows a minor injury or excessive eating or drinking, but there may be no accounting for the attack. The joint has the typical signs of inflammation: pain, heat, swelling, and redness, and walking is very difficult.

Various medications may be administered to reduce the uric acid level in the blood. The patient should stay off his or her feet until the inflammation subsides to prevent further irritation. Recurrent attacks are common, but if diagnosed early and treated properly, the development of chronic gout can be prevented. Chronic gout damages the affected joints, causing deformities. A complication of chronic gout is kidney damage from the uric acid deposits.

■ Herniation of Intervertebral Disks (Slipped Disk)

Cartilaginous pads or disks alternate with the vertebrae to form the spine. The disks act as shock absorbers between the vertebrae and accommodate the movement of the spine. Figure 16–6 illustrates the vertebral column. The inner core of each disk is rubbery and is surrounded by fibrous cartilage.

The intervertebral disks are subjected to constant strain. They may be injured or degenerate and lose their cushioning ability. The fibrous walls of the disk can weaken, and the inner core will bulge outward. This **herniation,** or rupture, of an **intervertebral disk** is commonly called a *slipped disk.*

The rupture of a disk most commonly occurs in the lower lumbar region and sometimes in the neck. The complication of a slipped disk is the pressure exerted on the spinal cord or a spinal nerve, as shown in Figure 16–7. Muscle spasms result often from the nerve stimulation.

A slipped disk in the lumbar region causes severe pain in the lower back. The pain radiates down the sciatic nerve to the back of the thigh and lower leg, making walking very difficult.

Diagnosis of a slipped disk is made principally by x-ray examination and the myelogram. The treatment depends on the nerve involvement and the age of the patient. In mild cases, bed rest on a firm mattress with an underlying board for support may be adequate. Muscle relaxants are administered to reduce muscle spasms. Careful application of heat is advantageous, and the patient is sometimes fitted with a surgical support. Some cases of slipped disk require traction. Exer-

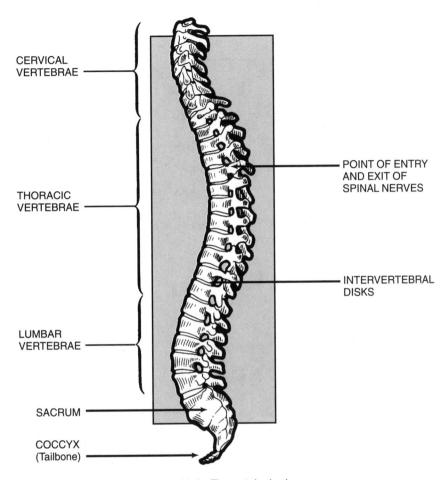

CERVICAL
VERTEBRAE

THORACIC
VERTEBRAE

LUMBAR
VERTEBRAE

SACRUM

COCCYX
(Tailbone)

POINT OF ENTRY
AND EXIT OF
SPINAL NERVES

INTERVERTEBRAL
DISKS

Figure 16–6. The vertebral column.

cises that improve posture and develop the proper use of muscles help to reduce stress on the vertebral column. Surgery is sometimes required to correct this condition.

A slipped disk in the cervical region causes severe pain in the neck, which radiates down the arm; neck movements are restricted by the pain. Treatment is similar to that for the lower back. A collar that supports the neck often gives relief from the pain.

■ Bursitis

Bursae are small fluid-filled sacs located near the joints that reduce friction on movement. **Bursitis** is an inflammation of these bursae, and it is a very painful condition. The bursae of the shoulder joint are the most frequently affected, although bursitis can develop at any joint. Repeated irritation of a bursa or an in-

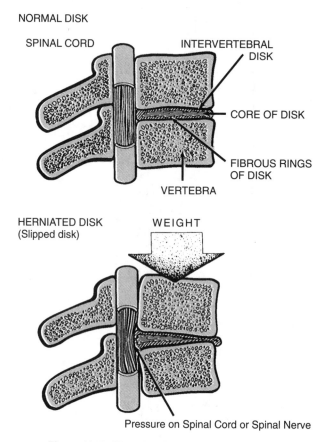

Figure 16–7. Normal and herniated (slipped) disk.

jury to it can cause bursitis. Limitation of movement results from the pain of the inflammation. Treatment includes resting the joint and applying moist heat. Steroids are sometimes injected into the joint to reduce the inflammatory response.

On the Practical Side

WHAT CAUSES TENNIS ELBOW?

Not necessarily tennis. The pain in the upper forearm near the elbow is due to tiny tendon tears. Activities that require wrist extension or forearm rotation can cause the injury and pain.

DISEASES OF MUSCLES

Skeletal muscles cannot function unless they are stimulated by nerves. In the previous chapter, diseases in which the nerves fail to innervate muscles were discussed. Muscles themselves can also be diseased and lose their ability to contract. Another cause of muscle failure is the improper transmission of the impulse for contraction at the myoneural junction.

■ Muscular Dystrophy

The term **muscular dystrophy** includes several forms of the disease, all of which are hereditary. The various forms are transmitted differently and affect different muscles, but the result is the same for all forms, muscle degeneration, which totally disables the individual. The most common and serious type is Duchenne, which is caused by a sex-linked gene affecting males.

Muscle fibers become necrotic, and the dead muscle fibers are replaced by fat and connective tissue. Neither of these tissues has the property of muscle cells, which is the ability to contract. Skeletal muscles are weakened by the degeneration.

Muscular dystrophy can appear at any age, but generally signs appear in the second or third year. A severe form can progress rapidly and affect the muscle of the heart, causing death; other forms progress slowly.

In the most severe form of muscular dystrophy, the calf muscles enlarge as a result of fat deposition. The shoulder muscles are weak, which causes the arms to hang limply. A child with this form of muscular dystrophy is very weak and thin and does not usually live to adulthood.

The genetic defect, in some way not yet known, interferes with protein metabolism. Creatine, formed from amino acids, is normally stored in muscle as **creatine phosphate.** Creatine phosphate assists in providing the necessary energy for muscle contraction. The muscular dystrophy patient is unable to store and use creatine; as a result, it is lost in the urine. Elevated serum creatinine phosphokinase confirms muscular dystrophy. Treatment includes physical therapy and orthopedic procedures.

■ Myasthenia Gravis

Myasthenia gravis is a neuromuscular disorder in which neither the nerves nor the muscles are diseased. The failure is in the transmission of the impulse from the nerves to the muscles at the myoneural junction. Myasthenia gravis affects women more often than men, and the cause is unknown.

The principal symptom of this disease is fatigue and the inability to use the muscles. All the voluntary muscles of the body are affected, including the muscles of facial expression. The lack of contraction in the facial muscles makes the patient's face expressionless. Simple actions such as chewing and talking become difficult.

Myasthenia gravis may be classified as an **autoimmune disease,** in which antibodies are produced against the body's own tissue. Such antibodies have been found in the serum of these patients. The antibodies attach near the myoneural junction and destroy acetylcholine, the neurotransmitter. Muscle contraction weakens as a result. Drugs that decrease the normal destruction of acetylcholine make the transmitter more available.

The thymus gland, which is involved in antibody production, at least in children, is often enlarged in myasthenia gravis patients. Removal of this gland sometimes brings about a remission but not a cure. The greatest danger in this disease is respiratory failure, because the muscles of respiration are unable to contract.

■ Tumors of Muscle

Muscle tumors are rare, but when they occur they are usually highly malignant. A malignant tumor of skeletal muscle is a **rhabdomyosarcoma.** The tumor requires surgical removal, and the prognosis is poor. The rhabdomyosarcoma metastasizes early and is usually an advanced malignancy when it is diagnosed.

DIAGNOSTIC TESTS FOR BONE, JOINT, AND MUSCLE DISEASES

Physical examination can indicate improper gait, decreased joint mobility, and/or deformities or masses. Primary laboratory tests for diseases of bones, joints, and muscles are x-ray procedures. Serum tests can show metabolic bone activity by measuring levels of calcium, phosphorus, and an enzyme, alkaline phosphatase, which is elevated in destructive bone diseases such as osteomalacia, hyperparathyroidism, and Paget's disease.

Serum test for the rheumatic factor and an elevated erythrocyte sedimentation rate are indicative of rheumatoid arthritis. Muscle biopsies, electromyography, and family histories are important in diagnosing muscular dystrophy.

CHAPTER SUMMARY

Bodily movements result from the interaction of muscles, bones, and joints. Diseases of these components of the musculoskeletal system cause pain and limit movement, and they can lead to structural deformities.

Pyogenic microorganisms cause bone infections and abscess formation. Tuberculosis can spread from the lungs to bone and destroy it. Other bone diseases result from mineral and vitamin deficiencies manifesting themselves by soft and deformed bones. Bone is also decalcified in hyperparathyroidism. Fractures occur under excessive stress, but when bones break spontaneously, a bone disease is indicated. A metastasized carcinoma, for example, causes pathologic fractures.

Dislocations, sprains, and strains are painful injuries of joints. A strain of the wrist which has become very common is carpal tunnel syndrome.

The most common joint disease is arthritis, which has several forms. Rheumatoid arthritis is the most progressive, severe, and crippling form. Osteoarthritis affects most people to some extent with age.

Muscular dystrophy is a degenerative disease in which muscles lose the ability to contract. They are unable to store creatine phosphate, an energy source for contraction. Another disease in which the muscles lose the ability to contract is myasthenia gravis, but, in this case, the failure is in the neuronal transmitter rather than in the muscles themselves. Tumors are rare in muscles, but when they occur they are usually highly malignant.

■ Self-Study

Multiple Choice

_____ 1. Bones are soft in rickets due to a _____ deficiency.
a. vitamin A
b. vitamin C
c. vitamin D

_____ 2. Osteomalacia affects _____.
a. children
b. adults

_____ 3. Bone penetrates the skin in a _____.
a. compound fracture
b. comminuted fracture
c. greenstick fracture

_____ 4. Herniation of intervertebral disks occurs most frequently in the _____.
a. thoracic region
b. lumbar region

_____ 5. _____ accompanies aging.
a. Rheumatoid arthritis
b. Osteoarthritis

Match

_____ 6. Pott's disease   a) estrogen level reduction
_____ 7. rickets   b) uric acid crystal deposits
_____ 8. gout   c) hyperparathyroidism
_____ 9. osteitis fibrosa cystica d) tuberculosis
_____ 10. osteoporosis   e) vitamin D deficiency

True or False

_____ 11. Osteomyelitis affects principally children and adolescents.

_____ 12. Women with large bone mass are most prone to osteoporosis.

_____ 13. An osteoma is a malignant bone tumor.

_____ 14. Rheumatoid arthritis is the most crippling form of arthritis.

_____ 15. Osteomyelitis is a local and systemic infection.

_____ 16. Osteoarthritis is the most common form of arthritis.

_____ 17. Muscular dystrophy is a hereditary disease.

_____ 18. Myasthenia gravis is an infectious disease of the muscles.

_____ 19. Rhabdomyosarcoma is a malignant bone tumor.

_____ 20. There is no cure for osteoarthritis.

(Answers on page 450)

Chapter 17

Diseases of the Skin

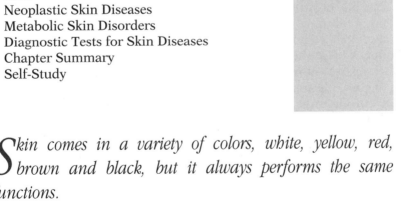

Chapter Outline

- Functions of the Skin
- Structure of the Skin
- Classification of Skin Diseases
- Infectious Skin Diseases
- Hypersensitivity Diseases of the Skin
- Neoplastic Skin Diseases
- Metabolic Skin Disorders
- Diagnostic Tests for Skin Diseases
- Chapter Summary
- Self-Study

*S*kin comes in a variety of colors, white, yellow, red, brown and black, but it always performs the same functions.

FUNCTIONS OF THE SKIN

The skin, or integument, has many characteristics that make it an extremely effective body covering. Unbroken skin acts as a barrier to prevent microorganisms

On the Practical Side

CORNS AND CALLUSES A VALUE?

Corns and calluses are layers of firm thick tissue which protect skin exposed to friction. They may become enlarged or painful but can usually be treated with over-the-counter products.

from entering the body, and the pigment of the skin, **melanin,** protects the body from harmful rays of the sun. The skin acts as a waterproof coat, preventing excessive water loss by evaporation, whereas the sweat glands and blood vessels of the skin regulate body temperature. Nerve endings in the skin sense temperature changes, pressure, touch, and pain, triggering the appropriate responses through the central nervous system. The oil glands of the skin provide a lubricant to keep it soft. The skin continually regenerates itself by sloughing off dead surface cells and forming new ones to replace them. This is significant in the healing of wounds.

The skin indicates malfunctionings within the body by color changes. **Cyanosis,** a blue coloration seen particularly in the lips, nose, or extremities, signals a lack of oxygen—a cardiac or pulmonary inadequacy. **Jaundice** indicates liver disease, bile obstruction, or hemolysis of red blood cells, in which case an accumulation of bilirubin in the blood produces the yellow coloration. An abnormal redness accompanies polycythemia (Chapter 6), carbon monoxide poisoning, and fever. **Pallor,** a whitening of the skin, may indicate anemia.

A total absence of melanin results from the hereditary condition of **albinism.** Melanin at times disappears from patches of skin once normally pigmented, signaling an **autoimmune disease** in which the **melanocytes,** melanin-producing cells, are being destroyed. The loss of pigmentation is called **vitiligo.**

Diseases of the skin are numerous, and the lesions of different diseases often resemble each other. Diagnosis requires the consideration of many factors: the patient's history of disease, inherited disorders, allergies, and emotional state as well as physical examination. Many skin diseases require laboratory tests or biopsies.

STRUCTURE OF THE SKIN

The outermost layer of skin is the epidermis, consisting of stratified, or layered, squamous epithelium. Cells of the bottom epithelial layer divide, forming new cells that gradually move up to the surface. Cells at the surface die and become

On the Practical Side

EVALUATION OF BURN DEPTH

Burns are classified on the skin depth involvement. First-degree burns affect the epidermis and are caused by sunburn or low-intensity flash. Recovery is complete within a week and peeling of the dead epidermis occurs.

Second-degree burns are caused by scalds or flash flame and affect the dermis or true skin. The epidermis is blistered, red, and broken, and the area is very painful. Recovery requires 2 to 3 weeks and some scarring and depigmentation usually occurs. If infection develops, a major problem with burns, it may convert to a third-degree burn.

Third-degree burns result from fire and prolonged exposure to hot liquids. Subcutaneous tissue is affected and the burn appears pale or charred. Broken skin exposes underlying fat tissue. The patient shows symptoms of shock. Healing requires time and grafting is necessary. Scarring and loss of contour results.

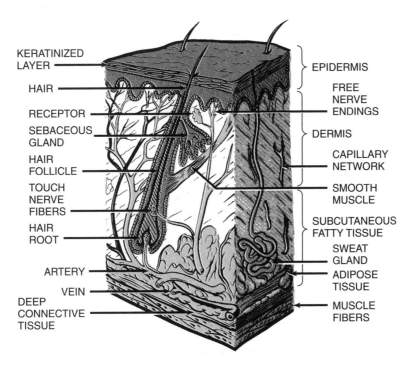

Figure 17–1. Structure of the skin.

keratinized, or scalelike, providing the waterproof layer of the skin. **Keratin** is a tough fibrous protein produced by cells called **keratinocytes;** the keratinized cells are continually being shed. Melanocyte cells that produce the protective melanin pigment that gives color to the skin are also found in the **epidermis.** There are no blood vessels in the epidermis.

The **dermis,** or "true skin," underlies the epidermis. The dermis is composed of connective tissue supporting the blood and lymph vessels, elastic fibers, and nerves. Hair follicles, sweat glands, and **sebaceous,** or oil, **glands** pass through the dermis.

The subcutaneous tissue under the dermis connects it to underlying structures. Numerous adipose, or fat cells are in the subcutaneous tissue, and they provide a food reserve and insulation. The sebaceous glands and hair follicles arise in this tissue. Figure 17–1 shows the structure of the skin.

CLASSIFICATION OF SKIN DISEASES

The skin can be affected by diseases in numerous ways. Skin infections are caused by bacteria, viruses, fungi, and parasites, and many skin diseases result from allergies, or hypersensitivities, to various proteins. Neoplasia, or uncontrolled growth of certain cells, results in the formation of skin tumors. Hyperactivity of the sebaceous glands causes other skin diseases.

The range of lesions in skin diseases is broad. They may be small, blisterlike eruptions called **vesicles** or larger fluid-containing lesions called **bullae.** Lesions containing pus are referred to as **pustules,** and nodules and tumors are lesions that are hard to the touch. Lesions that are flat are called **macular,** whereas those that are raised are termed **papular.** An area of skin reddened by congested blood vessels resulting from injury or inflammation is said to be **erythematous. Pruritus,** or itching, accompanies many skin diseases, especially those caused by allergies or parasitic infestation.

INFECTIOUS SKIN DISEASES

Skin diseases caused by bacteria, viruses, fungi, and parasites are generally contagious. Care must be taken to prevent the spread of the infection from one part of the body to another and from one person to another.

■ Bacterial Skin Infections

Impetigo. **Impetigo** is an acute, contagious skin infection common in children. It is caused by streptococcal and staphylococcal organisms carried in the nose that are passed to the skin. The face and hands are most frequently affected. **Erythema,** a reddened area, develops and oozing vesicles and pustules form. These rupture, and a yellow crust covers the lesion. Fever and enlarged lymph nodes may accompany the infection. The lesions should be washed with soap and water, kept dry, and exposed to the air. Antibiotic ointment may be used and oral antibiotics are sometimes prescribed to treat the infection systemically.

Erysipelas. **Erysipelas** is an inflammatory skin infection caused by streptococci that affects primarily the face. The strep organisms are probably transferred from respiratory discharges to the skin, entering through minute abrasions. Erysipelas can also develop if streptococci enter a surgical incision or wound.

Early symptoms of erysipelas include a sudden fever and shaking chills; reddened patches develop on the face, usually on the bridge of the nose. The redness spreads laterally, and the border is sharply defined and slightly elevated due to edema of the skin. The erythematous areas are hot to the touch and tender. If the eyelids are affected they become very swollen. Antibiotics are generally prescribed, but erysipelas is eventually self-limiting.

Abscess. Small, solitary skin abscesses are called boils or **furuncles.** They are usually caused by *Staphylococcus aureus.* Abscesses commonly develop around traumatized skin, embedded foreign substances, such as splinters, and in obstructed hair follicles. The lesion is elevated, red, and very painful. The core becomes necrotic and liquifies forming pus. The abscess is walled off and ruptures, releasing the purulent exudate.

Lyme Disease. An unusual "bull's eye" skin rash is a common early symptom of **Lyme disease.** This classic sign is an expanding red circle surrounded by a lighter area; a small welt is often present in the center of the rash. Flu-like symptoms may accompany the rash, general **malaise** (vague feeling of weakness), headaches, chills and fever, joint and muscle aches and/or extreme fatigue. The rash can appear any time from two days to five weeks after the patient is infected.

Lyme disease is caused by a bacteria, a spirochete, which is transmitted to humans by the bite of tiny deer ticks. Blood tests are used to diagnose the disease which responds well to antibiotic treatment. Left untreated, serious problems can result.

Lyme disease is named for Old Lyme, Connecticut where it was first recognized in 1975. Research has shown, however, that the Lyme bacteria had existed long before that time. Cases of the disease are concentrated in the northeastern states and Wisconsin and Minnesota although it has been diagnosed throughout the country.

Precautions to prevent Lyme disease include covering one's arms and legs when walking, hiking, or camping in wooded or grassy areas, and using a tick repellent. Showering immediately after leaving the wooded area is advantageous as ticks often remain on the skin before biting and can be washed off.

■ Viral Skin Infections

Cold sores or fever blisters are caused by the virus **herpes simplex.** The lesions generally form near the mouth or lips, as in Figure 17–2. The virus may be har-

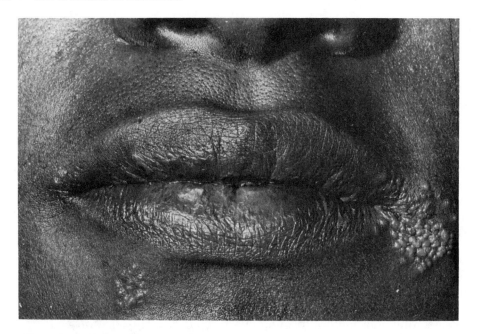

Figure 17–2. Typical cold sores or fever blisters caused by the virus herpes simplex. (*From Feinstein*, Dermatology. *Courtesy of Robert J. Brady Co.*)

bored in the body for a long time with no ill effect, but suddenly it becomes active and the infection develops. Cold sores frequently form when a person's resistance to infection is low or at a time of emotional stress. They often accompany a respiratory infection such as the common cold, or they develop during menstruation. A bad sunburn sometimes triggers the formation of cold sores. Antiviral drugs are effective for certain viral infections such as cold sores, and antibiotics are sometimes applied topically to treat secondary bacterial invasion.

Warts, called **verucca vulgaris,** are caused by viruses affecting the keratinocytes of the skin, causing them to proliferate. A benign neoplasm develops with a rough keratinized surface. Warts are most common in children and young adults, developing particularly on the hands. They are often multiple and are contagious, being spread by scratching. Warts sometimes disappear spontaneously, but they should be removed only by a physician. If the virus remains in the body, the warts tend to recur.

Warts are not serious or painful except when they form on the soles of the feet. These warts are called **plantar warts,** and, in contrast to warts elsewhere on the body, which appear as an elevation from the skin, plantar warts grow inward. Pressure on the soles of the feet make them very painful, and they are often difficult to remove permanently. **Genital** or **venereal warts** (see Chapter 14) are very serious and difficult to remove.

■ Fungal Skin Infections

Ringworm is a highly contagious, inflammatory skin infection caused by fungi. It usually affects children and is spread by scratching. Ringworm is sometimes contracted from infected pets. One form of ringworm develops on the scalp and the hairy skin of arms and legs. The lesions are red patches that are scaly or blistered. They are itchy and sore, and excessive scratching can lead to scarring and permanent hair loss.

Many different fungi cause ringworm infection on nonhairy skin, and any number of red, ring-shaped lesions can develop in an infected person. The fungi feed on perspiration and dead skin, particularly in body folds. Antifungal drugs are effective, but the disease can be prevented through cleanliness and thorough drying of the skin. Fungi thrive in a warm, damp environment.

Dermatophytosis, or athlete's foot, which thrives in damp, warm conditions, is such a fungal infection. In this disease the fungi attack the skin between the toes, making it red, cracked, itchy, and sore. Dermatophytosis spreads, if untreated, to other parts of the feet and even to distant sites on the body such as the armpits and groin. Athlete's foot is highly infectious and is often acquired from locker room floors or contaminated towels harboring the fungi.

Antifungal agents are effective in treating dermatophytosis, but it tends to recur if the fungi survive under the toenails. Drying the feet well between the toes and applying dusting powder to absorb moisture are good preventive measures against acquiring athlete's foot. Selecting shoes that are well ventilated, alternating shoes to allow drying, and wearing cotton socks rather than synthetic ones, also help to prevent the fungus.

■ Parasitic Infestations

Pediculosis or louse infestations are classified into three categories, head lice, pubic lice, and body lice.

Head lice are common among school children, and although annoying, these parasites are not dangerous and do not carry epidemic disease. Lice are spread from head to head directly or indirectly by shared combs, scarves, hats, and bed linen. Itching, the first symptom, results from the saliva of lice as they penetrate the scalp and engorge on human blood. The scratching that follows can open the skin to other invading organisms. Adult head lice are difficult to see, but their white eggs, called nits, can be located on the hair shaft. Treatment includes use of medicated shampoos followed by use of a finetoothed comb. Over-the-counter medications are also available.

Pubic lice infest pubic hair of both men and women and are generally spread by sexual contact. The lice do not spread other sexually transmitted diseases. Treatment includes use of a prescription cream.

Body lice are most common among underprivileged, transient people. This type of infestation can be prevented with good grooming and hygiene. Body lice can spread serious disease, and they have been responsible for typhus epidemics among soldiers during wartime.

Scabies, commonly called "the itch," is a contagious skin disease usually associated with poor living conditions. It is caused by a parasite called a mite. The female mite burrows into skin folds in the groin, under the breasts, and between fingers and toes. As she burrows she lays eggs in the tunnels, the eggs hatch, and the cycle starts again. The intense itching is caused by hypersensitivity to the mite. Blisters and pustules develop, and the tunnels in the skin appear as grayish lines. Scratching opens the lesions to secondary bacterial infection. Scabies is transmitted by close personal contact and can be linked to a venereal disease. Epidemics of scabies are common in camps and barracks.

To recover from scabies, the mites and eggs must be totally destroyed by hot baths, scrubbing, and medications to eliminate them. Underwear and bedding that harbor the eggs must be changed frequently. The itch may persist while treatment is being administered; applying calamine lotion provides relief.

HYPERSENSITIVITY DISEASES OF THE SKIN

Allergic or hypersensitivity reactions are frequently manifested by the skin. This fact serves as the basis for the **patch tests** given to determine specific allergies. Some diseases of the skin develop in **atopic people,** persons with a genetic predisposition to allergies. Others occur in anyone who has been sensitized to an allergen such as poison ivy. Emotional stress frequently triggers or exacerbates an allergy-caused skin disease.

■ Urticaria (Hives)
Urticaria, or hives, results from a vascular reaction of the skin to an allergen. The word *urticaria* is derived from a Latin word that means "plants covered with stinging nettles." The lesions are **wheals,** rounded elevations with red edges and pale centers. Wheals develop most often at pressure points like those under tight clothing, but they may appear anywhere on the skin or mucous membranes. The lesions are extremely pruritic, or itchy.

The allergic response causes damage to mast cells, which then release histamine. Histamine causes blood vessels to dilate and become more permeable. Blood proteins and fluid ooze out of the capillaries into the tissues and result in edema. This irritation to the tissues causes intense itching.

Urticaria is generally treated with steroids, antihistamines, and calamine lotion applied topically to reduce the itching. If the cause of the allergic reaction can be determined, that allergen should be avoided. Foods that are a common cause of hives include certain berries, chocolate, nuts, and seafood. Other allergens discussed in Chapter 2 frequently cause hives in the hypersensitive person. An attack of hives can also be brought on by emotional stress.

■ Eczema
Eczema, also called **contact dermatitis,** is a noncontagious inflammatory skin disorder. Eczema results from sensitization that develops from skin contact with

various agents, plants, chemicals, and metals. **Poison ivy** (to be described) and poison oak, dyes used for hair or clothing, and metals, particularly nickel, used in costume jewelry are examples of allergens that can cause eczema.

Eczema is a delayed type of allergic response in which lymphocytes are sensitized by an antigen, such as poison ivy, and react with it on subsequent exposure. The typical inflammatory reaction occurs: dilated blood vessels, reddened skin, and edema. Vesicles and bullae develop from the excess tissue fluid, and the lesions are very itchy. Scratching causes the vesicles to burst and ooze, and the eczema is thus spread. Scaly crusts form on the ruptured lesions. A patient with contact dermatitis is shown in Figure 17–3.

Contact dermatitis can affect anyone and is not limited to the genetically allergic person. Skin that has been damaged is more easily sensitized by contact with allergens than healthy skin. Emotional stress can also be a factor in sensitization. Corticosteroids are sometimes used to reduce the inflammatory reaction.

■ Poison Ivy

Contact with poison ivy can cause an extremely itchy rash with blisters and hive-like swelling; the response is a typical example of allergic contact dermatitis. Severity of the condition depends on the amount of plant resin on the skin and the

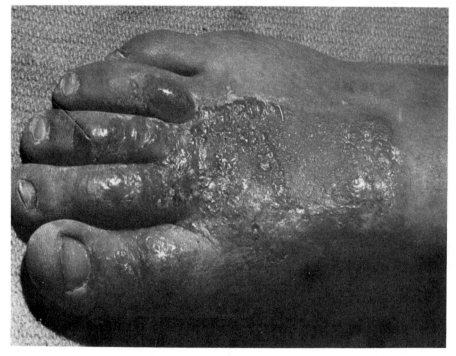

Figure 17–3. A patient with contact dermatitis from leather shoes. (*From Feinstein*, Dermatology. *Courtesy of Robert J. Brady Co.*)

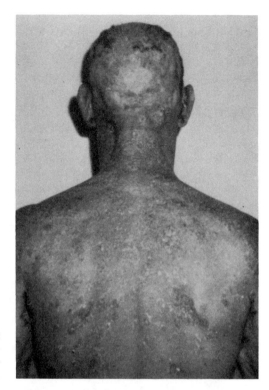

Figure 17–4. Patient experienced allergic drug eruption because of gold administration for rheumatoid arthritis. (*From Feinstein*, Dermatology. *Courtesy of Robert J. Brady Co.*)

individual's sensitivity to it. Some people are apparently immune to the resin. An initial exposure to the poison ivy plant produces no visible effect but sensitizes the person to subsequent exposure. The rash usually develops a few hours or a few days after contact. Treatment to lessen the inflammation is use of a topical cortisone-type cream, gel, or spray.

◼ Drug Hypersensitivity

Adverse drug reactions in an atopic person are very common. The reaction may be manifested by various skin lesions, vesicles, and itchy rash, or erythema. The patient seen in Figure 17–4 was treated with gold for rheumatoid arthritis and developed the allergic skin reaction shown. The drug reaction may be severe enough to cause anaphylactic shock and death.

Penicillin, effective in treating bacterial infections, is an antigen to some atopic patients that triggers serious vascular reactions. Patients allergic to penicillin should never receive it and should carry identification warning of their sensitivity.

NEOPLASTIC SKIN DISEASES

Tumors of the skin range in seriousness from the benign mole to melanoma, a potentially fatal disease. The development of skin cancer is frequently linked to excessive sun exposure in the fair-skinned. Irritating chemicals and various radiations have also been associated with skin cancer.

■ Nevus (Mole)

Melanocytes in the epidermis produce the pigment melanin that gives color to the skin and protects the body against harmful rays of the sun. The neoplastic growth of melanocytes causes an excessive production of melanin, resulting in a **nevus,** or mole. A nevus is a benign skin tumor that is not present at birth but develops later. Most people have several nevi. The moles themselves are harmless but they can become malignant, as was described in Chapter 3.

■ Basal Cell Carcinoma

The most common skin cancer is **basal cell carcinoma**—a slow-growing, generally nonmetastasizing tumor. It generally develops on the face of people with light skin who do not tan in the sun but have been exposed to the sun. Figures 17–5 A, B, and C show patients with basal cell carcinoma. The lesion begins as a pearly nodule with rolled edges that may bleed and form a crust. Ulceration occurs and size increases if it is neglected. This tumor is treated by surgical removal, cauterization, or radiation therapy.

■ Squamous Cell Carcinoma

Squamous cell carcinoma is more serious than basal cell carcinoma because it grows more rapidly, infiltrates underlying tissues, and metastasizes through lymph channels. Squamous cell carcinoma is a malignancy of the keratinocytes in the epidermis of people who have been excessively exposed to the sun. The lesion is a

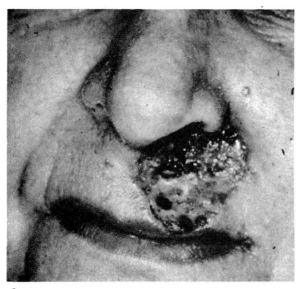

Figure 17–5A. Basal cell carcinoma removed by Moh's microscopically controlled excision for skin cancer. Reconstruction planned because of loss of lip function. (*Courtesy of Dr. Barry A. Goldsmith.*)

A

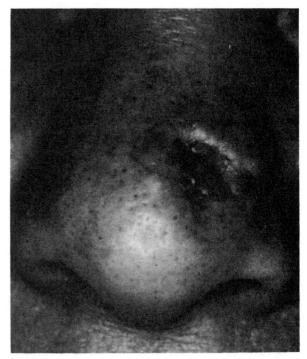

Figure 17–5B. A 48-year-old woman with progressive growth of whitish plaquelike lesion with central indentation over a 5-year period. Patient underwent three stages of microscopically controlled surgical excision. Wound extended down to cartilage layer. A skin graft was applied. (*Courtesy of Dr. Barry A. Goldsmith.*)

B

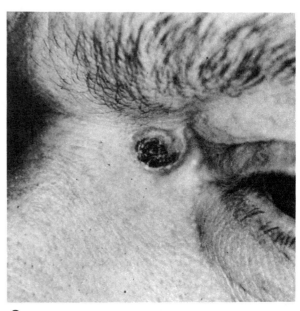

Figure 17–5C. A 62-year-old man with basal cell carcinoma recurrent after prior treatment with electric needle. Gross tumor was excised. Margins clear after one layer of Moh's microscopically controlled surgical excision. Excellent healing in this area. (*Courtesy of Dr. Barry A. Goldsmith.*)

C

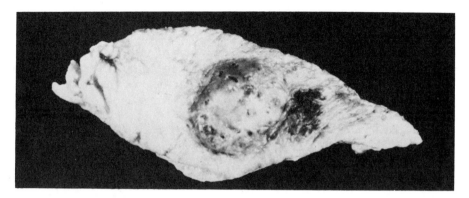

Figure 17–6. A malignant melanoma of the skin. (*Courtesy of Dr. David R. Duffell.*)

crusted nodule that ulcerates and bleeds. This cancer develops in any squamous epithelium of the body, including the skin or mucous membranes lining a natural body opening. It should be completely excised surgically or treated with radiation.

■ Malignant Melanoma

The most serious skin cancer is **malignant melanoma,** which arises from the melanocytes of the epidermis. It is highly malignant and metastasizes early. A ma-

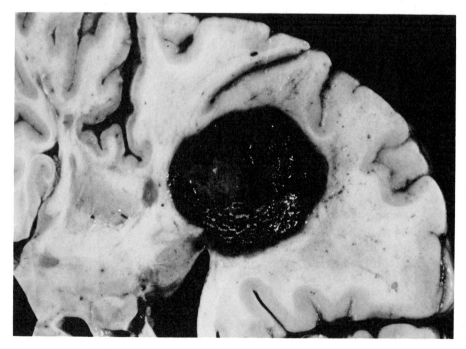

Figure 17–7. Malignant melanoma that metastasized to the brain. (*Courtesy of Dr. David R. Duffell.*)

lignant melanoma of the skin is seen in Figure 17–6. Melanoma sometimes develops from a mole that changes its size and color and becomes itchy and sore. It is usually excised with the surrounding lymph nodes to reduce metastasis. Prognosis depends on the depth of infiltration, previous spread, and how completely the tumor is excised. Figure 17–7 shows a malignant melanoma that metastasized to the brain.

METABOLIC SKIN DISORDERS

Hyperactivity of the sebaceous glands causes acne and chronic dandruff. Raised, horny lesions result from an excessive production of keratinocytes.

■ Acne (Vulgaris)

Many adolescents suffer at some time or another from acne: blackheads, pimples, and pustules. Acne is the result of hormonal changes that occur at puberty. The increased level of estrogen and testosterone stimulates not only growth at this time but also glandular activity. The sebaceous glands increase their secretions of **sebum,** the oily fluid that is released through the hair follicles. If the duct becomes clogged by dirt or make-up, the sebaceous secretion accumulates, causing a little bump or white head. Sebaceous accumulation at the surface becomes oxidized and turns black, causing the familiar blackhead. Blackheads should not be squeezed or picked because the broken skin offers an entry to bacteria that are always present on the skin surface. Once pyogenic bacteria enter the skin, pus forms and a pimple or pustule results. Squeezing the pimple spreads the infection.

There is no cure for acne, but various treatments can control the lesions. Acne generally corrects itself with maturity, but it may persist as a chronic condition that is aggravated by stress. Severe chronic acne as seen in Figure 17–8, can lead to disfiguring and scarring. The most important measure for controlling acne is frequent, thorough washing of the skin to remove excess oil and bacteria. Creams and heavy makeup that clog the pores should be avoided. Severe cases of acne are best treated by a dermatologist, who may prescribe topical steroids or antibiotics to prevent secondary bacterial infection.

■ Seborrheic Dermatitis (Chronic Dandruff)

The cause of dandruff is similar to that of acne: the excessive secretion of sebum from the sebaceous glands. The person with **seborrheic dermatitis** has an oily scalp, and the excessive secretion of sebum forms the familiar scales of dandruff. This condition can spread to the face and ears, and the eyebrows are often affected. Frequent shampooing, particularly with medicated shampoo, is the most effective treatment. Thorough brushing of the hair loosens the dandruff scales, and they will wash out easily.

■ Sebaceous Cysts

Sebaceous cysts form when a sebaceous gland duct becomes blocked, and the sebum accumulates under the surface of the skin, forming a lump. Sebaceous cysts are not considered serious but they can rupture, allowing bacteria to enter the

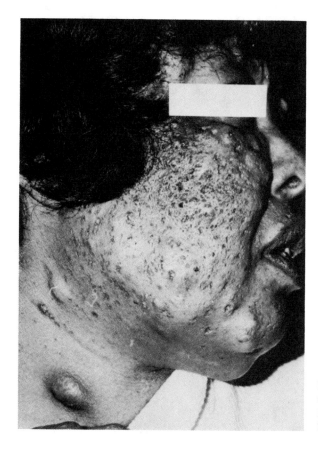

Figure 17–8. A patient with severe chronic acne. Note deep scarring and prominent cysts. (*From Feinstein*, Dermatology. *Courtesy of Robert J. Brady Co.*)

body. These cysts can be incised and drained, although they tend to recur, or they can be removed surgically.

A cyst that forms in the crease between the buttocks is the **pilonidal cyst.** This cyst begins as an ingrown hair and is very painful if it becomes infected and abscessed. A pilonidal cyst should be removed surgically.

■ Seborrheic Keratosis

The keratinocytes produce the fibrous protein keratin in the surface layers of the epidermis, making it waterproof. Proliferation of the keratinocytes, with resultant keratin excess, produces a benign, raised, horny lesion. This hyperplastic condition is called **seborrheic keratosis** and occurs with aging. The lesions, which are harmless, vary in color from yellow to brown, with edges that are sharply marked. No treatment is necessary.

■ Psoriasis

Psoriasis is a chronic skin disease with a hereditary basis, but the cause is unknown. The lesions are red patches with sharply marked edges, covered with white

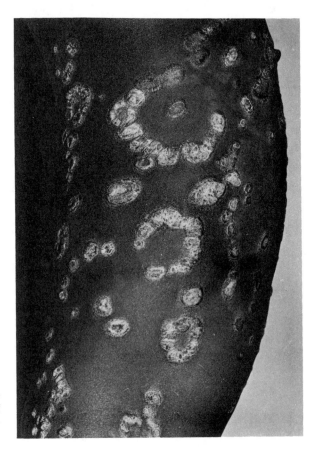

Figure 17–9. Psoriasis patient. Note the silvery scaling and the definite borders of individual lesions. (*From Feinstein*, Dermatology. *Courtesy of Robert J. Brady Co.*)

or silvery scales. Psoriasis lesions primarily form on the elbows and knees (the extensor surfaces of joints), but other parts of the body, such as the trunk, arms, legs, and scalp, can be affected. Typical lesions of psoriasis are seen in Figure 17–9.

There is no permanent cure for psoriasis, but the lesions can sometimes be controlled. The application of medications, some of which contain coal tar, cortisone-type drugs, and the use of ultraviolet light are the most effective treatments. Periods of exacerbation and remission are characteristic. Psoriasis can be aggravated by injury to the skin, infections, certain drugs, lack of sunlight, and stress.

DIAGNOSTIC TESTS FOR SKIN DISEASES

Biopsies are the usual tests for neoplastic lesions, chronic eruptions, and nodular lesions. Laboratory tests are used in certain conditions where it is necessary to culture a purulent lesion to identify bacteria or to examine a microscopic smear for a fungal infection. Blood tests may be ordered if a systemic infection is indicated.

CHAPTER SUMMARY

The skin, which protects the body from various elements in the environment, can become diseased in numerous ways. Streptococci and staphylococci cause such bacterial infections as impetigo, erysipelas, and boils. Cold sores and warts result from viral infections. Ringworm and athlete's foot are caused by a fungus. Even parasites such as the louse and mite can infest the skin.

Allergies are frequently manifested by skin diseases. Hives and eczema are examples of skin eruptions caused by hypersensitivity to various antigens. Allergic drug reactions often result in the development of skin lesions. Abnormal growth or neoplasia of the skin cells causes malignant and benign tumors, ranging from the common mole to malignant melanoma, a potentially fatal disease. Hyperactivity of the sebaceous glands results in acne and chronic dandruff.

Skin lesions take many forms, each of which is significant in diagnosing the disease. The lesions may be reddened areas, indicating inflammation and congested blood vessels. They may be fluid-filled, due to edema in the skin, or pus-filled, a result of a pyogenic bacterial infection. The location of the lesion, whether it tends to recur, and whether it itches, are also factors in the diagnosis.

■ Self-Study

True or False

_____ 1. Impetigo can involve a systemic infection.
_____ 2. Basal cell carcinoma metastasizes rapidly.
_____ 3. Fever blisters are examples of a bacterial infection.
_____ 4. Seborrheic keratosis is a malignant skin tumor.
_____ 5. Warts are benign neoplasms.
_____ 6. A mole is a nevus.
_____ 7. Ringworms are viral infections.
_____ 8. Athlete's foot is treated with antibiotics.
_____ 9. Dermatophytosis results from a fungal infection.
_____ 10. Seborrheic dermatitis is an infectious disease.

Match

_____ 11. scabies   a) bacterial
_____ 12. ringworm   b) viral
_____ 13. verucca vulgaris   c) fungal
_____ 14. urticaria   d) hypersensitivity
_____ 15. impetigo   e) parasitic

Match

_____ 16. erysipelas   a) wheals
_____ 17. vitiligo   b) malignant tumor
_____ 18. warts   c) benign skin tumors
_____ 19. melanoma   d) disappearance of melanin
_____ 20. hives   e) reddened patches on nose

(Answers on page 450)

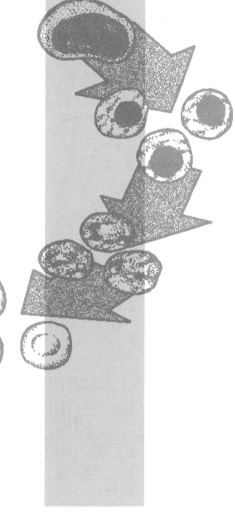

Chapter 18

Stress and Aging

Chapter Outline

- Homeostasis and Adaptation to Stress
- Effects of Stress on the Body
- Function of the Autonomic Nervous System in Response to Stress
- Stress and the Adrenal Cortical Hormones
- Treatment with Cortical Hormones
- Stress-Related Diseases
- Effects of Aging
- Chapter Summary
- Self-Study

*U*nder stress," and "stressed out" are common terms in today's fast-paced society, but few people realize the toll that stress takes on the human body.

HOMEOSTASIS AND ADAPTATION TO STRESS

The body is constantly striving to maintain a constant internal environment in the midst of ever-changing conditions. For example, excess acidity or alkalinity that develops in the blood and body fluids is removed through the kidneys. Normal body temperature is maintained despite climate extremes, and the proper amount of water is conserved to prevent dehydration or overhydration of tissues. This maintenance of a steady state is called **homeostasis.**

The regulation of the internal functioning of the body is controlled by the hypothalamus of the brain, which governs the autonomic nervous system and the master endocrine gland, the pituitary. Not only does the hypothalamus control homeostasis, it senses when the body or a body part is under stress and directs the proper response through nerves and glands.

How are the maintenance of homeostasis and the response to stress related to disease? The body is frequently subjected to forces requiring greatly increased internal activity. In responding or adapting to the stress, abnormal conditions can result.

Consider the phenomenon of inflammation previously described in Chapter 2. Although it produces pain that may be severe and the typical characteristics of swelling, heat, and redness, inflammation is a positive protective body response. It prevents the spread of an infection by barricading it and attempting to overcome foreign invaders such as pathogenic organisms or toxic substances.

Closely related to the mechanism of inflammation is the allergic reaction, or hypersensitivity. In this case, the inflammatory response is against a generally harmless invader such as pollen, dust, or a particular food, and the patient suffers from the disease of hay fever, asthma, or hives. The inflammation is more harmful than helpful under these conditions. Some diseases represent inappropriate responses to a stimulus.

Disease involves more than being overcome by a disease-producer. It includes the body's fight against it. The symptoms of respiratory tract diseases, coughing and sneezing, are reflex actions that aid in ridding the throat and nose of irritants. Vomiting, a symptom of gastrointestinal distress, is a reflex action to relieve the distress. The seriousness of any disease largely depends on the patient's defenses against it.

EFFECTS OF STRESS ON THE BODY

Many diseases have been described throughout this book as being stress related. Diseases of the gastrointestinal system, the respiratory system, and the skin are often aggravated, if not caused, by stress. Hypertension is another disease greatly affected by stress.

A wide range of situations in a person's life may be stressful, including living conditions, occupation, injury, inadequate diet, and prolonged exposure to cold. Worry, fatigue, and alcoholism also cause stress. Signs of damage caused by stress are often the result of the body's defense against or adaptation to it.

What are some changes that occur in the body when it is subjected to stress such as an injury? The blood sugar level rises, providing an additional energy supply needed for repair of the damaged tissue. The injured site becomes inflamed due to the increased blood flow to the area. The neutrophil count increases, enabling the phagocytic cells to engulf foreign matter and cellular debris.

If the injury is severe and blood loss results, the patient may go into shock (Chapter 8). The reduced blood volume lowers the blood pressure, and venous return to the heart is poor. Cardiac output then becomes inadequate to meet the demands of the body, and the patient loses consciousness because insufficient blood reaches the brain.

The response of the body to this stress is to increase blood pressure. Specialized neural receptors sense the low pressure, and through a neural mechanism, which will be explained, the blood pressure increases. The kidneys, sensing the reduced blood pressure due to the loss of blood, release a substance called renin that aids in restoring proper pressure. The adrenal glands are stimulated to release adrenalin, which also increases blood pressure and heart activity.

FUNCTION OF THE AUTONOMIC NERVOUS SYSTEM IN RESPONSE TO STRESS

We are all familiar with our bodily response to a stressful situation, a frightening experience, or an emotional upset. Our heart beat increases to the point of pounding, blood pressure rises, respiration quickens, and perspiration increases. These changes, which occur through the action of the autonomic nervous system, provide us with additional energy to meet the stress.

Large portions of the sympathetic nervous system are stimulated simultaneously by stress. The first response is redistribution of blood to where it is most needed: the heart, the brain, and the muscles of respiration. This is accomplished by a constriction of skin and gastrointestinal blood vessels and a dilation of those to the heart, brain, and active muscles. The constriction of the blood vessels elevates blood pressure, causing greater venous return to the heart and increased cardiac output.

The liver releases stored glucose into the blood when stimulated by the sympathetic nervous system, thus providing an increased energy source for actively metabolizing cells. The rate of cellular metabolism increases as the thyroid gland is stimulated under stress to secrete additional thyroxine. The adrenal medulla releases adrenalin (epinephrine), enhancing the stimulatory effect of the sympathetic nervous system. Glucocorticoids from the adrenal cortex also increase the level of blood glucose. This overall excitation of the body in response to stress is known as the alarm reaction. Figure 18–1 illustrates the function of the autonomic nervous system in stress.

STRESS AND THE ADRENAL CORTICAL HORMONES

Signals of an alarm reaction are sent to the hypothalamus, which in turn sends releasing factors to the pituitary gland (Chapter 13). The pituitary secretes ACTH

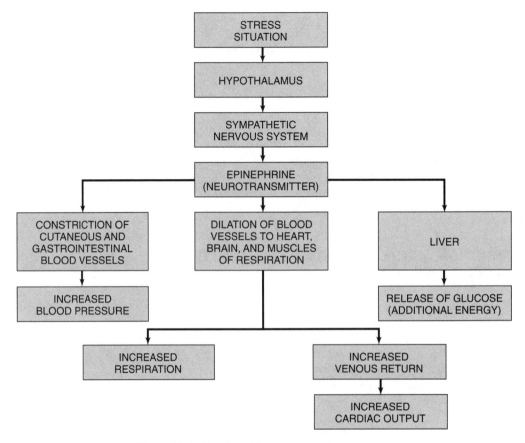

Figure 18–1. Function of the nervous system in stress.

(adrenocorticotropic hormone) and thyrotropin, which stimulate the thyroid gland and the adrenal cortex to release thyroxine and the corticosteroids. This hormonal response to stress is illustrated in Figure 18–2.

Cortisol, a glucocorticoid, is anti-inflammatory and inhibits unnecessary defense reactions. In the case of hay fever or rheumatoid arthritis, inflammation is actually the disease. In diseases of this type there are no pathogens or toxins to be barricaded, and the inflammatory response is harmful rather than beneficial.

It is necessary that a proper balance of aldosterone and anti-inflammatory cortisol be maintained. An excess of **anti-inflammatory hormones** produced during stress can actually cause the spread of an infection by weakening the barricade around infectious organisms. Stress can be a predisposing factor in the spread of tuberculosis for this reason. Tubercle bacilli can be held at bay until excessive cortisol is circulated. Nonpathogenic organisms that normally live in the respiratory tract, the intestines, or on the skin become dangerous when the defense mechanism against them is reduced.

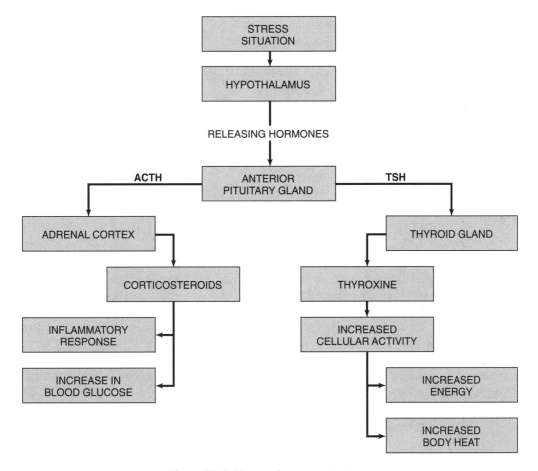

Figure 18–2. Hormonal response to stress.

The anti-inflammatory cortical hormones not only suppress the immune reaction against microorganisms, but they also suppress the tendency to reject foreign tissue in graft or transplantation procedures. These hormones are extremely important in preventing unnecessary inflammation in the typical inflammatory diseases.

TREATMENT WITH CORTICAL HORMONES

The effectiveness of corticosteroids as treatment for many inflammatory diseases has been described throughout the book. Caution is always required because of the side effects from these hormones. High dosages or prolonged use of cortisol or cortisone reduces a patient's response to infection, which can therefore go unnoticed and become very widespread in the absence of inflammatory symptoms.

STRESS-RELATED DISEASES

The symptoms, causes, and treatment of many of the diseases aggravated by stress have already been described. This section will try to explain how the stress or alarm reaction affects a particular disease.

■ Gastrointestinal Diseases Affected by Stress

The gastrointestinal system (Chapter 10) is particularly affected by stress, as most people have experienced. An emotional upset, worry, or fear can cause vomiting, diarrhea, or constipation. Some people under stress lose their appetite, whereas others eat compulsively.

Certain ulcers, called "stress ulcers," develop suddenly after a shock or trauma, such as severe burns or surgery. These ulcers differ from the chronic types and usually manifest themselves by bleeding rather than by pain.

Ulcerative colitis, an inflammation and ulceration of the colon, is a disease of unknown origin that is aggravated by stress. Severe diarrhea with blood and mucus accompanies the disease. Treatment for this inflammation includes a nonirritating diet, antibiotics to prevent infection of the lesions, and rest. The patient should be kept free from emotional stress, and psychological counseling should be offered to help the person cope with anxieties and tensions. Corticosteroids are frequently prescribed for their anti-inflammatory effect.

Regional enteritis or Crohn's disease is similar to ulcerative colitis. It is not caused by a pathogenic organism but is aggravated by stress, such as emotional upsets. Regional enteritis is an inflammation of the large or small intestine. The patient experiences abdominal pain, diarrhea, and weight loss. Corticosteroids are used with caution to prevent side effects from over-dosage.

■ Migraine Headaches

The migraine sufferer knows the effect of the disease on the body is more extensive than periodic headaches. A migraine headache usually begins in the temple on one side, spreads to the other side, and becomes generalized. It can last for a short time or for days, and the range of severity is very broad. Gastrointestinal disturbances frequently accompany the headache, including nausea or vomiting, and diarrhea or constipation. Visual changes including **photophobia,** abnormal sensitivity to light, may occur.

Frequently, stress or emotional upset precedes the onset of the headache. Migraines often occur during a woman's menstrual period because of hormonal changes. Attacks are sometimes triggered by such factors as high altitude, weather changes, polluted air, or smoking. Substances in the diet such as chocolate, aged cheese, food additives, and alcohol, especially red wine and beer, can trigger an attack.

Certain symptoms often precede the migraine headache: visual changes such as a sensation of flickering lights, dizziness, numb feelings in the arms and legs, and a flushing or paling of the skin. A warning signal of this type is referred to as an **aura.** Changes occur in the cranial arteries before the onset of the headache with a vasoconstriction, followed by a vasodilation, which causes the throbbing, aching pain. The eyes may become red, swollen, and show excessive tearing.

The exact cause of migraine headaches is not known but it is now thought to be due to an imbalance in brain chemicals and altered nerve activity which causes dilation of cerebral blood vessels. **Serotonin** is one of the neurotransmitters involved in regulating pain messages. Studies have shown that the serotonin level drops during a migraine headache when blood vessels are dilated.

Better understanding of migraine headaches has led to improved medications to stop the pain. Some of these are vasoconstrictors and mimic serotonin activity. **Analgesics,** medications which reduce pain, can be prescribed. Anti-depressants also affect serotonin levels and are sometimes prescribed even if the patient is not depressed.

The migraine sufferer should be aware of factors that can trigger an attack and avoid them. Counseling to deal with stress may be advantageous.

Cluster headaches (which are a variation of migraines), are named for their tendency to occur in clusters, often several within a day or longer period of time. The intense, throbbing pain of these headaches is generally confined to one side and may last for a few hours. Men are more often affected by cluster headaches than are women, who are more prone to migraines. The treatment is similar to that of migraines.

■ The Cardiovascular System and Stress

The response of the sympathetic nervous system to stress is a constriction of peripheral blood vessels that elevates the blood pressure. The adrenal cortex, responding to stress, also causes blood pressure elevation by excessive secretion of aldosterone. Sodium and water are retained under the influence of aldosterone, and the increased fluid volume causes increased blood pressure. A person predisposed to hypertension and subjected to prolonged stress will probably develop chronic high blood pressure. This is usually accompanied by arteriosclerosis (discussed in Chapter 8), which overworks the heart. The risk of a heart attack under these circumstances increases, particularly if the person is obese, smokes, and is sedentary in life-style.

A special case of hypertension is eclampsia of pregnancy, in which there is a sudden, intense increase in blood pressure. Eclampsia usually occurs in the third trimester and is accompanied by an increase in the level of serum albumin, which appears in the urine. Convulsions develop that can lead to a coma. The cause of eclampsia is unknown, but it is thought to be aggravated by stress (see Chapter 14).

■ Sexual Abnormalities Related to Stress

Prolonged and intense stress causes changes in the sex organs. The ovaries and testes shrink and decrease their activity. Menstruation becomes irregular and may even stop, as often experienced by women subjected to the stress of prison. In men, sperm production is decreased, and both men and women may experience a decline of libido (sex urge). The depressed activity of the gonads may result from decreased stimulation by the gonadotropic hormones of the pituitary gland. During prolonged periods of stress, the pituitary may secrete an excessive amount of ACTH at the expense of the gonadotropins.

■ The Respiratory System and Stress

The respiratory system is frequently affected by disease when a person's defenses against it are lowered by stress. The cause of the stress may be emotional factors like worry, depression, and conflict or physical factors such as trauma, prolonged exposure to cold, or inadequate nutrition. Stress reduces the body's ability to fight infection, as previously mentioned in the case of tuberculosis.

Development of the common cold during a time of stress is within the experience of most people. The alarm reaction, with its release of the cortical hormones, is probably related to this phenomenon. Infectious diseases of the respiratory system are not the only conditions affected by stress.

Asthma (Chapter 12), a disease characterized by marked changes in the diameter of the bronchi and obstruction of the air passageways, usually has an allergic basis. A wide variety of allergens or irritants can precipitate an asthma attack. The antigen–reagenic antibody complex (Chapter 2) attaches to the surface of the bronchial mast cells, causing the release of histamine and other **spasmogens,** substances that cause spasmodic contractions of the bronchial musculature.

An asthma attack—with its coughing, wheezing, and shortness of breath—can be aggravated by emotional or psychological stress. The asthmatic manifests a hyperactivity of the bronchi through an exaggerated response to autonomic nervous activity.

Other factors that aggravate an asthmatic condition are overexertion and viral respiratory tract infections. A young child's asthma can appear to be worse for a combination of reasons as school begins. The new experience is emotionally stressful, the school environment increases the child's exposure to respiratory infections, and school play can involve overexertion.

The treatment of asthma begins by reducing exposure to allergens or irritants wherever possible. Allergy shots aimed at desensitization are helpful for some people. The use of a bronchodilator such as epinephrine is generally quite effective. Severe cases may require administration of corticosteroids or ACTH to reduce the inflammatory reaction, edema, and excessive mucous secretion.

■ Skin Diseases Affected by Stress

Diseases of the skin may be caused by infectious agents, allergies, or abnormal cellular activity, but many of them are affected by stress (Chapter 17). A cold sore or fever blister, which is a viral infection, often develops when resistance to infection is low. The virus may be present and silent for a long time, only to become actively infective at the time of an emotional or physical stress.

Hives are an allergic skin disease that can be aggravated by stress. The relationship between hypersensitivity and stress has already been discussed. Treatment for hives often includes the administration of corticosteroids to reduce the inflammatory response. Eczema is another inflammatory skin disease of an allergic nature that is affected by emotional stress.

The cause of psoriasis is unknown, but it does have a hereditary basis and can be aggravated by stress. Application of corticosteroids and other medications is quite effective in controlling the lesions.

■ Systemic Changes Produced by Stress

Various stress-related diseases or diseases of adaptation have been discussed: cardiovascular, respiratory, and gastrointestinal disorders, as well as allergies and the migraine syndrome. Experimentation has shown other marked changes resulting from prolonged stress. The adrenal cortex becomes enlarged from overwork by excessive stimulation to secrete its hormones. Lymphoid tissue, which is important in immune reactions and the removal of foreign invaders, atrophies. Ulceration of the gastric and duodenal lining frequently develops.

EFFECTS OF AGING

Aging is not a process that begins at retirement but one that occurs continuously throughout a lifetime. The body constantly replaces worn-out cells but the rate of replacement gradually slows down in adulthood. Cellular activity is reduced, tissues lose moisture, and flexibility declines. Noticeable body changes occur in the eyes, the skin, and the endocrine glands as early as the 30s and 40s. Distance vision may remain good, but the ability to accommodate for close vision decreases. Connective tissues lose their elasticity, and muscles lose their speed of response and strength, making the body less agile. Hair often begins to gray as less melanin pigment is produced for the hair follicles.

Heredity and environment greatly affect the aging process. A person's ability to withstand or adapt to stress significantly influences the rate at which the aging process occurs. The diseases that a person has had, the amount of activity and exercise he or she engages in, and his or her nutritional habits all affect the physiologic changes that accompany aging.

Many diseases that make old age difficult begin in the middle years. Diagnosis and treatment of such diseases as diabetes, hypertension, and arthritis early in their course can prevent much discomfort and suffering in later life.

■ Common Diseases of the Elderly

The elderly patient frequently has a combination of several diseases, some of which are interrelated. Hip fractures are common, and most aged people develop some degree of arteriosclerosis, which affects circulation to the heart, brain, and legs. As coronary arteries become atherosclerotic, the risk of myocardial infarction, a heart attack, increases. Hypertension, which frequently accompanies arteriosclerosis, is a predisposing factor for stroke. Poor blood flow through narrowed, hardened cerebral arteries causes a form of senility.

On the Practical Side

STRETCHING FOR HEALTH

The body loses flexibility with aging, and "range of motion," the extent to which one can move muscles and joints, is reduced. A program of daily stretching (with physician approval) can help maintain flexibility and range of motion, and prevent injuries. Physicians can give specific directions on appropriate stretching techniques.

Debilitating changes occur in the musculoskeletal system. Osteoarthritis, a degenerative joint disease (Chapter 16), generally develops in the normal aging process, affecting those joints most subjected to stress during a lifetime. The pain and stiffness of the disease tend to restrict movement, and the immobility increases the risk of thrombosis and embolism. Lack of exercise causes muscles to become thin and weak, a condition known as disuse atrophy. An elderly person may become more accident prone as sight and hearing fail and the reflexes slow. Bones become more brittle and fracture easily under slight stress, and they heal slowly.

Gastrointestinal complaints stem from a number of diseases: gallbladder malfunction, diverticulitis, ulcers, and various malignancies. Decayed teeth, poorly fitting dentures, or the inability to wear dentures makes chewing difficult or impossible.

Prostatic hyperplasia (Chapter 14) in males causes urinary complaints. The inability to eliminate urine adequately results in stasis and predisposes to cystitis, inflammation of the bladder, and other urinary tract infections. Symptoms of painful urination, a change in frequency, and nocturia are common in elderly men.

The prevalence of cancer in the elderly is high. Many malignancies go undetected and are only discovered at autopsy. The exposure to carcinogenic agents through a lifetime no doubt takes its toll.

Visual acuity can diminish from a number of causes, but one eye disease that particularly affects the elderly is **cataracts.** Cataract formation is a clouding of the eye lens to the point of opacity. The patient experiences blurred and dimmed vision and may see double. These symptoms do not necessarily signal a cataract, but the eyes should be examined. Removal of cataracts has become a simple procedure, one that can often be performed on an outpatient basis. Intraocular lens implants have been very successful, eliminating the need for thick glasses.

In addition to the physical diseases that are common to the elderly, **senility** often causes a loss of memory, disorientation, and personality changes. Senility is defined as the loss of mental, physical, or emotional control and is manifested by

On the Practical Side

CATARACTS

Some degree of cataract formation affects about 50% of adults over 65. Several conservative procedures often eliminate the need for surgical removal. New prescription lenses, better lighting, and in some cases, eyedrops may be adequate treatment.

   If surgery is chosen, the procedure is fast, simple, and requires only local anesthesia. A small incision allows the removal of the clouded lens.

delusions of persecution, apathy, slovenliness, and at times sudden emotional outbursts. The patient's recent memory may be poor but long-standing memories are very vivid. The past is confused with the present, and the patient may fail to recognize loved ones.

The cause of senility may be physical, such as brain damage resulting from inadequate blood flow through hardened cerebral arteries. Psychological factors may also foster senility. A feeling of worthlessness, loss of interests, and the stress of worrying about health and future security may be underlying causes of senility. Lack of interest and attention can account for the failure to recall recent events.

Many of the problems of aging can be prevented through preparation for retirement time. Maintaining an interest in life by engaging in hobbies, community service activities, and part-time employment are effective in preventing withdrawal from society and in fulfilling the need to be useful.

Alzheimer's Disease. **Alzheimer's disease** is the most common form of senility, affecting 1 1/2 to 2 1/2 million Americans. The cause of Alzheimer's disease is not known; however, there is some familial tendency to develop it, perhaps because of a combination of acquired genes. Women are slightly more susceptible to the disease than are men. The disease usually manifests itself in persons over age 65, but it can occur in the late 40s or 50s. Alzheimer's disease manifests itself in the early stages by forgetfulness, failing attention, and declining mathematical ability, such as the inability to balance a checkbook. Later, the patient exhibits personality changes, speech difficulties, and general confusion. There is a tendency toward depression, irritability, and severe anxiety. Symptoms may be more noticeable to the casual observer than to family members. When the disease becomes severe, the patient experiences hallucinations at night, and the resulting sleeplessness causes the person to wander aimlessly.

Extensive research on the changes that take place in the nerve cells of these patients' brains has been done on autopsy findings. Abnormalities include a loss of neurons in regions essential for memory and understanding, and accumulations of twisted filaments and nerve tangles in the cortex. Aggregates of protein interfere with cerebral circulation, and degenerating nerve endings, referred to as **plaque,** disrupt transmission of nerve impulses. A deficiency in enzymes required to produce neurotransmitters has also been found. A protein **(amyloid)** is found in the plaque. This protein is associated with abnormal antibodies that may indicate an autoimmune disease.

There is no known prevention, treatment, or cure for Alzheimer's disease. Symptoms may be reduced, however, through physical activity—walking, dancing, rocking in a chair—which reduces the patient's restlessness. Counseling and support for family members is extremely important in dealing with this irreversible and progressive disease that leads to complete mental and physical disability of loved ones.

Diagnosis of Alzheimer's disease is based on family histories and interviews with family members. Tests are used to determine the patient's orientation and mood, recent and old memory, and the ability to solve problems and make judgments.

■ Care of the Elderly

Advances in medical science enabling people to live longer than in the past, and a decrease in the birth rate, have raised the median age in our society. A higher percentage of people are in an older age bracket and require proper attention and health care. **Geriatrics** is the branch of medicine that deals with the problems of aging and the diseases of the elderly.

Research in **gerontology,** the study of aging problems, has revealed the need for psychological support and counseling as well as physical care of the elderly. The aging patient must experience a sense of dignity, worth, and acceptance, whether the person is living with relatives or friends, at home, or in a health-care facility. The elderly should be supervised carefully to prevent accidents and should be kept alert and aware of their surroundings.

An important physical need of the elderly is proper nutrition: a diet that includes an adequate supply of protein, vitamins and minerals, fruits, vegetables, and milk. If a digestive problem exists, small and more frequent meals may be desirable. Food may have to be chopped or strained because of the inability to chew.

Another need of the aged is a rest and exercise program that helps maintain circulation. The elderly person should be encouraged to engage in a walking program that takes into account the person's strength limitations and does not cause exhaustion. Rest should include short naps or sitting in a chair with the feet elevated. Staying in bed for long periods is harmful, and anemia can develop in the absence of exercise since the mechanism for red blood cell production is not stimulated (Chapter 6).

A good understanding of the changes that occur in the aging process makes one better able to give proper health care to the elderly patient. The slowed rate of metabolism, with its decreased production of energy, makes the aged very sensitive to temperature changes. The elderly may require warmer clothing or extra blankets.

Resistance to infection is reduced in the elderly as the activity of lymphoid tissue decreases. Bronchopneumonia caused by staphylococci commonly develops in the aged after the flu. Early signs of infection should be noted and the proper medication prescribed. The chance of death naturally increases with age, and although many of the diseases that have been mentioned in this chapter do not cause death themselves, the slightest stress can bring it about.

CHAPTER SUMMARY

The body responds to stress in a variety of ways in the attempt to maintain homeostasis or adapt to the stress. The autonomic nervous system is extensively stimulated, and its response provides the body with additional energy to meet the emergency. Blood pressure is elevated, heart activity is increased, and blood rich in oxygen is provided to active muscles. The liver releases stored glucose needed by the actively metabolizing cells. Adrenalin is secreted by the adrenal medulla, enhancing the effect of the sympathetic nervous system.

The hypothalamus responds to stress by stimulating hormonal activity of the pituitary gland, which in turn stimulates the thyroid gland and the adrenal cortex. The rate of cellular metabolism and that of concurrent energy production is greatly increased by the elevated thyroxine level.

Hormones of the adrenal cortex have important functions in responding to stress. The mineralocorticoids such as aldosterone cause retention of sodium and water, increasing the volume of body fluid—an effect that elevates blood pressure. Aldosterone stimulates the inflammatory response that walls off infection and attempts to counteract it.

The glucocorticoids such as cortisol increase the level of circulating glucose and prevent an unnecessary inflammatory and immune response. This is important in allergic reactions and rheumatoid arthritis, in which no pathogen is present. Cortisol also suppresses the immune reaction that causes rejection of tissue grafts and transplants. Excessive cortisol can cause the spread of infection by reducing the protective barrier around an infectious agent and preventing the symptoms which signal an infection. Administration of cortisol, cortisone, or ACTH to reduce the inflammatory response in such diseases as regional enteritis, asthma, and rheumatoid arthritis must be done with caution to prevent side effects.

Many diseases are aggravated by stress, particularly those of the cardiovascular system, the skin, the respiratory, and digestive systems. Psychological and emotional factors, as well as physical factors, can trigger the alarm reaction, and the response to it exacerbates the disease. The treatment of these diseases includes identification of the source of stress and removing it where possible or counseling, which can enable the patient to adapt to the stress. Medication is prescribed as warranted.

Physiologic changes that are part of the aging process begin early in life. Heredity and environment significantly affect the rate at which these changes occur. A person's ability to withstand stress or adapt to it influences the manner in which aging occurs.

Elderly patients often suffer from cardiovascular problems: heart conditions, hypertension, and arteriosclerosis, which are interrelated. Wear and tear on the body cause degenerative diseases such as osteoarthritis, the pain and stiffness of which decrease mobility and predispose to circulatory problems, muscle atrophy, and anemia. The incidence of cancer is high among the elderly, although many malignancies are detected only at autopsy.

Mental changes also occur with aging. Memory may fail in the elderly patient, and the person then becomes disoriented. Personality changes, inappropriate behavior, and the inability to recognize loved ones indicate the altered mental state of senility. Senility can have a physical basis of brain damage owing to the lack of blood flow through cerebral arteries or Alzheimer's disease, or it can stem from psychological factors such as depression, worry, or a sense of uselessness. Thoughtful preparation for retirement age and suitable counseling can help to maintain an interest in life and provide a feeling of worth.

■ Self-Study

True or False

_____ 1. Blood sugar level rises when the body is subjected to stress.
_____ 2. Stress triggers increased glucocorticoid production.
_____ 3. Skin and gastrointestinal blood vessels dilate resulting from stress.
_____ 4. Stress elevates blood pressure.
_____ 5. The pituitary gland is regulated by the hypothalamus.
_____ 6. Cortisol stimulates defense reactions.
_____ 7. Gonadotropin production may decrease during stress.
_____ 8. Prolonged bed rest is recommended for the elderly.
_____ 9. Stress may affect the aging process.
_____ 10. Cancer is prevalent in the aging.

Match

_____ 11. asthma
_____ 12. Alzheimer's disease
_____ 13. peptic ulcer
_____ 14. migraines
_____ 15. cataracts

a) clouding of the eye lens
b) excessive dilation of cranial arteries
c) increased gastric secretion
d) hyperactivity of the bronchi
e) abnormal neurons of the brain

(Answers on page 450)

Chapter 19

Wellness: Diet and Exercise

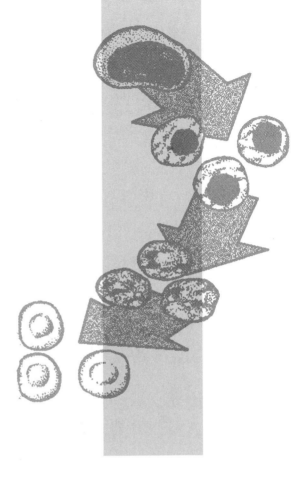

Chapter Outline

- Wellness
- Importance of Diet
- Value of Exercise
- Chapter Summary
- Self-Study

*W*e *hear much today about **holistic health** and **holistic medicine.** What do these comprehensive terms really mean? Holistic health focuses on the overall well-being of an individual to accept responsibility for self-care. It begins with an acceptance of one's self and a feeling of worth. Holistic medicine treats the whole person considering his or her physical, emotional, and spiritual needs.*

WELLNESS

An individual's health and well-being are greatly influenced by genetic make-up, family environment, and psychological characteristics. The external physical environment, food, water, and air, has its effect on wellness. It is important to see the relationship between these factors and disorders and diseases of the body.

One has the choice to select a lifestyle that promotes well-being. This includes proper diet, regular exercise, avoidance of smoking, and abuse of drugs and alcohol. A positive attitude about one's self, a feeling of self-worth, helps one to deal with emotions in a way that promotes health.

Unresolved negative emotions have a destructive effect on the body. They often lead to various psychosomatic illnesses in which the symptoms are real but aggravated by emotional stress. However, when the negative emotions are recognized as such, they can be worked out, often by a physical outlet. For some people it might be a brisk walk or run, a bike ride, or a cleaning project which gives satisfaction. Doing something to improve one's appearance, a manicure, a haircut, can have a very positive effect.

On the Practical Side

SKIN PATCH TO STOP SMOKING

The stick-on nicotine patch is helping many smokers quit the habit. The prescription patch reduces the craving for cigarettes and decreases withdrawal symptoms by delivering nicotine through the skin in decreasing doses over time.

Love and friendship are important factors in feeling good about one's self. A visit with a friend, a phone call, or writing a letter can be a great way of reducing the stresses of life.

Laughter has been shown to have effects on mind and body. It alters the respiratory rate, increasing it and bringing more oxygen into the blood. A good laugh temporarily increases heart rate and blood pressure and thus increases circulation to all the tissues.

Medical researchers are examining the connection between state of mind and body chemistry. It has been proposed that laughter and humor increase the body's natural pain fighters, brain chemicals called **endorphins** and **encephalins.** Everyone knows his or her own preference for humor, be it a book, a favorite comedian, a cartoon, or funny sayings of children. These ought to be sought as having a positive value in one's life.

Holistic practitioners recognize the value of a spiritual aspect of life. This may take many different forms but includes a belief in something or someone greater than self.

IMPORTANCE OF DIET

Research continues to show that a well-balanced diet together with regular exercise is the best form of preventive medicine. Eating a wide variety of foods including fruits, vegetables, grain products, milk and milk products, and lean meat provides all of the body's nutritional requirements. Food is the ideal source of vitamins and minerals, some of which have been found to reduce the risk of certain cancers. However, these same vitamins and minerals taken in excess as supplements can actually be toxic and cause cancer.

■ High Fiber–Low Fat Diet

The most healthful diets are high in fiber and low in fat. The National Cancer Institute recommends 20 to 30 grams of fiber daily. The recommendation stems from evidence suggesting that a high fiber–low fat diet lowers the risk of colon and rectal cancer. Five servings a day of fruits and vegetables, either fresh or cooked, and two slices of whole wheat bread meet this fiber requirement. **Legumes,** various kinds of peas and beans, are rich in protein, provide fiber, and contain virtually no fat.

■ Functions of Vitamins

In addition to providing fiber, fruits and vegetables provide a variety of vitamins, minerals, and other chemicals which may be related to cancer protection. One such example is **beta carotene** which the body uses to make vitamin A. It is contained in deep yellow and dark green vegetables. Good sources are carrots, spinach, sweet potatoes, winter squash, and tomatoes.

Vitamins C and E are **antioxidants** which fight **free radicals,** molecules that may cause disease by injuring cells. Vitamin C is present in oranges and grapefruit, strawberries, baked potatoes, and broccoli. Vegetable oils, leafy greens, and whole grains contain vitamin E.

Vitamin D is necessary for proper absorption of calcium and phosphorus from the gastrointestinal tract. These are the minerals that give hardness to bone. Calcium may be adequate in the diet but in the absence of vitamin D it cannot be utilized. Vitamin D fortified milk is a good source of this vitamin. Exposure to sunlight also provides a source of vitamin D as ultraviolet light converts a substance in the skin (a sterol) to vitamin D.

The B vitamins are water-soluble and many play an essential part in the body's enzyme system. The B vitamins include thiamine, riboflavin, pyridoxine, niacin, pantothenic acid, cobalamin (vitamin B_{12}), and folic acid.

Vitamin B_{12} and folic acid are essential in the formation of red blood cells. Vitamin B_{12} is obtained only from animal products or from supplements derived from microbes. Lack of this vitamin over a number of years leads to severe anemia and neurologic damage. By including lean meat, eggs, or dairy products in the diet the deficiency can usually be prevented.

The B vitamins are widely distributed in nature and therefore eating a balanced diet, as mentioned, prevents any deficiency. Many breakfast cereals are fortified to provide the recommended daily allowance (RDA), and fruits and vegetables are rich sources of vitamins.

Occasionally severe vitamin deficiencies occur in the elderly who live alone and stop eating, and in drug addicts and chronic alcoholics in the absence of adequate nutrition. Vitamin B deficiencies most seriously affect the nervous system causing "pins and needles" sensations, mental confusion, and an unsteady walk. Signs of the deficiency can be reversed with an improved diet and appropriate doses of vitamin supplements, but acute brain damage is irreversible.

Vitamin and mineral supplements should only be used when medically recommended due to aging, illness, or stringent weight-loss programs. Careful reading of the label will indicate expiration date after which they are ineffective. The RDA should not be exceeded.

■ Hypervitaminosis

Severe liver damage, even cirrhosis, can result from extremely high consumption of the fat-soluble vitamins, A and D. The current RDA for vitamin A is 5000 IU (international units) for adult men or pregnant women, 4000 for other women, and 2,500 for young children. It is almost impossible for adults to achieve toxic levels of vitamin A from food, but supplements which come in a wide range of dosages, some far exceeding the RDA, should never be used for extended periods of time without medical supervision. A nutritious diet coupled with normal intestinal function never needs a vitamin A or beta carotene supplement. Common side effects of taking too much vitamin A include itching, hair loss, dry skin and mouth, nausea, fatigue, and headaches.

■ Phytochemicals

Phytochemicals are substances contained naturally in fruits, vegetables, and grains which may be related to cancer protection. **Cruciferous** vegetables (those with cabbage-like odors), brussels sprouts, cauliflower, broccoli, cabbage, kale, turnips, and rutabaga, are good sources of these chemicals.

Preliminary studies have shown that people who have survived a heart attack may minimize chances of a second heart attack with a diet high in fruits, vegetables, grains, and fish. These foods provide large amounts of soluble fiber, antioxidant vitamins, and beta carotene. Essential minerals such as magnesium and potassium are also contained in these foods.

■ Triglycerides and Cholesterol

It is known that fatty cholesterol deposits in the arteries block them and deprive the heart, brain, and other organs of oxygen and nutrients. Let us consider the fat and fatty-like substances that cause blockages, noting their composition, their source, and manner of transport within the blood. The general name for these substances is lipid and includes **triglycerides** and **cholesterol.**

Triglyceride is the chemical name for fat. Body fat, for instance, is a triglyceride deposit. Animal fats such as lard and butter as well as fat in meat, poultry, and fish are triglycerides. Fat in vegetables, fruits, nuts, and cereals are all triglycerides. Blood tests for triglycerides measure the amount of fat present.

Triglycerides are compounds formed by joining fatty acids to glycerol, which is chemically an alcohol. If three fatty acids are joined, the compound is a triglyceride; if only one fatty acid is attached it is a monoglyceride; and if two, a diglyceride. These terms appear on common food labels.

The terms **saturated, unsaturated,** and **polyunsaturated** refer to the component fatty acids in a triglyceride. Fatty acids are long chains of carbon atoms connected together, and when the carbon atoms hold all the hydrogen atoms they can, they are saturated, and tend to be solid fats. When hydrogen atoms are missing they are called unsaturated fatty acids; polyunsaturated when several hydrogen atoms are missing, and these tend to be more liquid.

There is no unanimous agreement about the level of triglycerides in the blood and the potential for causing fatty cholesterol deposits in arteries. However, studies have shown that people with a triglyceride level below 180 mg/100 ml of plasma or serum had no increased risk of heart disease but the risk doubled for individuals in the range of 180 to 300 mg/100 ml of plasma. Triglyceride level can generally be reduced with weight reduction, increased exercise, and decreased alcohol intake.

■ Cholesterol: Good and Bad

Cholesterol is not a fat, chemically, but rather an alcohol. The large size of the cholesterol molecule gives it the solid, waxy characteristic. The name means "bile solid" and it is this that makes up most of the fatty cholesterol deposits (plaque) which block arteries. Cholesterol is an animal product found in meats and dairy products.

Total cholesterol values refer to the amount of cholesterol found in blood serum or plasma. Laboratory methods differ in accuracy, and an individual's cholesterol level may be affected by various factors. Recommended values have differed, however, it is generally agreed that a reduction in the total cholesterol level significantly reduces the risk of heart attacks and strokes. A level of 180 mg/100 ml (dL) of serum for individuals under 30 years of age and below 200 mg/dL for those over 30 is a suggested goal.

A person's total cholesterol value is not sufficient to evaluate cardiovascular risk. A breakdown into "good" and "bad" cholesterol levels is essential. To appreciate the difference one has to understand how cholesterol is transported through the blood. Lipids, fats (including triglycerides), and fatty-like substances (cholesterol) are not water-soluble and therefore cannot mix with blood plasma. In order to be water-soluble they are packaged into particles that contain blood proteins which do mix with water. These particles are classified **lipoproteins** according to their size as small, large, and very large. The size varies according to the amount of triglycerides they contain. The smallest particles are dense and are therefore called **high-density lipoproteins (HDL).** These particles do not contribute to the fatty cholesterol deposits in the arteries. They help to carry cholesterol and fat to the liver for reprocessing and thus reduce the amount of circulating fat. This HDL component is called "good" cholesterol.

The larger fatty cholesterol particles are less dense lipoproteins and are called **low-density lipoproteins (LDL).** These molecules tend to lodge in arterial walls forming the plaque that leads to heart attacks, strokes, and other problems. Hence LDL cholesterol is called "bad" cholesterol. Lipoproteins that contain the most triglycerides are the largest and least dense and are known as **very-low-density lipoproteins (VLDL).**

An individual's HDL cholesterol measurement indicates the number of fatty-cholesterol particles present in a serum sample and the LDL measurement indicates the number of larger fatty particles. The higher the LDL cholesterol, the greater the risk of coronary artery disease. The higher the HDL cholesterol, the lower the risk.

Dietary cholesterol in the small intestine is absorbed into the bloodstream but not all cholesterol in the body comes from food. The major source is the liver which manufactures it.

A recycling of cholesterol occurs as it drains with the bile into the small intestine. The chief way the body rids itself of cholesterol is through the bowel with the elimination of feces.

Cholesterol is used to form bile salts which enhance fat absorption and help keep cholesterol in solution. A low level of bile salts can cause the cholesterol to form crystals, cholesterol gallstones.

The best way to reduce the "bad" cholesterol (LDL) level is by diet and exercise. Dietary fat enhances the absorption of cholesterol and stimulates the liver to form more of it; therefore fat intake should be restricted. Regular endurance-type exercise, walking, running, swimming, and so forth, tends to reduce LDL and increase HDL cholesterol. This is the greatest protection against fatty deposits in the arteries. For some individuals with various risk factors medications are prescribed to reduce the cholesterol level.

VALUE OF EXERCISE

Regular aerobic exercise improves the body's ability to utilize oxygen which is necessary to burn calories for the production of energy. The efficiency of the heart and lungs is improved; the resting heart rate is lowered and blood pressure is reduced.

Oxygen, unlike food, cannot be stored but it is readily available for ordinary action. The secret is to distribute it throughout the entire body, often to meet increased demands for it. During exercise the lungs are working hard to take in more oxygen, the heart is pumping strongly to circulate the blood, and the blood vessels are carrying the blood to active muscles for the energy production that is needed. How well these systems function determines endurance fitness.

When the body is not used it deteriorates. Symptoms of inadequate exercise include fatigue, falling asleep after a heavy meal, and experiencing exertion from climbing stairs.

■ Aerobic Exercise

Aerobic exercises are those which force the body to take in and distribute oxygen such as running, walking, swimming, and cycling. Exercise of this type enables the lungs to process more air with less effort. The heart becomes stronger, pumping out more blood with each stroke and therefore reducing the number of strokes per minute. The conditioned athlete has a very low resting heart rate because of the heart's efficiency. The number and size of blood vessels is increased to better distribute blood. As calories are being burned for energy, weight loss follows with the development of a leaner body.

Walking for fitness is the fastest growing participant sport in the country. Brisk walking on a regular schedule offers cardiovascular benefits, promotes weight loss, improves muscle tone, and prevents age-related illnesses. The walking must be brisk, last for at least 20–30 minutes without interruption, and be done at least three days a week to attain the aerobic benefits. The walk must be brisk enough to sufficiently elevate the heart and respiratory rate. Kenneth H. Cooper, M.D., the father of Aerobics, provides tables in his book, *Aerobics*, which give the amount of exercise optimum for one's age, sex, and conditioning. Before beginning an exercise program a person should check with his or her medical doctor to assure that it is appropriate. This applies even to children who may have a condition that would preclude the exercise.

CHAPTER SUMMARY

Today's focus on health is wellness or preventive medicine through proper diet and exercise. Holistic health and holistic medicine consider the well-being of the individual, physically, emotionally, and spiritually.

One has the choice to select a lifestyle that promotes health. This includes a positive attitude about one's self, a feeling of worth, and the willingness to accept responsibility for well-being.

The importance of a diet high in fiber, low in fat, and rich in vitamins was discussed in terms of cancer prevention. The danger of excessive fat intake was described and "good" and "bad" cholesterol were distinguished.

The value of regular aerobic exercise to increase the efficiency of the heart and lungs was explained.

■ Self-Study

Match

_____ 1. beta carotene

_____ 2. encephalins

_____ 3. legumes

_____ 4. antioxidants

_____ 5. phytochemicals

a) fight free radicals

b) peas and beans rich in protein and fiber

c) found in fruits, grains and vegetables

d) pain-fighting brain chemicals

e) used to make vitamin A

Multiple Choice

_____ 6. _____ is essential in the formation of red blood cells.
   a. Thiamine
   b. Riboflavin
   c. Vitamin B_{12}

_____ 7. Vitamin B deficiency most seriously affects the _____ system.
   a. digestive
   b. nervous
   c. urinary

_____ 8. Severe liver damage can result from excessive consumption of _____ vitamins.
   a. fat-soluble
   b. water-soluble

_____ 9. _____ fats tend to be solid.
   a. Saturated
   b. Unsaturated

_____ 10. _____ is the chemical name for fat.
   a. Triglyceride
   b. Cholesterol

True or False

_____ 11. Vitamins C and E are antioxidants.

_____ 12. Vitamin A is necessary for proper absorption of calcium and phosphorus from the digestive tract.

_____ 13. The B vitamins are water-soluble.

_____ 14. High-density lipoproteins (HDL) contribute to plaque deposits within arterial walls.

_____ 15. Regular endurance-type exercise reduces low-density lipoprotein (LDL).

(Answers on page 450)

Glossary of Terms

Abdominal muscles. Muscles of abdominal wall which assist in respiration

Abscess. Collection of pus in a cavity

Acetylcholine. Neuronal transmitter substance

Achlorhydria. Absence of hydrochloric acid from gastric juice

Achondroplasia. Disorder of cartilage formation in the fetus

Achondroplastic dwarf. Undersized person with short arms and legs but normal trunk

Acidosis. Excessive acidity of the blood and body fluids (pH of blood less than 7.3)

Acquired immune deficiency syndrome (AIDS). Viral infection of certain white blood cells that destroys a person's immune system

Acromegaly. Disease caused by excessive growth hormone in an adult

ACTH. See Adrenocorticotropic hormone

Activated lymphocytes. A type of white blood cell which provides cell-mediated immunity

Active immunity. Bodily produced antibodies

Acute. Sudden onset, short duration

Addison's disease. Disease of adrenal cortical hypoactivity

Adenocarcinoma. Cancer of a gland

Adenohypophysis. Anterior pituitary

Adenoma. Benign glandular tumor

Adenomatous or nodular goiter. Enlargement of thyroid due to tumors

ADH. See Antidiuretic hormone

Adhesions. Union of two surfaces normally separate

Adrenal diabetes. Hyperglycemia due to hyperadrenalism

Adrenocorticotropic hormone (ACTH). Hormonal stimulant of adrenal cortex

Adrenogenital syndrome. Adrenal virilism; excessive masculinization

Aerobic exercise. Physical exercise that increases heart and lung activity

Agglutination. Clumping of red blood cells

AIDS. See Acquired immune deficiency syndrome

Albinism. Congenital absence of melanin

Albuminuria. Plasma protein (albumin) in the urine

Aldosterone. Principal mineralocorticoid of adrenal cortex

Alkalosis. Excessive alkalinity of the blood and body fluids (pH of blood more than 7.4)

Alleles. One of two or more alternative forms of a gene at the same site on a chromosome

Allergen. Foreign protein causing an allergic reaction

Allergy. Hypersensitivity to normally harmless proteins

Alpha cells. Glucagon-producing cells of pancreas

ALS. See amyotrophic lateral sclerosis

Alveoli. Tiny, thin-walled air sacs of the lung

Alzheimer's disease. Premature senility

Amenorrhea. Absence of menstruation

Amphetamines. Drugs sometimes used as an appetite depressant

Amylase. Carbohydrate enzyme

Amyloid. Abnormal protein often found at autopsy in brain tissue of Alzheimer's disease patients

Amyotrophic lateral sclerosis (Lou Gehrig's disease). Degenerative disease of the motor neurons characterized by atrophy of muscles

Anaerobic. Absence of air or oxygen

Anaphylactic shock. Circulatory failure resulting from an allergic reaction

Anaphylaxis. Exaggerated hypersensitivity reaction to a previously encountered antigen

Anaplasia. Lacking differentiation and form

Androgens. Male hormones

Anemia. Disease of insufficient hemoglobin

Aneurysm. A dilation or saclike formation in a weakened blood vessel wall

Angina pectoris. Acute chest pain due to inadequate cardiac oxygen supply

Angiocardiography. X-ray examination of the heart using opaque dyes

Angioma. A benign tumor of blood vessels

Angioplasty. Opening of blood vessels by insertion of a small balloon through a catheter

Ankylosis. Fixation of a joint, often in an abnormal position

Anomaly. Deviation from the normal

Anorexia. Loss of appetite

Anorexia nervosa. Nutritional disease of psychoneurotic origin

Antibody. Molecule produced by the body in response to the presence of an antigen

Anticoagulants. Substances that prevent blood clotting

Antidiuretic hormone (ADH). Hormone of posterior pituitary affecting kidney tubules

Antigen. Protein not normally found in the body

Antihistamine. Drug that counteracts the effect of histamine

Anti-inflammatory hormones. Hormones that inhibit the inflammatory or immune response, e.g., cortisol

Antineoplastic agents. Substances that inhibit the growth of cancer cells

Antioxidant. Agent which fights cell-destroying free radicals

Anuria. Absence of urine formation

Aorta. Main trunk of the systemic circulation: largest artery that carries blood away from the heart

Aortic insufficiency. Valve to aorta does not close properly

Aortic stenosis. Narrowing of the valve leading to the aorta

Aphasia. Loss of speech

Aplastic. Lacking new development

ARC. AIDS-related complex

Areola. Darkly pigmented area surrounding the nipple

Arrhythmia. Abnormal rhythm of the heart beat

Arteriosclerosis. Hardening of the arteries

Ascites. Abnormal accumulation of fluid in the abdominal cavity

Ascorbic acid (Vitamin C). Vitamin essential for healthy membranes and night vision

Aseptic. Free from infectious material

Aspermia. Lack of formation or ejaculation of sperm

Aspirate. To withdraw fluid from a body cavity

Aspiration (pathogenic). Inhalation of regurgitated gastric contents into the pulmonary system

Astrocytoma. Benign, slow-growing brain tumor

Asymptomatic. Showing no symptoms

Atelectasis. A collapsed or airless state of the lung

Atherosclerosis. Development of lipid deposits in arterial walls

Atopic person. One with a genetic predisposition to allergies

Atresia. Absence or closure of a normal body opening

Atrial fibrillation. Rapid, uncoordinated impulse over the atria

Atrioventricular valves. Valves between the atria and ventricles that assure a one-way blood flow through the heart

Atrophy. Decreasing in size; wasting

Aura. Warning preceding an epileptic seizure and/or migraine headache

Auscultation. Listening for sounds inside the body, usually with a stethoscope

Autoimmune disease. Disorder in which antibodies act on a person's own tissue

Autonomic nervous system. Nerve network that controls smooth muscle and internal organs

Autosomes. All chromosomes other than sex chromosomes

Azotemia. Presence of nitrogen-containing compounds in the blood

Barium. Opaque substance used in some x-ray examinations

Basal cell carcinoma. A nonmetastasizing skin tumor

Basal ganglia. Areas deep in the cerebrum that control much automatic action

Benign. Nonmalignant

Beta-carotene. Precursor of vitamin A contained in deep yellow and dark green vegetables

Beta cells. Insulin-producing cells of the pancreas

Bicuspid valve. Also called mitral valve, situated between the left atria and ventricle

Bile. An emulsifier secreted by the liver to aid in fat digestion

Biliary calculi. Gallstones

Biliary cirrhosis. Liver degeneration due to chronic bile duct disease

Bilirubin. Orange pigment derived from hemoglobin

Biopsy. Microscopic examination of cells and tissues to detect the presence of cancer

Bleeding time. Screening test used in diagnosing coagulation disorders

Blood urea nitrogen (BUN). Indicator of kidney function

B-lymphocytes. Stimulate plasma cells to produce immunoglobulins

Bone callus. Network of woven bone formed between broken bone ends

Bowman's capsule. Site of initial urine formation

Bradycardia. Abnormally slow pulse rate

Bradykinin. Potent vasodilator

Bronchi. Branching air tubules from trachea to bronchioles

Bronchiectasis. Chronic dilation and distention of the bronchi with subsequent infection

Bronchioles. Smallest bronchi terminating in alveoli

Bronchogenic carcinoma. Most common type of lung cancer

Bronchoscope. Lighted tube designed to view bronchial interior

Bronchopneumonia. Acute inflammation of lungs and bronchioles

Bulbourethral glands. Pair of glands in the male that secretes into the urethra as it enters the penis

Bulimia. A gorge-and-purge syndrome

Bulla. A large, fluid-containing lesion

Bullae. Blisterlike structures formed by fusion of alveoli in emphysema

BUN. See Blood urea nitrogen

Bursa or bursae. Fluid-filled sacs that reduce friction near joints

Bursitis. Inflammation of a bursa

Cachexia. State of profound ill health; emaciation

Calcium. Mineral essential for bone formation, the blood clotting mechanism, and muscle contraction

Candida albicans. Fungus capable of causing vaginitis

Capillary fluid shift mechanism. Movement of fluid from the blood into tissue spaces

Carcinogenesis. Development of cancer

Carcinoma. A malignant tumor of epithelial or glandular tissue

Carcinoma in situ. Premalignant stage of cancer

Cardiac arrest. Sudden stoppage of heart action

Cardiac arrhythmia. Disturbance of heart rhythm

Cardiac catheterization. Procedure for examining the chambers of the heart

Cardiac cycle. Cycle of events during which an electrical impulse is conducted through the atria and ventricles causing alternate contraction and relaxation

Cardiac sphincter. Valve at entrance to stomach

Cardiogenic shock. Shock resulting from extensive myocardial infarction

Cardiopulmonary resuscitation (CPR). Emergency procedure for life support, which includes artificial respiration and manual external cardiac massage

Carotene. Plant pigment essential to the formation of vitamin A

Carotid arteries. Branches of the aorta sending blood to the head and upper extremities

Carotid phonoangiography (CPA) (Carotid audiofrequency analysis). Procedure to determine degree and location of carotid stenosis

Carpal tunnel syndrome. Repetitive strain injury of the wrist

Caseation. Destructive process forming cavities in lungs in tuberculosis

Caseous. Cheeselike mass resulting from destruction of tissue

Casts. Molds of kidney tubules consisting of protein and blood cells

Cataract. Opacity of the eye lens

Cell-mediated immunity (Cellular immunity). Acquired immunity characterized by T lymphocytes

Cerebral palsy. Muscular disorder caused by brain damage at or near the time of birth

Cerebral vascular accident (CVA). Stroke

Cerebrospinal fluid. Protective fluid around the brain and spinal cord

Cervix. Narrow lower end of the uterus adjoining the vagina

CGH. See Chorionic gonadotropic hormone

Chancre. Characteristic lesion of primary syphilis

Chemical carcinogens. Cancer-causing agents

Chemotaxis. Response involving movement to a chemical stimulus

Chemotherapy. Treatment of a disease with chemicals

Chlamydial infection. Prevalent venereal disease

Cholangiogram. X-ray films of bile duct system using radiopaque dyes

Cholecystectomy. Surgical removal of the gallbladder

Cholecystitis. Inflammation of the gallbladder

Cholecystogram. X-ray films of gallbladder using radiopaque dyes

Cholelithiasis. Formation or presence of gallstones

Cholesterol. Large waxy molecule which comprises artery-blocking plaque

Choriocarcinoma. Highly malignant tumor of the placenta

Chorionic gonadotropic hormone (CGH). Hormone secreted by the placenta

Chromosome. One of the thread-like structures in the nucleus of a cell that functions in the transmission of genetic information

Chronic condition. Gradual development, long term

Chronic obstructive pulmonary disease (COPD). Disorder in which the exchange of respiratory gases is deranged

Chronic ulcerative colitis. Inflammation of the large intestine due to unknown cause

Chymotrypsin. A proteolytic enzyme

Cilia. Hairlike structures that sweep the respiratory mucosa

Cirrhosis. Chronic degenerative liver disease with nodular regeneration and scarring

Clitoris. Small, elongated erectile body anterior to the urinary meatus in the female that is sensitive to sexual stimulation

Coarctation. Stricture or narrowing

Collagen. Fibrous protein in connective tissue

Collateral circulation. Accessory blood vessels

Colostomy. Artificial abdominal opening to allow evacuation of colon

Comminuted fracture. Bone fracture in which the bone is shattered or crushed

Complication. A new disease that develops concurrently with an existing one

Compound fracture. Bone fracture in which the skin is pierced

Computerized tomography (CT scan). Noninvasive x-ray technique for obtaining a cross-sectional view of the body

Concussion. Transient disorder of the nervous system resulting from a severe blow to the head

Congenital. Present at and existing from birth

Congenital disease. Disorder present at birth

Congestive heart failure. Inadequate heart action resulting in edema

Conjunctiva. Membrane that lines the eyelids and covers the eyeballs

Conn's syndrome. Disease of adrenal cortical hyperactivity

Consolidated. Solidified

Contusion. Injury to the brain from a severe impact

Convulsion. Involuntary contraction, or a series of contractions, of voluntary muscles

COPD. See Chronic obstructive pulmonary disease

Coronary arteriography. Selective injection of contrast material into coronary arteries for a film recording of blood-vessel action

Coronary thrombosis. Blood clot in coronary artery

Cor pulmonale. Right-sided heart failure due to chronic lung disease

Corpus luteum. Yellow glandular mass in the ovary formed from ruptured Graafian follicle

Cortisol. Principal glucocorticoid of adrenal cortex

Cortisone. Glucocorticoid usually converted to cortisol in humans

CPR. See Cardiopulmonary resuscitation

Creatine phosphate. Form of energy storage in muscles

Creatinine. Waste product of protein metabolism

Cretinism. Mental and physical retardation due to congenital thyroid deficiency

Cruciferous vegetables. Vegetables with cabbage-like odors which contain phytochemicals

Cryosurgery. Use of subfreezing temperature to destroy tissue

Cryptorchidism. Failure of the testes to descend into the scrotum

CT scan. See Computerized tomography

Cubic millimeter (mm^3). Unit of measure

Curettage. Scraping of material from the wall of a cavity or other surface such as scraping of the endometrium in a D&C

Cushing's syndrome. Disease of adrenal cortical hyperactivity

CVA. See Cerebral vascular accident

Cyanosis. Blue coloration of tissue due to lack of oxygen

Cyst. A fluid-filled sac

Cystic fibrosis. Disease of the exocrine glands

Cystic hyperplasia. Multiple cysts in the breast

Cystitis. Inflammation of the urinary bladder

Cystoscope. Instrument used to examine the bladder interior

Cytotoxic T cells. Cells capable of killing invading organisms and hence called killer cells

D&C. Dilation of the cervix and curettage, scraping of the endometrium

Debilitated. Totally weakened

Deciliter (dl). See Grams per 100 milliliter

Defibrillator. Device to correct ventricular fibrillation

Delirium tremens (DTs). An acute mental disturbance resulting from long-standing alcohol abuse, marked by shaking, delirium, and hallucinations

Dementia. Organic loss of intellectual function

Deoxyribonucleic acid (DNA). Blueprint for protein synthesis within the cell

Dermatophytosis. Athlete's foot

Dermis. The true skin

Dermoid cyst. Teratoma; ovarian cyst containing skin, hair, oil glands, and teeth

DES. See Diethylstilbestrol

Desensitize. To reduce sensitivity to an allergen, as in allergy shots

Detoxify. Make poisonous substances harmless

Diabetes insipidus. Disease resulting from antidiuretic hormone deficiency

Diabetes mellitus. Disease resulting from lack of insulin

Diabetic nephropathy. Kidney disease resulting from diabetes mellitus

Diabetic retinopathy. Vascular disorder of the retina that can result in blindness

Diagnosis. Determination of the nature of the disease

Dialysis. Method of artificially clearing blood of waste products

Diaphragm. Dome-shaped musculofibrous partition separating the thoracic and abdominal cavities; principal muscle of respiration

Diastole. Relaxing, filling phase of the heart

Diastolic pressure. Lowest pressure in the arteries

Diethylstilbestrol (DES). Synthetic hormone, formerly administered to prevent spontaneous abortion

Diffuse colloidal goiter. Endemic goiter caused by insufficient iodine in diet

Dilate. Enlarge

Dilantin. Anticonvulsant drug

Dilation. Widening

Disease. The unhealthy state of a body part or physiologic system

Disuse atrophy. Shrinkage or wasting through inactivity

Diuretic. Drug or other substance that promotes the formation and excretion of urine

Diverticulitis. Inflammation of diverticula (sacs)

Diverticulosis. Formation of pouches, or sacs, by the mucosa

Diverticulum. A small pouch or sac that forms in the intestinal wall

dl. See **Deciliter**

DNA. See Deoxyribonucleic acid

Dominant gene. Gene that will always be expressed

Dopamine. A neuronal transmitter substance that is deficient in Parkinson's disease

Doppler scanning. Technique used in ultrasound to monitor flowing blood or a beating heart

Down's syndrome. Mongolism

DTs. See Delirium tremens

Duodenal ulcer. Peptic ulcer of first segment of small intestine

Dysentery. Severe inflammation of the colon

Dysmenorrhea. Painful menstruation

Dyspareunia. Pain during sexual intercourse

Dyspepsia. Indigestion

Dysphagia. Difficulty in swallowing

Dysplasia. Abnormal development

Dyspnea. Shortness of breath

Dysuria. Painful urination

Ecchymosis. A bruise; superficial discoloration caused by escape of blood into the tissue

Echocardiography. Diagnostic procedure for studying the structure and motion of the heart

Eclampsia. Toxemia of pregnancy resulting in convulsions

E. coli. See *Escherichia coli*

Ectopic. Misplaced or malpositioned

Ectopic pregnancy. Implantation of fertilized ovum outside the uterus

Eczema or contact dermatitis. A noncontagious inflammatory skin disorder

Edema. Excess of fluid in the tissues

EEG. See Electroencephalogram

Ejaculatory ducts. Pair of ducts which penetrate the prostate gland to enter the male urethra

Electrocardiogram. Electrical recording of heart action that aids in the diagnosis of heart diseases

Electrocautery. Application of a needle heated by electric current for the destruction of tissue such as warts

Electroencephalogram (EEG). Electrical recording of brain waves

Electrolyte balance. Balance of salts: sodium, potassium, calcium, and others

Electromyogram (EMG). Record of electric activity in a skeletal muscle

Embolism. A detached thrombus

EMG. See Electromyogram

Emphysema. Inflation of the lungs with trapped air

Empyema. Accumulation of pus in the pleural cavity

Encephalin. Naturally occurring pain-relieving chemical

Encephalitis. Inflammation of the brain and meninges

Endarterectomy. Surgical procedure to remove blockage in carotid artery

Endocarditis. Inflammation of heart lining

Endocardium. Membrane lining the heart

Endocrine glands. Ductless glands of internal secretion

Endometriosis. Proliferation of endometrial tissue outside of the uterus

Endorphin. A body's natural pain fighter

Endoscope. Lighted instrument used to view interior of digestive tract

Endoscopic sclerotherapy. Procedure for treating esophageal varices

Epidermis. Outermost layer of skin

Epidermoid carcinoma. A cancer of epithelial tissue, skin, or mucous membranes

Epididymitis. Inflammation of epididymis

Epididymis. Coiled tube that lies along the outer wall of each testis and conducts sperm to the vas deferens or ductus deferens

Epilepsy. Disease of abnormal electrical discharges in the brain

Epinephrine (adrenalin). Bronchial dilator and hormone

Epistaxis. Bleeding from the nose

Epstein-Barr virus. Herpes virus that causes infectious mononucleosis

Erysipelas. An inflammatory skin infection caused by streptococci

Erythema. Skin area reddened by inflammation or infection

Erythematous. An area of skin reddened by congested blood vessels resulting from injury or inflammation

Erythroblastosis. Abnormal increase of erythroblasts, immature red cells

Erythroblastosis fetalis. Hemolytic anemia of the newborn

Erythrocytes. Red blood cells

Erythrocytosis. Abnormal increase of erythrocytes (red blood cells)

Erythropoiesis. The process of red cell development

Erythropoietin. Hormone stimulating red cell production

Escherichia coli (E. coli). Species of bacteria normally present in the intestines. Most frequent cause of urinary tract infections and a serious pathogen in wounds

Esophageal varices. Varicose veins of the esophagus

Esophagitis. Inflammation of the esophagus

Esophagoscope. Endoscope used to view interior of esophagus

Estrogen. Female hormone

Etiology. Cause of disease

Eunuchism. Loss of male hormones before puberty

Exacerbation. Period in which symptoms become more severe

Exfoliative cytology. Study of cells shed or scraped from a body surface

Exocrine glands. Glands of external secretion through ducts

Exophthalmos. Protrusion of eyeballs due to postocular edema

External intercostal muscles. Muscles between the ribs used in inspiration

Extracorporeal shockwave lithotripsy (ESWL). Procedure to shatter gallstones

Extradural hemorrhage. Hemorrhage outside the dura of the brain or spinal cord

Extrinsic factor. Vitamin B_{12}

Fallopian tubes. Pair of ducts opening at one end into the uterus and at the other end into the peritoneal cavity, over the ovary which convey the ova and sperm for fertilization

Familial polyposis. A hereditary disease in which numerous polyps develop in the intestinal tract

Fetal alcohol syndrome. Disease of babies born to alcoholic mothers

Fibrin. Plasma protein essential for blood clotting

Fibroblasts. Connective tissue cells capable of producing fibers

Fibrocystic disease. See Cystic hyperplasia

Fimbriae. Fringe-like projections at outer, open ends of fallopian tubes

Flatus. Gas of the intestinal tract

Fluoroscopy. Examination of form and motion of deep structures of the body by means of x-ray

Foramen ovale. Fetal opening between atria

Friable. Breakable

Fulminating. Disease of sudden onset and rapid progression

Functional disease. Abnormal condition in which there is no organic change

Furuncle. Suppurative staph infection originating in a gland or hair follicle

Galactosemia. Disease in which galactose cannot be used

Gangrene. Death of tissue due to loss of blood supply followed by bacterial invasion

Gastric ulcer. Peptic ulcer of the stomach

Gastritis. Inflammation of the stomach

Gastroscope. Endoscope used to view stomach interior

Gastroscopy. Inspection of stomach interior using a gastroscope

Gene. Unit of genetic material and inheritance

Genital herpes. Viral infection spread by intimate contact

Genital warts. Painful eruptions of the skin and mucous membranes of the genitalia caused by type 2 herpes simplex virus

Geriatrics. Branch of medicine dealing with the aged

Gerontology. Study of the problems of aging

Gigantism. Excessive size and stature usually caused by hypersecretion of growth hormone

Glioma. Malignant brain tumor

Glomerulonephritis. Kidney disease affecting glomeruli

Glomerulus. Tuft of capillaries through which blood filtration occurs

Glucagon. Hormone secreted by the pancreas to raise blood glucose level

Glucocorticoids. Steroid hormones of the adrenal cortex that increase synthesis of glucose and exert an anti-inflammatory effect

Glycogen. Storage form of glucose

Glycosuria. Sugar present in the urine

Goiter. Enlargement of the thyroid

Gonadotropins. Hormonal stimulant of sex glands

Gonococcus. Gonorrhea-producing organism

Gout. Joint disease resulting from excessive uric acid

Graafian follicle. Saclike structure containing ova

Grams per 100 milliliter (deciliter) (g/dl). Unit of measure

Grand mal epilepsy. Severe form of epilepsy

Granular contracted kidney. Shrunken condition of the kidney following long-standing kidney disease

Graves' disease. Disease of severe hyperthyroidism

Greenstick fracture. A cracked bone

Group A hemolytic streptococci. Organisms causing infection that leads to rheumatic fever

Gynecomastia. Enlargement of breasts in the male

HDL. See **High-density lipoprotein**

Heart block. Failure in the normal conduction of electrical impulses that control heart activity

Heart murmurs. Abnormal heart sounds indicating valve disease

Helper T cells. Cells which help the immune system by increasing the activity of killer cells, B cells, and suppressor T cells

Hematemesis. Bloody vomitus

Hematocrit. The volume percentage of erythrocytes in whole blood

Hematuria. Blood in the urine

Hemiplegia. Paralysis on one side of the body

Hemoglobin. Oxygen-carrying pigment of erythrocytes

Hemolysis. Rupture of red blood cells

Hemoptysis. Coughing up of blood

Hemorrhage. Large blood loss in a short period of time

Hemorrhoids. Varicose veins of the rectum

Heparin. Naturally occurring anticoagulant also used therapeutically

Hepatavax B. Vaccine providing immunity against virus type B hepatitis

Hepatic coma. State of unconsciousness due to liver dysfunction

Hepatitis. Inflammation of the liver

Hepatocarcinoma. Cancer of the liver

Hereditary. Genetically determined

Hermaphrodite. Person with ovarian and testicular tissue

Herniation of intervertebral disk. Slipped disk

Herpes simplex. Virus causing cold sores and a sexually transmitted disease.

Heterozygous. Having different alleles for a given trait

Hiatal hernia. Protrusion by part of the stomach through the diaphragm near the esophagus

High-density lipoprotein (HDL). Good cholesterol

Hirsutism. Abnormal hairiness, especially in women

Histamine. Substance released from damaged tissue causing dilation and increased permeability of blood vessels

HIV. See Human immunodeficiency virus

Hodgkin's disease. A malignant disease of the lymph nodes

Holistic health. Overall well-being of an individual

Holistic medicine. Treatment of the whole person including physical, emotional, and spiritual needs

Homeostasis. Maintenance of stability amidst changing conditions

Homozygous. Having identical alleles for a given trait

Hormones. Chemical messengers secreted by the endocrine glands

HPV. See Human papillomavirus

Human immunodeficiency virus. Virus that causes AIDS

Human papillomavirus (HPV). Virus responsible for genital warts and uterine cervical carcinoma

Humoral immunity. Immunity characterized by circulating antibodies (immunoglobulins) produced by plasma cells

Huntington's chorea. Hereditary disease causing mental and physical deterioration

Hydatidiform mole. Benign tumor of the placenta

Hydrocephalus. Excessive fluid in or around the brain

Hydrolithotripsy. Nonsurgical laser beam procedure that crushes kidney stones in patients who are immersed in a tank of water

Hydronephrosis. Dilation of renal pelvis with urine

Hydrosalpinx. Fluid-filled tube

Hydroureters. Distention of the ureters with obstructed urine

Hymen. Membranous fold that partly or completely closes the vaginal opening

Hyperactive. Excessively active functioning of an organism or body part such as an endocrine gland

Hyperactive bone marrow. Excessive production of blood cells

Hyperadrenalism. Overactivity of adrenal cortex

Hypercalcemia. Excessive calcium in the blood

Hyperemia. Increased amount of blood in an area

Hyperestrogenism. Hormonal imbalance that can cause feminization of males with cirrhosis of the liver

Hyperglycemia. Elevated blood glucose level

Hyperkalemia. An excess of potassium

Hypernephroma. Carcinoma of the kidney

Hyperparathyroidism. Overactivity of parathyroids

Hyperpituitarism. Overactivity of pituitary

Hyperplasia. Growth by increased number of cells

Hypersensitivity. Excessive reaction to a particular stimulus

Hypertension. High blood pressure

Hypertensive heart. Enlarged heart due to high blood pressure

Hyperthyroidism. Overactivity of thyroid

Hypertrophy. Enlargement of a structure

Hypervitaminosis. Excessive vitamin intake, particularly of vitamins A and D

Hypoactive. Diminished activity of an organism or body part such as an endocrine gland

Hypoadrenalism. Underactivity of adrenal cortex

Hypoalbuminemia. Albumin deficiency in the blood causing edema

Hypocalcemia. Abnormally low calcium level in the blood

Hypochromic. Lighter than normal color

Hypoglycemia. Abnormally low blood glucose level

Hypogonadism. Decreased functional activity of the gonads

Hypoparathyroidism. Underactivity of the parathyroids

Hypophysis. Pituitary gland

Hypopituitarism. Underactivity of the pituitary

Hypoplasia. Incomplete or underdevelopment of an organ or tissue

Hypoproteinemia. Deficiency of blood proteins

Hypotension. Low blood pressure

Hypothalamus. Portion of the brain which affects the autonomic nervous system, endocrine system and many body functions

Hypothyroidism. Underactivity of thyroid

Hypovolemic shock. Disruption of circulation due to severe blood volume reduction

Hypoxia. Decreased availability of oxygen to the tissues

Idiopathic. Cause of a disease is unknown

Idiopathic thrombocytopenia purpura (ITP). A severe platelet deficiency

Immune. Not susceptible to a particular disease

Immunoglobulin. Antibodies carried in plasma against a particular antigen; protective immunity

Immunoglobulins, IgE. Antibodies that cause allergic diseases; reagins

Impetigo. An acute contagious bacterial skin infection

Impotence. Inability to achieve and adequately maintain an erection

Infarct. Death of tissue

Infectious mononucleosis. Acute infection caused by the Epstein-Barr virus (EBV)

Inflammation. Tissue response to injury

Inflammatory exudate. Fluid that has oozed out of blood vessels as a result of inflammation

Influenza. Inflammation of the mucosa of the upper respiratory tract

Insulin. Hormone secreted by pancreas in order to regulate carbohydrate metabolism

Insulin-dependent diabetes mellitus (IDDM). Juvenile-onset diabetes

Insulin shock. Hypoglycemic shock

Intercostal muscles. Muscles between the ribs used in respiration

Interferon. Protective substance made by the body

Internal intercostal muscles. Muscles between the ribs used in expiration when breathing is difficult

Intima. Inner lining of blood vessels

Intravenous pyelogram (IVP). X-ray examination of kidney and ureters using contrast dye

Intrinsic factor. Substance in gastric juice

Intussusception. Telescoping of an intestinal segment into the part forward to it

Iodine. Mineral essential for the formation of thyroid hormone

Iron. Mineral essential to the formation of hemoglobin

Ischemia. Inadequate blood supply to an organ or tissue

ITP. See Idiopathic thrombocytopenia purpura

Jaundice. Yellowish discoloration of skin and tissues due to excessive bilirubin in the blood

Juxtaglomerular apparatus. Cells that secrete renin

Kaposi's sarcoma. Rare malignant, metastasizing neoplasm most often associated with AIDS

Karyotype. Chromosomal composition of the nucleus

Keloid. Hard, raised scar

Keratin. Tough fibrous protein produced by keratinocytes

Keratinize. To fill with keratin

Keratinocytes. Epidermal cells that synthesize keratin

Ketone bodies. Acetone and related byproducts of fat metabolism

Klinefelter's syndrome. Sexual anomaly due to an extra X chromosome

Kupffer's cells. Phagocytic cells lining blood spaces in the liver

Labia majora. Longitudinal folds of skin outside the labia minora

Labia minora. Small parallel folds of skin between the labia majora and the opening of the vagina

Lanoxin. Trademark for a medication to increase efficiency of heart contraction

Laparoscopy. Visualization of internal organs by means of a lighted tube inserted through a small abdominal incision

Larynx. Voice box

LDL. See **Low-density lipoprotein**

Legumes. Peas and beans rich in protein and fiber

Leiomyoma. A fibroid tumor, benign tumor of smooth muscle

Lesion. Structural abnormality

Lethargy. State of being indifferent, apathetic, or sluggish

Leukemia. Cancer of white blood cells and white blood cell forming tissue

Leukocytes. White blood cells

Leukocytosis. Excessive production of white blood cells

Leukopenia. Abnormal decrease in the number of white blood cells

Leukorrhea. Vaginal discharge other than blood

Libido. Sex urge

Ligament. Band of fibrous tissue connecting bones and strengthening joints

Ligate. To tie or bind together

Lipase. Enzyme which breaks down fat or lipid

Lipoma. A benign fatty tumor

Lipoprotein. Molecule consisting of fat and protein

Lithotripsy. Nonsurgical crushing of kidney stones or gallstones

Lobar pneumonia. Severe infection of one or more lobes of the lung

Low-density lipoprotein (LDL). Bad cholesterol

Lower respiratory diseases. Diseases of the trachea, bronchi, and lungs

Lues. Syphilis

Lumbar puncture. Spinal tap; removal of cerebrospinal fluid for diagnostic or therapeutic purposes

Lumen. Channel through a tube or tubular organ

Lumpectomy. Removal of tumor only

Lupus erythematosus (discoid). A noncontagious inflammatory skin disease

Lupus erythematosus (systemic). An autoimmune or collagen disease

Lyme disease. Acute inflammatory infection transmitted by a tickborne spirochete

Lymphadenopathy. Diseased lymph nodes

Lymphatic (lymphocytic). Pertaining to the lymph nodes

Lymphocytes. White blood cells produced in lymphoid tissue

Lymphocytic leukemia. Cancer of the lymph nodes

Lymphoid tissue. Lymph nodes, thymus gland, spleen

Lymphokines. Chemical factors produced by T lymphocytes to attract macrophages to the site of infection or inflammation

Lymphomas. Malignancies of lymphoid tissue

Lymph tissue. Specialized tissue for filtering out and removing bacteria

Macula. Spot or thickening distinguishable by color or otherwise from its surrounding

Magnetic resonance imaging (MRI). Non-invasive technique for internal visualization using magnetic fields

Malabsorption. Inability to absorb normal nutrients

Malaise. Vague feeling of weakness or discomfort

Malignant. An invasive tumor capable of metastasis

Malignant melanoma. A highly malignant skin tumor

Mammography. X-ray of the breast

Mast cells. Cells that release histamine in an inflammatory response

Medullary cavity. Cavity within long bones filled with yellow bone marrow

Melanin. Naturally occurring black pigment that gives color to hair, skin, and iris of the eye depending on the amount of pigment

Melanocytes. Epidermal cells that produce the pigment melanin

Melena. Stools darkened by blood pigments

Memory cells. T cells that cause a potent and rapid antibody response to an antigen

Menarche. Onset of menstruation

Meninges. Protective coverings on the brain and spinal cord

Meningitis. Inflammation of the meninges

Meningocele. Saclike protrusion of meninges and cerebrospinal fluid through a vertebral opening

Meningomyelocele. Protrusion of nerve fibers into a blind sac through a vertebral opening

Menopause. Time during which menstrual cycle wanes and stops

Menorrhagia. Excessive or prolonged bleeding during menstruation

Metaplasia. Conversion of normal tissue into abnormal

Metastasis. Spread of cancer to a distant site

Metrorrhagia. Bleeding between menstrual periods

mg. See Milligram

Migraine. Recurring headache caused by vascular changes and an imbalance in neurotransmitters, particularly serotonin

Milligram (mg). One-thousandth of a gram

Milliliter (ml). One-thousandth of a liter

Millimeter (mm). One-thousandth of a meter

Millimeter of mercury (mm Hg). Unit of measure (e.g., blood pressure)

Mineralocorticoid. Hormone secreted by the adrenal cortex; aldosterone, for example

Mitral insufficiency. Abnormally large opening in the mitral valve causing the valve to be incompetent

Mitral stenosis. Abnormally small opening in the mitral valve

Mitral valve. Atrioventricular valve between the left atria and ventricle, also called bicuspid valve

ml. See Milliliter

mm. See Millimeter

mm Hg. See Millimeter of mercury

Monocytes. Macrophages; large phagocytic leukocytes

Mons pubis. Rounded fleshy prominence over the pubic symphysis which becomes covered with hair at puberty

Motor neurons. Neurons that carry impulses to muscles and glands

MRI. See **Magnetic resonance imaging**

MS. See Multiple sclerosis

Mucosa. Mucous membrane lining digestive tract

Mucus. Thick fluid secreted by mucous membranes

Multiple sclerosis (MS). Demyelinating disease of the central nervous system

Muscular dystrophy. Degenerative muscle disease

Mutation. Permanent change in the DNA structure

Myasthenia gravis. Disease of the neuromuscular junction

Myelin. Lipid sheath on neuronal fibers, destroyed in multiple sclerosis

Myelocele. Open neural tube with disordered nerve fibers

Myelogenic (myelocytic). Produced in the bone marrow

Myelogenous leukemia. Cancer of the bone marrow

Myocardial infarction. Dead portion of heart muscle tissue

Myocardium. Cardiac (heart) muscle

Myoma. A benign tumor of muscle

Myxedema. Disease of severe hypothyroidism

Necrotic. Dead cells or tissue

Negative feedback mechanism. Control of hormonal secretion by inhibition of the stimulator

Neisseria meningitidis. Most common causative organism of meningitis

Neoplasia. New and abnormal growth

Neoplasm. A tumor

Nephron. Functional unit of the kidney where urine is formed

Nephrotripsy. Nonsurgical laser beam procedure in which kidney stones are crushed without use of a water tank

Neurogenic shock. Circulatory failure due to generalized vasodilation

Neurohypophysis. Posterior pituitary

Neurons. Nerve cells

Neurotropic. Organisms having an affinity for the nervous system

Nevus. A mole, a benign, pigmented skin tumor

Niacin. Vitamin essential to the enzyme system of cells

Night blindness. Inability to see in dim light

Nitroglycerine. Medication generally administered for angina pectoris to dilate coronary arteries

Nocturia. Need to urinate during the night

Nondisjunction. Failure of chromosomes to separate during cell division

Nonhemolytic streptococci. Organisms causing infectious endocarditis

Non-insulin-dependent diabetes mellitus (NIDDM). Maturity-onset diabetes

Nonsuppurative. Inflammation with no pus involvement

Normoblasts. Nucleated red blood cells

Nosocomial diseases. Acquired from a hospital environment

Nystagmus. Involuntary, rapid movement of the eyeball

Occluded. Closed

Occult blood. Blood in stools observed by means of chemical tests

Oliguria. Diminished urine secretion

Orchitis. Inflammation of the testes

Organic brain syndrome. Impaired brain function caused by long-term excessive consumption of alcohol

Organic obstruction. Material blockage

Osteitis fibrosa cystica. A decalcifying bone disease caused by hyperparathyroidism

Osteoarthritis. Chronic joint disease

Osteoblasts. Bone-forming cells

Osteoclasts. Bone-dissolving cells

Osteogenic sarcoma. Primary bone malignancy

Osteoma. Benign bone tumor

Osteomalacia. A decalcifying bone disease in adults due to a dietary deficiency

Osteomyelitis. Infectious bone inflammation

Osteopenia. Subnormally mineralized bone

Osteoporosis. Deterioration of the bone

Oxytocin. Hormone of posterior pituitary

Pacemaker. Patch of tissue setting heart rate; sinoatrial node

Paget's disease. (1) Cancer of the nipple and areola; (2) disease of excessive bone formation

Pallor. Paleness

Palpitations. Noticeably rapid heartbeat

Pancreatitis. Inflammation of the pancreas

Panhypopituitarism. Total absence of anterior pituitary hormones

Papilloma. A polyp or a benign epithelial tumor

Pap smear. Specimen of epithelial cells and cervical mucus obtained during a pelvic exam for cytologic evaluation

Papule. Small, solid raised skin lesion

Paralytic obstruction. Blockage due to failure of peristalsis

Parathormone. Parathyroid hormone

Paresis. Partial paralysis associated with organic loss of intellectual function

Parkinson's disease. Degenerative disease of the basal ganglia

Passive immunity. Administration of preformed antibodies in immune serum

Patch test. Skin test for identifying allergens

Patent ductus arteriosis. Congenital heart disease in which the ductus arteriosis, a fetal blood vessel, fails to close after birth

Pathogenesis. Development of abnormal condition

Pathogenic organisms. Disease-producing organisms

Pathologic aspiration. Drawing of vomitus or mucus into the respiratory tract

Pathologic fracture. A fracture due to a diseased bone

Pathology. Branch of medicine that studies the characteristics, causes, and effects of disease

Pediculosis. Louse infestation of the hair

Peptic ulcer. Gastric or duodenal ulcer

Pericardium. Double membranous sac enclosing the heart

Periosteum. Vascular connective tissue layer covering the surface of bone

Peripheral resistance. Resistance encountered by the blood from the walls of the vessels

Peristalsis. Rhythmical waves of smooth muscle contractions

Peritonitis. Inflammation of abdominal cavity lining

Petechiae. Small, flat, red spots caused by spontaneous hemorrhages in the skin

Petit mal epilepsy. Mild form of epilepsy

Phagocytic cells. Cells capable of digesting bacteria and other harmful substances

Pharynx. Throat

Phenobarbital. Anticonvulsant and sedative drug

Phenylketonuria. Disease in which phenylalanine cannot be used

Phlebitis. Inflammation of a vein

Phlebotomy. Incision of a vein for letting of blood

Phytochemicals. Substances contained in fruits, vegetables, and grain which may prevent cancer

Pilonidal cyst. A sebaceous cyst formed in the buttocks

Pipe-stem colon. Appearance of the colon in chronic ulcerative colitis in which the normal pouch-like markings are lacking

Placenta. Structure joining fetus and mother in the uterus

Plantar warts. Common warts on the sole of the feet caused by a virus

Plaque. Fatty deposit on blood vessel walls in atherosclerosis

Platelets. Formed elements of the blood that initiate the clotting mechanism

Pleura. Delicate membrane enclosing the lung

Pleural cavity. Space between lungs and inner chest wall

Pleural membrane. Double-layered membrane forming pleural cavity

Pleurisy. Inflammation of the pleural membranes

Pleurocentesis. Surgical puncture and drainage of the pleural space

Pneumothorax. Entrance of air or gas into the pleural cavity

Poison ivy. Plant that causes severe allergic contact dermatitis in many people

Poliomyelitis. Viral disease affecting motor neurons

Polycystic kidney. Congenital kidney disease associated with multiple cyst formation

Polydactyly. Extra fingers or toes

Polydipsia. Excessive thirst

Polymorphs. Polymorphonuclear leukocytes, neutrophils

Polyuria. Excessive urination

Portal vein. Vein that conveys nutrient-rich blood to the liver

Potassium. Mineral essential to heart and muscle action

Pott's disease. A form of tuberculosis affecting the vertebral column of children

Preeclampsia. First phase of toxemia of pregnancy

Premature ventricular contraction (PVC). A cardiac arrhythmia

Premenstrual syndrome (PMS) also called premenstrual tension (PMT). Syndrome of nervous tension, irritability, weight gain, edema, and clumsiness preceding onset of menstruation

Prepuce (foreskin). Flap of loosely attached skin covering the glans penis that is often removed shortly after birth in the procedure called circumcision

Primary atypical pneumonia. An acute inflammation of the upper respiratory tract caused by a variety of viruses

Primary follicle. Ova surrounded by a single layer of cells already present in high numbers in females at birth

Primary hypertension. Elevated blood pressure not caused by another disease

Proctoscope. Lighted tube used to examine rectum

Proerythroblasts or **erythroblasts.** Primitive red blood cells

Progesterone. Female hormone

Prognosis. Predicted course and outcome of the disease

Prolactin. Gonadotropic hormone

Prolapse. Falling or sliding of an organ from its normal position in the body

Prostate gland. Firm structure in males that surrounds the neck of the urinary bladder and urethra and contributes to the formation of semen

Prostatic hyperplasia. Benign enlargement of the prostate

Prostatitis. Inflammation of the prostate

Prothrombin. Enzyme essential to blood coagulation

Pruritus. Itching

Psoriasis. A chronic hereditary skin disease

Psychogenic factors. Emotional or psychological factors

Puerperal sepsis. Infection of the endometrium after childbirth or abortion

Puerperium. Period after childbirth

Pulmonary edema. Accumulation of fluid in lung tissues and alveoli

Pulmonary hypertension. Condition of abnormally high pressure within the pulmonary circulation

Pulmonary stenosis. Abnormally small opening to pulmonary artery that prevents proper oxygenation of the blood

Purpura. Petechiae; flat, red spots caused by small hemorrhages

Pustule. Pus-containing lesion

Pyelitis. Inflammation of the renal pelvis

Pyelonephritis. Suppurative inflammation of the kidneys and renal pelvis

Pyloric sphincter. Valve at entrance to small intestine

Pyloric stenosis. Narrowing of the pyloric sphincter at the outlet of the stomach causing an obstruction

Pyogenic organisms. Pus-forming bacteria

Pyosalpinx. Pus-filled tube

Pyuria. Pus in the urine

Rabies. Hydrophobia, fatal viral disease transmitted by a rabid animal

Radical mastectomy. Removal of breast, chest muscles, and axillary lymph nodes

Radiopaque dyes. Dyes used to show contrast on x-ray films

Rales. Abnormal respiratory sounds heard on auscultation of the chest

Rapid plasma reagin (RPR) test. Diagnostic procedure for syphilis

Raynaud's disease. Disease characterized by poor blood flow to fingers or toes brought on by cold or stress

Reagins. Antibodies formed by allergy sufferers

Recessive gene. Gene that is expressed in the homozygous condition

Reduction. Alignment of broken bone ends to promote healing

Reflux. Backward flow

Regeneration. Replacement of damaged or diseased cells

Regional enteritis. Inflammation of the intestine due to unknown cause

Regurgitation. Abnormal back flow of fluid

Relapse. Return of a disease

Releasing factors. Stimulatory substances sent from hypothalamus to anterior pituitary

Remission. Period in which symptoms subside

Renal pelvis. Juncture between the kidneys and ureters

Renin. Enzyme secreted in kidney to raise blood pressure

Resolution. Return to normal state, as in a lung after lobar pneumonia

Respiratory epithelium. Mucous membrane lining respiratory tract

Resuscitation. Restoration to consciousness after respirations have ceased

Reticulocytes. Red blood cells with endoplasmic reticulum

Reye's syndrome. Potentially serious neurologic illness that sometimes develops in children following a viral infection

Rhabdomyosarcoma. Malignant muscle tumor

Rh factor. A protein factor; an antigen present on the red blood cells of about 85 percent of the population

Rhinitis. Inflammation of mucous membranes of the nose

Rhodopsin. Light-absorbing pigment in the rods of the retina

Riboflavin. Vitamin essential for cellular metabolism

Rickets. Bone disease of infancy and early childhood caused by a vitamin D deficiency

Ringworm. A contagious skin infection caused by fungus

RPR. See Rapid plasma reagin

Salmonella. Bacteria causing typhoid fever, some forms of gastroenteritis, and food poisoning

Salpingitis. Inflammation of the fallopian tubes

Sarcoma. A malignant tumor of connective tissue

Scabies. A contagious skin disease caused by a parasite

Sclera. White of the eye

Sclerotic. Hard

Scrotum. Sac-like structure outside the body wall containing the testes

Sebaceous glands. Oil glands

Seborrheic dermatitis. Chronic dandruff

Seborrheic keratosis. Horny lesions of excess keratin

Sebum. Oil secretion of sebaceous glands

Secondary hypertension. Elevated blood pressure due to another disease

Seizures. A form of convulsions

Seminal vesicle. Either of the paired sac-like glandular structures that lie behind the male urinary bladder and contribute to the formation of semen

Seminiferous tubules. Site of sperm development within the testes

Seminoma. Highly malignant tumor of the seminiferous tubules

Senility. Loss of mental, physical, or emotional control associated with aging

Sensory neurons. Neurons that convey impulses to the central nervous system

Septic embolism. A detached clot containing pus-forming bacteria

Septicemia. Systemic infection of the blood

Sequela. One disease condition resulting from another

Sequestrum. Piece of dead bone separated from sound bone by necrosis

Serotonin. A neurotransmitter substance and vasoconstrictor

Sex-linked inheritance. Acquisition of traits on the sex chromosomes

Shingles. Herpes zoster; viral infection of sensory neurons

Shock. Failure of circulatory system to meet tissue needs

Sickle cell anemia. An inherited red blood cell deficiency generally confined to blacks

Signs. Objective evidence of disease

Simmond's syndrome. A premature senility

Sinoatrial node (S.A. node). Specialized patch of tissue also called the pacemaker

Sinuses (paranasal). Spaces within the skull bones lined with mucous membrane and opening to the nasal cavity

Sodium. Mineral essential for the transmission of nerve impulses and muscle contraction

Somatotropin. Growth hormone of the anterior pituitary

Somnolence. Unnatural sleepiness or drowsiness

Spasmogen. Substance that causes spasmodic contraction of the bronchial musculature; histamine

Spastic colon. Irritable bowel; colitis

Specific gravity. Measure of fluid concentration

Spheroidal. Round

Spider veins. Small, red, wavy networks of superficial veins

Spina bifida. Incomplete closure of the vertebral column

Spina bifida occulta. Defect of the vertebral column hidden by intact skin and evident only by radiologic examination

Spirometer. Instrument used to measure ability of lungs to move air in and out

Spirometry. Laboratory test of lung capacity by means of a spirometer

Splenectomy. Removal of the spleen

Splenomegaly. Enlargement of the spleen

Sprain. A joint injury resulting from wrenching or twisting

Spur. Spicule of projecting bone formed in arthritic joints

Squamous cell carcinoma. A malignant skin tumor

Staghorn calculus. Kidney stone named for its shape as it completely blocks the renal pelvis

Staphylococci. Microorganisms always present on the skin; may cause infection

Stasis. Stoppage or slowing of flow

Status asthmaticus. Severe asthma attack that does not respond to usual treatment

STD. Sexually transmitted disease

Stenosis. Narrowing of an opening

Strabismus. Crossed eyes

Strains. Pulled muscles

Streptococci. Microorganisms normally present in the throat; may cause infection

Streptokinase. Enzyme present in hemolytic streptococci used to dissolve blood clots

Striae. Streaks or lines that often result from tension in the skin as seen in the abdomen following pregnancy. Classic sign in hyperadrenalism (also called stretch marks)

Stroke. Cerebrovascular accident (CVA)

Subarachnoid hemorrhage. Hemorrhage between the arachnoid and pia mater layers covering the brain

Subdural hemorrhage. Hemorrhage between the dura mater and arachnoid layers covering the brain

Suppressor T cells. Cells that suppress B cell activity

Suppurative. Inflammation with pus formation

Symptoms. Subjective evidence of disease

Syncope. Fainting due to cerebral anemia

Syndrome. Symptoms occurring concurrently

Synovial membrane. Lining of joint capsule

Systole. Contracting phase of the heart

Systolic pressure. Highest pressure in the arteries

Tachycardia. Rapid heart beat

Tay-Sachs disease. Autosomal recessive condition

T-cells. Whole cell antibodies

Tendon. Band of strong fibrous tissue that connects muscle to bone

Teratoma. Highly malignant tumor of the testes, whereas in the female, benign tumor of the ovary

Tetanus. Lockjaw; disease characterized by muscle spasms and convulsions

Tetanus antitoxin. Passive immunization against tetanus

Tetanus toxoid. Active immunization against tetanus

Tetany. Sustained contraction of muscle

Tetralogy of Fallot. Serious congenital heart defect consisting of four (tetra) abnormalities

Thiamin-Vitamin B$_1$. Coenzyme necessary for carbohydrate metabolism, the lack of which affects the cardiovascular and nervous systems

Thrombocytopenia. Scarcity of blood platelets

Thrombolytic drugs. Medication to dissolve blood clots

Thrombophlebitis. Blood clot in an inflamed vein

Thrombosis. Development of blood clots on the inner wall of a blood vessel

Thyrotropin. Anterior pituitary stimulant of thyroid gland

Thyroxine. Thyroid hormone (T$_4$)

TIA. See Transient ischemic attack

Tissue plasminogen activator (TPA). Thrombolytic (blood-clot dissolving) drug used in the treatment of heart disease

T lymphocytes. Lymphocytes processed by the thymus gland to provide immunity against specific antigens

Toxic shock syndrome (TSS). Infection of *Staphylococcus aureus*

Toxins. Poisonous substances produced by pathogenic organisms, certain animals, and some plants

Toxoid. Chemically altered toxin

TPA. See Tissue plasminogen activator

TPI. See *Treponema pallidum* immobilization

Trachea. Windpipe

Tracheobronchitis. Inflammation of the trachea and bronchi

Tracheostomy. Opening into the trachea through which a tube may be inserted and the airway suctioned

Tracheotomy. Surgical opening of the trachea to free the air passageway

Transient ischemic attack (TIA). Period of cerebrovascular insufficiency

Trauma. Wound or injury

Tremor. Purposeless, quivering motions

Treponema pallidum. Spirochete causing syphilis

Treponema pallidum **immobilization (TPI).** Test for the presence of antibodies against *Treponema pallidum*

Trichomonas. Parasite causing vaginitis

Tricuspid valve. Atrioventricular valve between right atria and ventricle

Triglyceride. Chemical name for fat

Triiodothyronine. Thyroid hormone (T_3)

Trisomy 21. Chromosome 21 in triplicate

Trypsin. Proteolytic enzyme

TSS. See Toxic shock syndrome

Tubercle. Small, rounded nodule characteristic of tuberculosis

Tubercle bacillus. Organism causing tuberculosis

Tuberculin test. Test to determine past or present tuberculosis infection based on a skin reaction to a purified protein of the tubercle bacilli

Turner's syndrome. Sexual anomaly due to missing one sex chromosome

Ultrasonography. Process of imaging deep structures of the body by measuring and recording the reflexion of pulsed or continuous high-frequency sound waves

Ultrasound. Sound waves of the very high frequency of over 20,000 vibrations per second which can be used diagnostically and therapeutically

Ultrasound arteriography. Noninvasive test to measure velocity of blood and degree of carotid stenosis

Upper respiratory diseases. Diseases of the nose and throat

Urea. Waste product of protein metabolism

Uremia. Toxic condition of the blood resulting from kidney failure

Ureterocele. Prolapse of the terminal portion of the ureter into the bladder

Ureters. Pair of urinary tubes connecting kidneys to bladder

Urethra. Single urinary tube from the bladder to body exterior

Urethritis. Inflammation of the urethra

Uric acid. Product of metabolism of nucleic acids present in the blood and excreted in the urine

Urinalysis. Physical, chemical, or microscopic examination of urine

Urinary calculi. Stones in the kidney system

Urticaria. Hives

Uterus. Hollow, pear-shaped internal organ of reproduction in which the fertilized ovum is implanted and the fetus develops

Vaccine. Dead or deactivated pathogens that can engender immunity

Vagina. Part of the female genitalia that forms a canal from the opening in the vestibule to the uterine cervix

Vaginal opening. Entrance to the vagina

Vaginitis. Inflammation of the vagina

Valvular insufficiency. Inability of a valve to close

Varicose veins. Swollen, dilated veins

Vas deferens. Duct of the testes which conveys sperm through the inguinal canal into the abdominal cavity where it helps to form the ejaculatory duct

Vasopressin. Antidiuretic hormone

VDRL test. Screening procedure for syphilis

Vegetations. Small growths on diseased heart valves

Ventricles. Spaces within the brain in which cerebrospinal fluid is made

Ventricular fibrillation. Rapid, irregular, ineffective twitches of ventricles

Verucca vulgaris. Warts

Vesicle. Small, blisterlike lesion

Vitamin K. Essential to blood-clotting mechanism

Vitiligo. Loss of skin pigmentation

Volvulus. Twisting of the intestine on itself

Vulva. Female external genitalia

Wernicke's encephalopathy. Brain disease associated with chronic alcoholism

Wheal. Lesion of hives

Wheezing. Respiratory sound indicating narrowed air passageways

Whiplash. Neck sprain

Wilms' tumor. Malignant tumor of the kidney occurring in young children

Yeast infection. Vaginal infection caused by a fungus

References

Barlow AL, et al: Set-up and administration of Moctanin™ (Monoctanoin) for retained cholesterol stones in the common bile duct. Soc Gastrointest Assist J 9(3):112–14, Winter 1987.

Becker CD, et al: Treatment of retained cystic duct stones using extracorporeal shockwave lithotripsy. Am J Roentgen 148(6):1121–22, June 1987.

Bradley WG: Recent views on amyotrophic lateral sclerosis with emphasis on electrophysiological studies. Muscle Nerve 10(6):490–50, July-August 1987.

Brown P: How does HIV cause AIDS? New Scientist 31–35, July 18, 1992.

Expanded Surveillance Case Definition for AIDS among Adolescents and Adults. CDC Morbidity and Mortality Weekly Report, Vol. 41, Dec. 18, 1992, 4–11.

Fitzpatrick TB, et al: Dermatology in General Medicine, 3rd ed. New York, McGraw-Hill, 1987.

Fragile X Southeast Network, C/O Child Advocacy Commission of Durham, P.O. Box 1151, Durham, NC 27702.

Gallo RC, and Montagnier L: AIDS in 1988. Sci. Am. 259(4):41–48, ct. 1988.

Groer ME, and Skekleton ME: Basic Pathophysiology, 3rd ed. St. Louis, C.V. Mosby, 1989.

Guyton AC: Human Physiology and Mechanisms of Disease, 5th ed. Philadelphia, W.B. Saunders, 1992.

Guyton AC: Textbook of Medical Physiology. Philadelphia, W.B. Saunders, 8th ed., 1991.

Farber E: Cancer Development and Its Natural History. Proceedings of the Second National Conference on Cancer Prevention and Detection, Seattle, Wash., 1676–1679, June, 1987.

Hillet AD, and Miller RN: Management of bulbar symptoms in amyotrophic lateral sclerosis. Adv Exp Med Biol 209:201–21, 1987.

Holmes BC: Sexual Lifestyles and Cancer Risk. Cancer Prevention and Detection: Lifestyles. Fifth National Conference on Cancer Nursing, American Cancer Society, September 1987.

Hudson AJ, Jr: Outpatient management of amyotrophic lateral sclerosis. Semin Neurol 7(4):344–51, December 1987.

Kent TH, and Hart MN: Introduction to Human Disease, 3rd ed. Norwalk, Connecticut, Appleton-Century-Crofts, 1993.

Konradi D, and Stockert P: A close-up look at leukemia. Nursing 19(6):34–42, June 1989.

Kosowicz J: Atlas of Endocrine Diseases. Bowie, Maryland, Charles Press, 1978.

Koutsky LA, et al: Underdiagnosis of Genital Herpes by Current Clinical and Viral-Isolation Procedures. New England J. of Med. 326:1533–1539, June 4, 1992.

Le Maistre CA: Reflections on Disease Prevention. Proceedings of the Second National Conference on Cancer Prevention and Detection. Proceedings of the Second National Conference on Cancer Prevention and Detection, Seattle, Wash., June, 1987.

Maddox J: Where the AIDS virus hides away. Nature, 362:287, March 25, 1993.

National Fragile X Foundation, 1441 York Street, Suite 215, Denver, CO 80206.

Netter FH: Ciba Collection of Medical Illustrations. West Caldwell, New Jersey, Ciba Pharmaceutical Co. Vols 1–8, 1993.

1993 Revised Classification System for HIV Infection. CDC Morbidity and Mortality Weekly Report, Vol. 41, Dec. 18, 1992, 1–3.

Palca J: AIDS: The Evolution of an Infection. Research News 941, November, 1991.

Pinsky PF, et al: Reye's syndrome and aspirin: Evidence for a dose response effect. JAMA, 657(5): August 5, 1988.

Price SA, and Wilson L: Pathophysiology: Clinical Concepts of Disease Processes, 4th ed. New York, McGraw-Hill, 1992.

Purtilo DT: A Survey of Human Disease, 2nd ed. Menlo Park, California, Addison-Wesley, 1989.

Ross SO, and Krieger JN: The latest studies on occupational exposure to HIV. AJN 89:1424–5, November 1989.

Sheldon H: Boyd's Introduction to the Study of Disease, 11th ed. Philadelphia, Lea & Febiger, 1992.

Sloane E: Biology of Women, 3rd ed. Albany, Delmar, 1993.

Sochurek H: Medicine's New Vision. Easton, Pennsylvania, Mack Publishing Co, 1988.

Solomon J, et al: When the patient suffers from esophageal bleeding. RN 50(2):24–27, February 1987.

Stalheim-Smith A, and Fitch GK: Understanding Human Anatomy and Physiology. Minneapolis/St. Paul, West Publishing Company, 1993.

Temin HM, and Bolognesi DP: Where has HIV been hiding? Nature 362:292–293, March 25, 1993.

Tilkian SM, et al: Clinical Implications of Laboratory Tests, 4th ed. St. Louis, C.V. Mosby, 1987.

Tortora GJ, and Grabowski SR: Principles of Anatomy and Physiology, 7th ed. New York, Harper and Row, 1993.

Walter JB: An Introduction to the Principles of Disease, 3rd ed. Philadelphia, W.B. Saunders, 1992.

Warden-Tamparo C, and Lewis MA: Diseases of the Human Body, Philadelphia, F.A. Davis, 1989.

Answers to Self-Study Questions

Chapter 1
1. T
2. F
3. T
4. F
5. T
6. F
7. F
8. T
9. F
10. T
11. b
12. e
13. a
14. d
15. c

Chapter 2
1. F
2. T
3. F
4. F
5. T
6. F
7. T
8. F
9. T
10. T
11. T
12. F
13. F
14. T

15. T
16. d
17. b
18. c
19. a
20. e
21. b
22. a
23. b
24. b
25. a

Chapter 3
1. F
2. T
3. T
4. T
5. T
6. F
7. T
8. T
9. T
10. F
11. F
12. F
13. F
14. T
15. T
16. F
17. T
18. T
19. T
20. F

21. c
22. a
23. b
24. d
25. e

Chapter 4
1. E
2. C
3. A
4. B
5. D
6. A
7. B
8. C
9. E
10. A
11. F
12. T
13. T
14. F
15. T
16. T
17. F
18. T
19. T
20. F

Chapter 5
1. T
2. T
3. T

4. F
5. T
6. F
7. T
8. F
9. F
10. T
11. d
12. e
13. c
14. b
15. a
16. c
17. b
18. a
19. e
20. d

Chapter 6
1. T
2. F
3. F
4. F
5. T
6. F
7. T
8. T
9. F
10. T
11. d
12. c
13. e
14. b

15. a
16. c
17. b
18. c
19. c
20. c

Chapter 7
1. T
2. T
3. F
4. F
5. F
6. F
7. F
8. T
9. F
10. F
11. b
12. d
13. c
14. b
15. c
16. b
17. b
18. b
19. b
20. b

Chapter 8
1. b
2. b

3. a
4. c
5. b
6. b
7. a
8. a
9. b
10. a
11. T
12. T
13. T
14. F
15. F
16. d
17. a
18. b
19. e
20. c

Chapter 9
1. F
2. F
3. T
4. F
5. T
6. T
7. T
8. F
9. T
10. T
11. T
12. F
13. T

14. T
15. F
16. c
17. a
18. d
19. b
20. e
21. d
22. e
23. c
24. d
25. a

Chapter 10

1. F
2. T
3. F
4. T
5. F
6. T
7. T
8. T
9. T
10. F
11. T
12. F
13. T
14. F
15. F
16. a
17. b
18. b
19. a
20. c
21. b
22. b
23. a
24. b
25. a

Chapter 11

1. T
2. T
3. T
4. T
5. T
6. F
7. F
8. T
9. T
10. T
11. b
12. a
13. a
14. a
15. b
16. a
17. b
18. a
19. a
20. c

Chapter 12

1. T
2. T
3. T
4. F
5. F
6. F
7. T
8. T
9. F
10. F
11. F
12. T
13. T
14. F
15. F
16. e
17. a

18. c
19. b
20. d
21. d
22. d
23. c
24. b
25. c

Chapter 13

1. T
2. F
3. F
4. F
5. F
6. F
7. T
8. F
9. T
10. T
11. F
12. F
13. F
14. F
15. T
16. e
17. c
18. d
19. b
20. a
21. b
22. b
23. b
24. b
25. b

Chapter 14

1. F
2. F
3. F

4. F
5. T
6. T
7. T
8. F
9. F
10. T
11. c
12. e
13. b
14. a
15. d
16. a
17. b
18. a
19. b
20. a
21. e
22. d
23. a
24. b
25. c

Chapter 15

1. T
2. T
3. F
4. T
5. F
6. F
7. F
8. F
9. T
10. F
11. F
12. T
13. T
14. F
15. T
16. e

17. b
18. d
19. a
20. c

Chapter 16

1. c
2. b
3. a
4. b
5. b
6. d
7. e
8. b
9. c
10. a
11. T
12. F
13. F
14. T
15. T
16. T
17. T
18. F
19. F
20. T

Chapter 17

1. T
2. F
3. F
4. F
5. T
6. T
7. F
8. F
9. T
10. F
11. e
12. c
13. b

14. d
15. a
16. e
17. d
18. c
19. b
20. a

Chapter 18

1. T
2. T
3. F
4. T
5. T
6. F
7. T
8. F
9. T
10. T
11. d
12. e
13. c
14. b
15. a

Chapter 19

1. e
2. d
3. b
4. a
5. c
6. c
7. b
8. a
9. a
10. a
11. T
12. F
13. T
14. F
15. T

Index

A

abdominal muscle(s), in respiration, 217
abscess
  Bartholin's gland, 297
  brain, 335, 336*f*
  pulmonary. *See also* empyema
    in bronchiectasis, 227
  skin, 377
acetylcholine, in myasthenia gravis,
    367–368
achlorhydria, 178
achondroplasia, 48
achondroplastic dwarfism, 48, 49*f*
acid–base balance, 148
acidosis, 148
  in diabetes mellitus, 283
acne, 386, 387*f*
acquired immune deficiency syndrome, 20
  causative agent of, 20
  diagnosis of, 319
  latency period of, 20
  prevention, precautions for health-care
    professionals, 21–22
  risk groups for, 20
  symptoms of, 20
  transmission of, 20
  vaccine, development of, 22
acquired immunity, 15
acromegaly, 252, 253*f*
ACTH. *See* adrenocorticotropic hormone
activated lymphocyte(s), 15, 17, 17*f*
active immunity
  versus passive immunity, 23*f*
  vaccination and, 22–23
acute disease, definition of, 8

Addison's disease, 67, 276–278
adenocarcinoma, 36
  of breasts, 301
  of pancreas, 210
  of stomach, 37*f*, 176*f*
  vaginal, 300–301
adenohypophysis, 250, 250*f*. *See also* pituitary gland, anterior
adenoma(s), 41–42, 42*f*
  pituitary, 252
adenomatous goiter, 264–266
ADH. *See* antidiuretic hormone
adhesion(s), 15
  effects on fallopian tubes, 295–296,
    296*f*
  intestinal, 184
adrenal cortex, 272, 272*f*, 273
  diseases of, 274–278
adrenal cortical hormones, in response to
    stress, 393–395, 395*f*
adrenal diabetes, 274
adrenal gland(s)
  function, 272–274
    assessment of, 287
  structure of, 272, 272*f*
adrenalin (epinephrine), 25, 226, 393
adrenal medulla, 272, 272*f*, 273–274
adrenal virilism, 274, 276, 277*f*
adrenocorticotropic hormone, 252, 272
  deficiency, 254
  in response to stress, 393–394
adrenogenital syndrome, 274–275, 276*f*
aerobic exercise, 413
Aerobics (Cooper), 413
agglutination, 25
aging, effects of, 399–403

AIDS. *See* acquired immune deficiency syndrome
alarm reaction, 393
albinism, 374
albumin, 161, 194
    production, 202
albuminuria, 150, 161–162
alcohol
    effects on nervous system, 76–77
    and pregnancy, 78–79
alcoholic cirrhosis of liver, 199–203
Alcoholics Anonymous, 80
alcoholism, 75–80
    complications of, 79f
    effects on cardiovascular system, 78
    effects on digestive system, 77–78
    signs and symptoms of, 76
    treatment of, 79–80
aldosterone, 273
    actions of, 149
alkaline phosphatase, 368
alkalosis, 148
alleles, 46
allergen(s), in asthma, 224
allergic reaction, 24f
allergic rhinitis, 220–221
allergies, 23–27. *See also* hypersensitivity
    inflammation due to, 12f
allergy shots, 24
alpha cells, 280–281
ALS. *See* amyotrophic lateral sclerosis
alveoli, 217, 228
    in disease, 235, 235f
    in emphysema, 228
Alzheimer's disease, 401–402
amenorrhea, 69–70, 302–303
amphetamines, and weight loss, 74
amylase, 208, 210
amyloid protein, 402
amyotrophic lateral sclerosis, 337
anabolic steroids, 273
anaerobic bacteria, 333
analgesics, 397
anaphylactic shock, 25–26, 26f, 142, 142f
    vascular events in, 25–26, 27f
anaphylaxis, 24–25
    treatment for, 25
anaplasia, 36–37
androgen(s), adrenal, 273

anemia, 87–93. *See also* blood, diseases of
    aplastic, 5, 92
    causes of, 92f
    diagnosis of, 99
    hemolytic, 88–92
        jaundice in, 197
    hypochromic, 88
    iron-deficiency, 67
    pernicious, 64, 88, 176, 188
    secondary, 92–93
    sickle cell, 51, 88–89
    spheroidal (spherocytic), 89
aneurysm(s), 135–136, 137f
    cerebral, 344, 344f
angina pectoris, 111, 141
angiocardiography, 125
angiography, cerebral, 347–348
angioma, 41, 42f
angioplasty, 111
angiotensin, 148
ankylosis, 362
anomalies
    genetic, 4, 7
    sex chromosome, 55–56
anorexia
    cancer and, 36
    definition of, 68
    in regional enteritis, 181
anorexia nervosa, 68–70, 69f
antibiotic resistance, 6–8
antibodies, 15, 17–18. *See also* immunoglobulin(s)
anticoagulant(s), 133
antidiuretic hormone, 258
    actions of, 149, 258f
    deficiency, 259, 259f
antigen(s), 15, 17, 220
antihistamine, 221
anti-inflammatory hormone(s), in response to stress, 394–395
antineoplastic agents, 40
antioxidant(s), 409
anuria, 152
aorta, 130–131
    normal anatomy of, 116, 118f
aortic coarctation, 116, 117f
aortic insufficiency, 120
aortic stenosis, 119–120, 120f
aphasia, 345

aplasia, 5, 5*f*
aplastic anemia, 5, 92
appendicitis, 178–179
appendix, 169, 179*f*
arachnoid, 324
areola, 294
arrhythmia(s)
  in alcoholism, 78
  cardiac, 124
arteriography, ultrasound, 143
arteriole(s), 130*f*, 131
arteriosclerosis, 131, 399
artery(ies), 130–131
  diseases of, 131–138
    effects on heart and brain, 133*f*
arthritis, 361–364
artificial sweeteners, 71
ascites, 201–202, 203*f*
  with hepatocarcinoma, 205
ascorbic acid. *See* vitamin C
ASD. *See* atrial septal defect
aseptic technique, 298
aspermia, 254–256
aspiration, 302
  pathologic, 337
assay(s), 287
asthma, 224–226, 225*f*
  and stress, 398
astrocytoma, 347
atelectasis, 231, 232*f*
atherosclerosis, 109, 110*f*, 131–132, 132*f*
  and obesity, 72
    thrombus formation in, 132–135,
      133*f*–134*f*
athlete's foot, 379
atopic people, 380
atresia, 58–59
atrial fibrillation, 124
atrial septal defect, 112, 114*f*
atrioventricular valve(s), 104
atrium/atria, cardiac, 104–105
atrophy, 4
aura
  migraine headache, 396
  seizure, 340
auscultation, 124
autoimmune disease(s), 19, 120, 367,
    374
autoimmunity, 19

autonomic nervous system, 326
  effects on heart, 106–108
  in response to stress, 393, 394*f*
autosomal dominant disorder(s), 47–48,
    48*f*
autosomal recessive disorder(s), 48–51
autosomes, 46
axillary nodes, 16*f*
axon, 324, 325*f*, 328
azidothymidine, 22
  for AIDS, 22
azotemia, 152, 153*f*
AZT. *See* azidothymidine

B

bacteria
  antibiotic resistance in, 6
  pyogenic, 15, 154, 223
bacterial infection(s)
  in cold, 220
  of skin, 376–377
barium, 188
barrel chest, 228
Bartholin's glands, 293*f*, 294
  abscess, 297
  inflammation, 297
basal cell carcinoma, 383, 383*f*–384*f*
basal ganglia, 325–326, 337–338
basal metabolic rate, 261
benign, definition of, 31
benign prostatic hyperplasia, 311, 311*f*,
    400
beta carotene, 409
beta cells, 73, 280
bicuspid valve, 104
bile, 168, 195–196
bile duct(s), 196, 196*f*
  obstruction, 205, 206*f*
biliary calculi, 206–207, 207*f*
biliary cirrhosis, 205, 206*f*
bilirubin, 88, 195–197
biohazard symbol, 21*f*, 21–22
biopsy, 38–39
  techniques of, 38–39
bladder, urinary, 149, 150*f*
  carcinoma of, 160, 160*f*
  diseases of, 159–160
bleeding, cancer and, 35
bleeding disease(s), 93–94

bleeding time, 99
blood, composition of, 86–87
blood disease(s), 85–100. *See also* anemia
  diagnostic procedures for, 99
blood-forming tissue, diseases of, 95–98
blood pressure
  control mechanisms, 140–141
  diastolic, 140
  normal, 140
  systolic, 140
blood test(s), 99
blood transfusion, incompatible, 26*f*
blood urea nitrogen, 152
blood vessel(s), 129–131
  diseases of, 129–143
  functions of, 131
  intima, 131
  structure of, 131
blue bloaters, 228–229
B lymphocytes, 17, 17*f*
body fat, 410–411
body lice, 379
body temperature, regulation, 4, 259, 261
  in elderly, 402
boil(s), 377
bone(s)
  compact, 352, 353*f*
  diseases of, 354–359
    diagnostic tests for, 368
    infectious, 354–355
    secondary, 356–357
    in vitamin and mineral deficiencies,
      355–356
  fractures, 357–359
  function of, 352
  infections, 354–355
  interaction with muscles and joints,
    352
  metabolism, 278
  neoplasia of, 359
  spongy, 352, 353*f*
  structure of, 352
  tuberculosis of, 355
  tumors of
    benign, 359
    malignant, 359
bone callus, 359
bone development, defective, 48
bone marrow, 352, 353*f*

bone marrow smear, 99
bone marrow transplantation, 98
bone spurs, 363
Bowman's capsule, 148
bradycardia, 124
bradykinesia, 337
bradykinin, 23
brain, 325–326
  abscess of, 335, 336*f*
  concussion of, 345
  contusion of, 346
  specialized areas of, 328–329, 329*f*
  traumatic disorders of, 345–346
brain damage, 343
brain tumor(s), 346–347
breast(s), 294
  benign tumors of, 301–302
  cystic hyperplasia, 301–302
  fibrocystic disease, 301–302, 302*f*
  neoplasms of, 301
  self-examination, 301
breast cancer, 301
breath-holding, 223
broad ligament, 292
bronchial asthma, 224–226, 225*f*
  and stress, 398
bronchial mucosa, 223
bronchial tree, 216*f*, 217
bronchiectasis, 226–227, 227*f*–228*f*
  in cystic fibrosis, 240
bronchiole(s), 216–217, 223, 225*f*
bronchitis, 223–224
bronchogenic carcinoma, 239*f*, 239–240
bronchopneumonia, 233–234, 234*f*
bronchoscope, 239
bronchus/bronchi, 216, 223
  dilation, 226–227
  obstructed, 223, 224*f*
bruise, 137. *See also* ecchymosis
buffalo hump, 274, 275*f*
bulbourethral glands, 307, 309*f*
bulimia, 70
bullae, 376
  in emphysema, 228–229, 230*f*
BUN, 152
bundle of His, 107
burn(s), depth, evaluation of, 375
bursae, 352
bursitis, 365–366

C

cachexia, 32
calcium, 67
    deficiency, bone disorders in, 355–356
calluses, 374
cancer
    causes of, 33–35, 34*f*
    development, 32, 33*f*
        stages of, 32
    diagnosis of, 37–39
    in elderly, 400
    prevention of, 35
    signs and symptoms of, 35–36, 36*f*
    staging, 39
    treatment of, 39–40
    types of, 36–37
    warning signs of, 36, 36*f*
cancer cachexia, 32
Candida albicans, 297
capillary(ies), 131
capillary fluid shift mechanism, 140–141
capillary permeability, 12–13
carbon dioxide, 217, 218*f*
carcinogenesis, 32, 33*f*
carcinoma, 36
    bladder, 160, 160*f*
    bronchogenic, 239*f*, 239–240
    cervical, 298
    endometrial, 298
    of liver, 203–205
    of prostate gland, 311–313
    renal, 155, 156*f*
    versus sarcoma, 38*f*
carcinoma in situ, 298
cardiac arrest, 124
cardiac catheterization, 125, 125*f*
cardiac cycle, 105
cardiac sphincter, 171
cardiogenic shock, 142, 142*f*
cardiopulmonary resuscitation, 110,
    124
cardiovascular system, in alcoholism, 78
carotene, 66
carotid artery(ies), 130–131
carotid audiofrequency analysis, 142
carotid phonoangiography, 142
carpal tunnel syndrome, 360–361
caseation, 238

caseous material, in tuberculosis, 238
cast(s), urinary, 150, 162
cataracts, 400–401
CAUTION acronym, for warning signs of
    cancer, 36, 36*f*
CDC. *See* Centers for Disease Control
cecum, 169, 179*f*
cell-mediated immunity, 17, 17*f*
Centers for Disease Control, 21
central nervous system, 327*f*
cerebral hemispheres, 325
cerebral hemorrhage, 343–344
cerebral palsy, 343
    atactic, 343
    athetoid, 343
    spastic, 343
cerebrospinal fluid, 325–326
    examination of, 347
cerebrovascular accident, 132, 343–345
cerebrum, 325
cervical nodes, 16*f*
cervix, 292, 292*f*
    carcinoma of, 298
chancre, syphilitic, 316, 316*f*
chemical agents, inflammation caused by,
    12*f*
chemical carcinogens, 34, 34*f*
chemotaxis, white blood cells and, 13
chemotherapy, 39–40
    consolidation stage, 96
    induction stage, 96
    for leukemia, 96
    maintenance stage, 96
chlamydia, 296
chlamydial infection, 318
    diagnosis of, 319
cholecystectomy, 207
cholecystitis, 205, 207*f*
cholelithiasis, 206–207, 207*f*
cholesterol
    dietary, 410–412
    metabolism, 412
    serum, 411
    total, 411
    transport, in blood, 411
chorea, 338
choriocarcinoma, 300
chorion, 295
chorionic gonadotropin, 300

chromosome(s), 46
  abnormalities, 53–55
chronic atrophic gastritis, 173
chronic disease, definition of, 8
chronic fatigue syndrome, 22
chronic obstructive pulmonary disease,
    222–226
chymotrypsin, 208
cilia, 218
circulation, 129–131
circulatory system, 130
circumcision, 307
cirrhosis
  biliary, 205, 206f
  of liver, 199–203, 204f
clitoris, 293f, 294
cluster headaches, 397
coagulation disorders, diagnosis of, 99
coagulation necrosis, 134
coarctation, of aorta, 116, 117f
cobalamin. See vitamin B₁₂
cold sore(s), 377–378, 378f, 398
collagen, 67
collateral circulation, in cirrhosis of liver,
    201
colon, 169
  carcinoma of, 183–186
  lumen of, 183
  in ulcerative colitis, 181, 182f
color blindness, 51–53
colostomy, 181
comminuted fracture(s), 357, 358f
common cold, 219–220
  and stress, 398
complications, 8–9
compound fracture(s), 357, 358f, 359
compression sclerotherapy, 139
computerized tomography scan, 8
  abdominal, 211
  of brain, 348
concussion, of brain, 345
congenital birth defects, 7
congenital diseases, 57–59
congenital heart disease, 112–116
congestive heart failure, 112, 113f
  in valvular heart disease, 119
conjunctiva, 65
Conn's syndrome, 274
constipation, 187

contact dermatitis, 380–381, 381f
contusion, of brain, 346
convulsion(s), 339–340
COPD. See chronic obstructive pulmonary
    disease
corns, 374
coronary arteriography, 125–126
coronary artery disease, 109–111
coronary blood supply, 105, 106f
coronary thrombosis, 109
cor pulmonale, 112
corpus luteum, 295
cortex, cerebral, 325
corticosteroids
  in response to stress, 394–395
  treatment with, 395
cortisol, 273, 275–276
  plasma, assay, 287
  in response to stress, 394
  treatment with, 395
cortisone, 273, 275–276
  therapy, 256, 395
cough
  in bronchitis, 223
  in lung cancer, 239
  as sign of cancer, 35–36
CPR. See cardiopulmonary resuscitation
cranial nerve(s), 324, 327f
creatine phosphate, 367
creatinine, 148–149, 152
cretinism, 267–272, 269f–270f
Crohn's disease, 180–181, 396
cruciferous vegetables, 410
cryptorchidism, 314, 314f
CTS. See carpal tunnel syndrome
CT scan. See computerized tomography
    scan
Cushing's syndrome, 274, 275f
CVA. See cerebrovascular accident
cyanosis, 113, 114f, 374
  in emphysema, 228–229
  in heart disease, 124
  in valvular heart disease, 118–119
cyst, 35
cystic fibrosis, 240
  complications of, 240, 241f
cystitis, 159
cystoscope, 160

cystoscopic examination, 162
cytotoxic T cells, 17*f*, 18

D

dandruff, chronic, 386
D&C. *See* dilation and curettage
debilitating disease, 227
defibrillator, 124
degenerative neural disease(s), 335–337
delirium tremens, 78, 203
dementia
    AIDS, symptoms of, 20
    in Huntington's disease, 339
demyelination, in multiple sclerosis, 336
dendrite(s), 324, 325*f*
deoxyribonucleic acid (DNA), 6, 46
dermatophytosis, 379
dermis, 375*f*, 376
dermoid cyst, 42, 299
DES. *See* diethylstilbestrol
desensitization, 221
diabetes insipidus, 258–259
diabetes mellitus, 64, 282–286
    complications of, 283, 284*f*
    insulin-dependent (type I), 282
    non-insulin-dependent (type II), 282
    and obesity, 73
    patient education, 286
    symptoms of, 282–283
    tests for, 285–286
    treatment of, 283–284
diabetic coma, 284–285, 285*f*
diabetic nephropathy, 153
diabetic retinopathy, 283
diagnosis, 8–9
diagnostic imaging techniques, 8
dialysis, 153
diaphragm, 217
diaphragmatic hernia(s), 185, 185*f*
    and obesity, 73
diarrhea, 187
    in regional enteritis, 181
diastole, 105
diastolic pressure, 140
diet(s)
    high fiber–low fat, 409
    importance of, 409–412
    weight-loss, 74–75

dietary deficiencies, 63–81
dietary excesses, 63–81
diethylstilbestrol, exposure in utero,
        300–301
digestion, 168–170
    disturbances of, 64
digestive tract, 168–169, 170*f*
    in alcoholism, 77–78
    diagnostic procedures for, 187–188
    diseases of, 167–189
    disorders of, 186–187
dilation, 226
dilation and curettage, 300
diphtheria toxoid, 333
discoid lupus erythematosus, 19
disease, mechanisms of, 3–4
dislocation(s), 360
disuse atrophy, 357, 400
diverticulitis, 180, 180*f*
diverticulosis, 180, 180*f*
diverticulum, 180
DNA. *See* deoxyribonucleic acid
dominant gene(s), 46–47
L-dopa, for Parkinson's disease, 338
dopamine, in Parkinson's disease, 338
Doppler imaging, 143
double pneumonia, 231
Down's syndrome, 53–54, 54*f*
drug(s)
    hypersensitivity to, skin manifestations,
        382, 382*f*
    and nervous system, 330
DTs. *See* delirium tremens
duodenal ulcer(s), 175
duodenum, 168
dura mater, 324
dwarfism
    achondroplastic, 48, 49*f*
    pituitary, 255*f*, 256–257
dysentery, 186
dysmenorrhea, 304
dyspareunia, 304
dyspepsia, 173
dysphagia, 36, 171
dysplasia, 5, 5*f*
dyspnea, 87, 114–115, 223
    in heart disease, 123–124
dysuria, 154, 161

E

ecchymosis/ecchymoses, 77, 94, 137
ECG. *See* electrocardiogram
echocardiography, 125
eclampsia, 307, 397
ectopic pregnancy, 305, 305*f*
eczema, 380–381, 399
edema, 15, 150, 161, 194
    hypersensitivity and, 23
    and hypervitaminosis, 67
EEG. *See* electroencephalography
ejaculation, 310
ejaculatory duct, 307, 309*f*
elderly
    care of, 402–403
    common diseases of, 399–402
electrocardiogram, 124–125
electroencephalography, 340, 348
electrolyte balance, 148
electromyography, 337, 348, 361
embolism, 134, 135*f*–136*f*
    cerebral, 344–345
    septic, 134
embolus, 134, 135*f*–136*f*
EMG. *See* electromyography
emphysema, 227–230, 229*f*
empyema, 235–236
encephalin(s), 408
encephalitis, 331–332
    lethargic, 331
encephalopathy, AIDS, symptoms of, 20
endarterectomy, 345
endocarditis, 120
    infectious, 121–123, 122*f*
endocardium, 104, 104*f*
endocrine disease(s), 247–290
    diagnosis of, 287
endocrine gland(s), 207–208, 248, 249*f*
    atrophy, 248
    functions of, 248–249
    hyperactive, 248
    hypoactive, 248
endometriosis, 304–305
endometrium, carcinoma of, 298
endorphin(s), 408
endoscope, 188
endoscopic sclerotherapy, 140, 201
environmental agents, cancer caused by, 34*f*

environmental factors, disease caused
    by, 7
enzyme(s), synthesis, in liver, 194–195
eosinophil(s), increased, conditions indi-
    cated by, 99
epidermis, 374, 375*f*, 376
epidermoid carcinomas, 36
epididymis, 307, 308*f*, 308, 309*f*
    cyst formation in, after DES exposure in
        utero, 301
epididymitis, 313
epidural hemorrhage, 346
epilepsy, 339–340
epinephrine, 25, 273–274
    for asthma, 226
    in response to stress, 393
epistaxis, 77
Epstein-Barr virus, 98
erysipelas, 377
erythema, 376–377
erythematous skin, 376
erythroblastosis, 92
erythroblastosis fetalis, 89–92
erythrocytes, 86–87
    sickled, 89*f*
erythrocytosis, 93
erythropoiesis, 86*f*, 87
erythropoietin, 87
esophageal varices, 77, 139–140, 171, 201,
    202*f*
esophagitis, 171, 172*f*
esophagoscope, 171
esophagus, 168
    cancer of, 171
    diseases of, 171–173
estrogen(s)
    adrenal, 273
    ovarian, 294
ESWL. *See* extracorporeal shock wave
    lithotripsy
etiology, of disease, 5–8
exacerbation, 8
excretory system, diseases of, 147–163
    diagnosis, 161–162
exercise(s)
    aerobic, 413
    for elderly, 402
    value of, 412–413
exfoliative cytology, 39

exocrine glands, 240
exophthalmos, 264, 266*f*
expiration, muscles of, 217
expiratory reserve, 242*f*
Exposure Control Plan, 21
extracorporeal shock wave lithotripsy, 207
extradural hemorrhage, 346
extrinsic factor, 88

F

fallopian tubes, 292, 292*f*–293*f*
familial diseases, 53
familial polyposis, 52*f*, 53, 183–184, 184*f*
fat(s), 410–411
    metabolism of, 282–283
    polyunsaturated, 411
    saturated, 411
    unsaturated, 411
fatty acids, 411
fatty liver, 73
fatty nutritional cirrhosis of liver, 199–203
fetal alcohol syndrome, 79
fetal–maternal relationship, 296
fever blister(s), 377–378, 378*f*, 398
fibrin, 15, 233
fibrinogen, 195
fibroadenoma, of breast, 301, 302*f*
fibroblasts, 14*f*, 15
    in wound healing, 14*f*
fibroids, 41
fibroid tumor(s), of uterus, 298–299, 299*f*
fight or flight mechanism, 274
fimbriae, 292
fingernails, and health problems, 7
fingerprints, identification by, 46
flatus, 185
fluoroscopy, 242
folic acid, 409
follicle(s)
    Graafian, 294
    primary, 294
follicle-stimulating hormone, 252
food poisoning, *Salmonella*, 181–183
foramen ovale, 112
foreign substances, inflammation due to, 12*f*
foreskin, 307

fracture(s), 357–359
    comminuted, 357, 358*f*
    compound, 357, 358*f*, 359
    in elderly, 399
    greenstick, 357, 358*f*
    reduction, 358–359
    simple, 357, 358*f*
fragile X syndrome, 54–55
free radicals, 409
friable, definition of, 123
frozen section, biopsy technique, 38–39
FSH. *See* follicle-stimulating hormone
functional condition, 5
fungal infection(s), of skin, 379
furuncles, 377

G

galactosemia, 49–51
gallbladder, 196
    diseases of, 205–207
        and obesity, 73
gallstones, 206–207, 207*f*
gangrene, 134–135
    in appendicitis, 179
    in diabetes mellitus, 283
gas exchange, respiratory, 217, 218*f*
gastric juice, 168
    analysis of, 173, 188
gastric ulcer(s), 175
gastritis, 173
    chronic atrophic, 173
gastroenteritis, 178
gastrointestinal disease(s)
    affected by stress, 396
    in elderly, 400
gastrointestinal system, malfunctioning of, 64
gastroscope, 173
gastroscopy, 173
gene(s), 46
    dominant, 46–47
    recessive, 47
genetic anomalies, 4, 7
genetic predisposition, and cancer, 34*f*
genital herpes, 317–318
genitalia, external, female, 293*f*, 294
genital wart(s), 318, 378
geriatrics, 402

gerontology, 402
GFR. *See* glomerular filtration rate
GH. *See* growth hormone
Ghon lesion, 237
giant cell tumor(s), of bone, 359
gigantism, 252
glandular tissue, cancer of, 36. *See also*
    adenocarcinoma
glioblastoma, 347
glioma(s), 347, 347f
glomerular filtration rate, 152
glomerulonephritis, 150–152
    acute, 150–151, 151f
    chronic, 151–152
glomerulus, 148
glucagon, 207
    secretion, 248, 280–282
glucocorticoid(s), 273
    in response to stress, 393
glucose
    blood. *See also* hyperglycemia; hypo-
        glycemia
        normal, 282
        regulation of, 281, 281f, 282
    metabolism, 194, 281
    urinary, 162, 282
glucose tolerance test, 285–287
glycogen, 194, 281
    storage of, 64
glycosuria, in diabetes mellitus, 282
goiter, 262–264, 265f
    adenomatous, 264–266
    diffuse colloidal, 263–264, 265f
    endemic, 263
    in iodine deficiency, 67
    multinodular, 265f
    nodular, 264, 265f
gonadotropins, 252
    deficiency, 254–256
    effects on female reproductive system,
        294–295, 295f
gonococcus, 296, 315
gonorrhea, 296, 310, 315–316
    diagnosis of, 319
gout, 364
Graafian follicle(s), 294
grand mal epilepsy, 339–340
granular contracted kidneys, 152, 154
Graves' disease, 264–266, 266f–267f

gray matter, 325
greenstick fracture(s), 357, 358f
group A hemolytic streptococci, 120
growth, abnormal patterns of, 5, 5f
growth hormone, 251–252
    assay, 287
    excess, 252
    therapy, 256
growth plate, 352, 353f
gynecomastia, 77, 203

H

hair follicles, 375f, 376
hair loss, and chemotherapy, 40
handwashing, 6
hay fever, 220–221
HDL. *See* high-density lipoprotein(s)
headache(s)
    cluster, 397
    migraine, 396–397
head lice, 379
heart
    action, abnormalities of, 124
    autoimmune diseases and, 19
    conduction system of, 106–107, 109f
    functions of, 104–105
    and lungs, relationship of, 105–106,
        107f–108f
    structure of, 104, 104f, 115f
heart block, 124
heart disease(s), 109–126. *See also* congeni-
    tal heart disease
    cyanotic, 113
    diagnosis of, 124–126
    hypertensive, 111–112
    symptoms of, 123–124
heart failure
    left-heart, 112, 113f
    right-heart, 112, 113f
heart murmur(s), 117
heart rate, regulation of, 107–108, 124
heart valve(s), 104–105, 105f
    diseases of, 117–120
    insufficiency, 117
    stenosis, 114, 117
    vegetations in
        in infectious endocarditis, 123, 123f
        in rheumatic fever, 121, 121f

Helicobacter pylori, 175
helper T cells, 17*f*, 18–19
  inhibition of, 20
hematemesis, 171, 176
  in cirrhosis of liver, 201
hematocrit, 86, 99
hematuria, 150, 162
hemiplegia, 345
hemoglobin, 87, 99
  breakdown, in bruise, 137
hemolysis, 25, 87
hemolytic anemia, 88–92
  jaundice in, 197
hemophilia, 93–94
hemoptysis, 238
  in lung cancer, 239
hemorrhage
  cerebral, 343–344
  extradural (epidural), 346
  subarachnoid, 346
  subdural, 346
hemorrhage(s), 136–137
hemorrhoid(s), 139, 187–188
  prolapsed, 187
heparin, 23, 110
Hepatavax B, 199
hepatic coma, 78, 203
hepatitis
  fulminating, 198
  infectious, 198–199
  serum, 198
  viral, 198–199
hepatitis virus
  type A, 198
  type B, 198
  type C, 199
hepatocarcinoma, 203–205
hereditary disease(s), 45–59. *See also* fa-
    milial disease(s)
  transmission of, 47–53
heredity, 46–47
hermaphrodite(s), 56
hernia(s)
  diaphragmatic, 185, 185*f*
  strangulated, 185, 185*f*
herpes, genital, 317–318
herpes simplex virus, 317–318, 377–378,
    378*f*
herpes zoster, 334–335

heterozygous, definition of, 46
hiatal hernia, 171–173, 172*f*
hiccoughs, 241–242
high-density lipoprotein(s), 411–412
hirsutism, 276, 277*f*
histamine, 12–13, 23, 220–221, 225, 380
HIV. *See* human immunodeficiency
    virus
hives, 380, 398–399
Hodgkin's disease, 39, 97–98
holistic health, 407
holistic medicine, 407
homeostasis, 3–4
  and adaptation to stress, 391–392
  definition of, 392
homozygous, definition of, 46
hormonal therapy, 39–40
hormone(s), 248
  in anorexia nervosa, 70
  of anterior pituitary, 251–252
  anti-inflammatory, in response to stress,
    394–395
  and cancer, 34, 34*f*
  secretion, 248
    negative feedback mechanism, 248
  tropic, 251
hot flashes, 304
human immunodeficiency virus, 20
  infection, 21
    classification of, 21
human papillomavirus, 35, 318
humoral immunity, 17, 17*f*
Huntington's chorea, 59, 338–339
Huntington's disease, 338–339
hydatidiform mole, 299–300
hydrocephalus, 326, 331, 341–343
  communicating, 342
  noncommunicating, 342
hydrochloric acid, 168, 173–175
  absence of, 178
hydrolithotripsy, 156–157
hydronephrosis, 157, 158*f*, 311, 311*f*
hydrosalpinx, 296
hydroureter(s), 157, 311, 311*f*
hygiene, and infection, 6
hymen, 293*f*, 294
hyperadrenalism, 274–276
hypercalcemia, 67, 279, 279*f*
hyperemia, 12

hyperestrogenism, 77
hyperglycemia, 274, 282
hypergonadism, 286–287
hyperkalemia, 152
hypernephroma, 155
hyperparathyroidism, 279f, 279–280, 356
    diagnosis of, 368
hyperpituitarism, 252
hyperplasia, 5, 5f
hypersensitivity, 23–27. *See also* allergies
    to drugs, skin manifestations, 382,
        382f
    skin manifestations, 380
hypertension, 111–112, 140–141
    effects of, 141
    in elderly, 399
    idiopathic, 141
    and kidney disease, 141
    pregnancy-induced, 307
    primary, 141
    pulmonary, 112
    secondary, 141
    stress-related, 397
    treatment of, 141
hypertensive heart disease(s), 111–112
hyperthyroidism, 264–266
hypertrophy, 4
hyperventilation, 217
hypervitaminosis, 67, 410
hypoadrenalism, 276–278
hypoalbuminemia, 202
hypocalcemia, 280
hypoglycemia, 286
hypogonadism
    in female, 287
    in male, 287
hypoparathyroidism, 280
hypophysis, 250
hypopituitarism, 253–258, 254f
hypoplasia, 5, 5f
hypoproteinemia, 162
hypothalamus, 248, 250, 250f
    in response to stress, 393, 394f
hypothermia, 4
hypothyroidism, 264, 266–267, 268f
    congenital, 267–272, 269f–271f
hypoventilation, and obesity, 72
hypovolemic shock, 142, 142f
hypoxia, 223–224

I

idiopathic, definition of, 7
idiopathic hypertension, 141
idiopathic thrombocytopenic purpura, 94
immune deficiency, 20–22
immune response, stimulation by antigens,
        15
immunity, 15–19. *See also* autoimmunity
    acquired, 15
    active
        versus passive immunity, 23f
        vaccination and, 22–23
    cell-mediated, 17, 17f
    humoral, 17, 17f
    innate, 16–17
    passive
        versus active immunity, 23f
        vaccination and, 23
immunoglobulin(s), 17f, 220
    hypersensitivity and, 23
    injection, protection against hepatitis A,
        198
    types of, 18
immunoglobulin E, 220, 225
impetigo, 376–377
impotence, 313–314
inborn errors of metabolism, 46
incontinence, 161
infarct, 51, 109, 134
infection(s)
    bacterial
        in cold, 220
        of skin, 376–377
    of bone, 354–355
    chlamydial, 318
        diagnosis of, 319
    in elderly, 403
    fungal, of skin, 379
    human immunodeficiency virus, 21
    hygiene and, 6
    nosocomial, 234
    of skin, 376–380
    viral, of skin, 377–378
infectious endocarditis, 121–123, 122f
infectious mononucleosis, 98
inferior vena cava, 131
inflammation, 11–28, 12f
    suppurative, 15
    vascular changes in, 13, 13f

inflammatory exudate, 13–15, 233
influenza, 222
influenzal pneumonia, 234–235
inguinal lymph nodes, 16*f*
initiation, of carcinogenesis, 32, 33*f*
innate immunity, 16–17
inspiration, muscles of, 217
inspiratory capacity, 242*f*
inspiratory reserve volume, 242*f*
insulin, 207
   secretion, 248, 280–281
   therapy
      for diabetes mellitus, 283–284
      patient identification card, 286
insulin shock, 284–285, 285*f*
integument. *See* skin
intercostal muscles, 217
interferon, 6
intervertebral disk(s), herniation, 364–365,
      366*f*
intestinal atresia, 58–59
intestinal lymph nodes, 16*f*
intestinal obstruction, 184–185, 185*f*
   organic, 184
   paralytic, 184
intestine(s). *See also* large intestine; small
      intestine
   diseases of, 178–186
intravenous pyelography, 162
intrinsic factor, 64, 88, 173
intussusception, 184, 185*f*
iodide, therapy, 264
iodide trap, 260
iodine, 67
iron, 67
irritable bowel syndrome, 185–186
ischemia, 109, 132
islands of Langerhans, 207, 280–281, 281*f*
-itis, 11
ITP. *See* idiopathic thrombocytopenic pur-
      pura
IVP. *See* intravenous pyelography

J

jaundice, 88, 196–197, 374
   causes of, 197
   in cirrhosis of liver, 202
   with hepatocarcinoma, 205

joint(s)
   diseases of, 359–366
      diagnostic tests for, 368
   function of, 352
   interaction with bones and muscles, 352
   range of motion, 352
   structure of, 352
juxtaglomerular apparatus, 148

K

Kaposi's sarcoma, in AIDS, 20
karyotype, 46
keloid, 15
keratin, 376
keratinized layer, of skin, 375*f*, 376
keratinocytes, 376
ketone bodies, 283
kidney(s), 149, 150*f*
   autoimmune diseases of, 19
   carcinoma, 155, 156*f*
   diseases of, 150–152
      hypertension and, 141
   failure, 152
   functions of, 148–149
   granular contracted, 152, 154
   polycystic, 157–159, 159*f*
   tuberculosis of, 238–239
kidney stones, 155–157, 157*f*
killer cells, 17*f*, 18–19
Klinefelter's syndrome, 55–56, 57*f*
knuckle cracking, 360
Kupffer's cells, 195

L

labia majora, 293*f*, 294
labia minora, 293*f*, 294
laboratory tests, 8
Laennec's cirrhosis of liver, 199–203
laparoscopy, 304
large intestine, 16*f*, 169
LDL. *See* low-density lipoprotein(s)
legume(s), 409
leiomyoma(s), 41
lesion(s), 5
lethargic encephalitis, 331
lethargy, 254

leukemia, 39, 95–96
  acute, 96
  chronic, 96
  lymphocytic, 96, 97f
  myelogenous, 96, 97f
  signs and symptoms of, 95f, 95–96
  types of, 96, 97f
leukocyte(s), 12, 86
  immune response and, 12
  increased, conditions indicated by, 99
leukocyte count, 95
leukocytosis, 15
  in osteomyelitis, 355
leukopenia, 40
leukorrhea, 297
LH. See luteinizing hormone
lice, 379
ligament(s), 352
ligation, 139
lipoma, 40, 42f
lipoproteins, 411
lithotripsy, 156–157
liver
  in alcoholism, 77–78
  blood supply to, 194, 194f
  carcinoma of, 203–205
  cirrhosis of, 199–203, 204f
  detoxifying function, 195
  diseases of, 196–205. See also hepatic
    coma
  functions of, 194–196, 195f
  hobnailed, 199, 201f
  normal anatomy of, 200f
  nutrient storage in, 64
  regeneration of, 194
liver function tests, 211
lobar pneumonia, 231–233
lockjaw, 332–333
long bone(s), structure of, 352, 353f
Lou Gehrig's disease, 337
low-density lipoprotein(s), 412
lower respiratory disease(s), 219, 222–240
lumbar puncture, 331
lumpectomy, 301
lung(s)
  blood supply to, 218
  consolidated, 233
  and pleural cavity, air pressure differ-
    ence between, 218, 219f

lung cancer, 239f, 239–240
lupus erythematosus, 19
luteinizing hormone, 252
Lyme disease, skin rash of, 377
lymphadenopathy, 95
  AIDS, 20
lymphatic system, 16
  anatomy of, 16f
lymph node(s), 17f
lymphocyte(s)
  activated, 15, 17, 17f
  increased, conditions indicated by, 99
lymphoid tissues, 17f
lymphokine(s), secretion of, 18–19
lymphoma(s)
  histiocytic, 97
  lymphocytic, 97
  malignant, 97–98
lymph tissue, 221

M

macrophage(s), 15. See also monocyte(s)
macular lesions, 376
magnetic resonance imaging, 8
  of brain, 348
malabsorption, 64–65
malabsorption syndrome, 179, 188
malaise, 377
malignant, definition of, 31
malignant melanoma, 41, 385f, 385–386
malignant tumors, 32–40
malnutrition, 7, 64–65
  causes of, 64–65, 65f
mammography, 301
mast cell(s), 23, 220, 225, 380
mastectomy, radical, 301
master gland, pituitary gland as, 248, 256
medical alert bracelet(s), 25
medullary cavity, of long bone, 352, 353f
melanin, 41, 374, 383
melanocytes, 374, 383
melanoma, 41
melena, 176, 188
  in regional enteritis, 181
memory cell(s), 17f
  action of, 18f
  reactivation of, 18
menarche, 294

meninges, 324
meningitis, 324, 331
meningocele, 341, 341*f*
meningomyelocele, 341, 341*f*
menopause, 294
menorrhagia, 88, 303
menstrual abnormalities, 302–303
menstruation, 295
mental retardation, in fetal alcohol syndrome, 79
metabolism, regulation of, 260–261
metaplasia, 5, 5*f*
metastasis, 32, 37, 38*f*
  to liver, 203–205
metrorrhagia, 303
migraine headache(s), 396–397
mineral(s)
  deficiency, 67
  functions of, 68*f*
  supplements, 410
mineralocorticoids, 273
miscarriage, 306
mitral insufficiency, 119
mitral stenosis, 117–118, 119*f*
mitral valve, 104
  cusps, sclerosis, 119
  in rheumatic heart disease, 120–121
  vegetations in, in rheumatic fever, 121, 121*f*
mole, 41, 41*f*, 383. *See also* nevus
monocyte(s), 15. *See also* macrophage(s)
  increased, conditions indicated by, 99
mons pubis, 293*f*, 294
moon-face appearance, 273
motion sickness, 186
motor nervous system, 329
mouth
  cancer of, 170–171
  diseases of, 170–171
MRI. *See* magnetic resonance imaging
MS. *See* multiple sclerosis
mucus, in bronchitis, 223
multidrug resistance, 6
multiple sclerosis, 335–337
muscle(s)
  diseases of, 367–368
    diagnostic tests for, 368
  function of, 352–354
  interaction with bones and joints, 352

  involuntary, 354
  structure of, 352–354
  tumors of, 368
  voluntary, 354
muscular dystrophy, 367
  diagnosis of, 368
mutation, 47
  disease and, 4
myasthenia gravis, 367–368
Mycobacterium tuberculosis, 236–237
myelin, 324, 325*f*
myelocele, 341, 341*f*
myelocyte(s), 96
myelography, 348
myocardial infarction, 109–110, 111*f*, 132, 399
  treatment of, 110–111
myocardial ischemia, 109
myocardium, 104, 104*f*
myoma, 41
myoneural junction, 328, 354
myxedema, 266–267, 268*f*

N

nausea, 186
necrosis, 134
  coagulation, 134
  gangrenous, 134–135
negative feedback mechanism, 248
Neisseria meningitidis, 331
neoplasia, 31–43
  definition of, 31
neoplasm, 31
  classification of, 31
nephron, 148, 149*f*
nephrotripsy, 156
nervous system, 323–349
  developmental errors of, 340–343
  diagnostic procedures for, 347–348
  diseases of, 330–339
  and drugs, 330
  function, 328–329
  infectious disease of, 330–335
  structure of, 324–327
neural disease(s), 330–339
  degenerative, 335–337
neural disorders, 324
neurogenic shock, 142, 142*f*

neurohypophysis, 251. *See also* pituitary
    gland, posterior
neuromuscular junction, 328
neuron(s), 324, 325*f*
    motor, 324
    sensory, 324
neurotropic disease, 330
neutrophil(s), 12–13
    increased, conditions indicated by, 99
nevus, 41, 42*f*, 383
niacin, 409
night blindness, and vitamin A deficiency,
    65
nipple, 294
    Paget's disease of, 301
nitroglycerin, 111
nocturia, 312
nondisjunction, 53
nonsuppurative, definition of, 150
normoblast(s), 86*f*, 87
nosocomial infection(s), 234
nutrient(s), improper absorption of, 64
nutrition, for elderly, 402
nystagmus, 77, 336

O

obesity, 70–74
    causes of, 72, 259
    complications of, 72–73, 73*f*
    diagnosis of, 73–74
    diseases aggravated by, 72–73, 73*f*
    treatment of, 73–74
occult blood, in stool, 188
Occupational Safety and Health Adminis-
    tration, 21
oliguria, 152
orchitis, 313
organic brain syndrome, in alcoholism, 76
organs, adaptation to stress, 4
OSHA. *See* Occupational Safety and
    Health Administration
osteitis fibrosa cystica, 356
osteoarthritis, 363–364, 400
    and obesity, 72
osteoblast(s), 278, 352
osteoclast(s), 278, 352
osteogenic sarcoma, 357, 359
osteoma, 359

osteomalacia, 66, 356
    diagnosis of, 368
osteomyelitis, 354–355
osteopenia, 356–357
osteoporosis, 356–357
ovaries, 292, 292*f*–293*f*, 294
    neoplasms of, 299
ovulation, 294
oxygen, 217, 218*f*
    metabolism, 412
oxytocin, 258

P

pacemaker, cardiac, 107–108, 124
packed cell volume, 99
Paget's disease
    of bone, 357, 368
    of nipple, 301
pain, phantom, 328
pallor, 7, 87, 374
pancreas
    anatomy of, 207–208, 209*f*
    cancer of, 210
    diseases of, 208–210
    endocrine, 207–208, 280–282
    exocrine, 208
    functions of, 207–208
    hyposecretion of, 282
    structure of, 207–208, 208*f*
pancreatitis, 77–78, 208–210
    acute hemorrhagic, 209, 210*f*
panhypopituitarism, 253–254, 257
pantothenic acid, 409
Papanicolaou, George N., 39
papillary muscle(s), 119
papilloma, 41, 42*f*. *See also* wart
Pap smear (Papanicolaou smear), 35, 39,
    298
    HPV and, 318
papular lesions, 376
paranasal sinuses, 220
parasitic infestations, 379–380
parathormone, 278–279
parathyroid gland(s)
    diseases of, 279–280
    function, 278–279
        assessment of, 287
    structure of, 278, 278*f*

paresis, 317, 345
Parkinson's disease, 325, 337–338, 338*f*
passive immunity
    versus active immunity, 23*f*
    vaccination and, 23
patch tests, 380
patent ductus arteriosus, 115–116, 116*f*
pathogenesis, 6
pathogenic organisms, inflammation due
        to, 12, 12*f*
pathology, 6–7
PDA. *See* patent ductus arteriosus
pediculosis, 379
pelvic bone, fracture, 358
pelvic inflammatory disease, 296, 315, 318
penicillin, allergy, 382
penis, 307, 309*f*
    erection of, 308–310
pepsin, 174–175
peptic ulcer(s), 173–175, 174*f*–175*f*, 188
pericardium, 104, 104*f*
periosteum, 352
peripheral resistance, 141
peristalsis, 168
peritonitis, 176
permeability, histamine effects on, 12–13
pernicious anemia, 64, 88, 176, 188
pertussis vaccine, 333
petechiae, 94, 123, 137
petit mal epilepsy, 339
pH, regulation of, 148
phagocytes, 13. *See also* neutrophil(s)
phagocytic cells, 221
phagocytosis, 16–17
phantom pain, 328
pharynx, 216
phenylketonuria, 48–49
    enzyme block in, 50*f*
phlebitis, 138
phlebotomy, 93
phosphorus, deficiency, bone disorders in,
        355–356
photophobia, 396
physical agents, inflammation due to, 12*f*
phytochemicals, 410
pia mater, 324
PID. *See* pelvic inflammatory disease
pilonidal cyst, 387
pink puffers, 228–229

pipestem colon, 181, 182*f*
pituitary dwarfism, 255*f*, 256–257
pituitary gland
    anterior, 250, 250*f*
        adenoma, 252
        diseases of, 252–253
        hormones of, 251–252
        target organs for, 251*f*, 251–252
    effects
        on female reproductive system,
            294–295, 295*f*
        on male reproductive system, 308
    failure, 253–258, 254*f*
    function, 249–251
        assessment of, 287
    insufficiency, 253–258, 254*f*, 256*f*
    as master gland, 248, 256
    and optic nerve, anatomical relation-
        ship, 255*f*, 256
    posterior, 251
        functions of, 258
        hyposecretion, 258–259
    structure of, 249–251, 250*f*
PKU. *See* phenylketonuria
placenta, 295–296
plantar warts, 378
plaque
    amyloid, 402
    arteriosclerotic, 109, 110*f*, 131–132,
        132*f*
plasma cells, 17*f*
    B lymphocyte transformation into, 18
platelet(s), 86
    in thrombosis, 132
pleura, 217
pleural cavity, 217
pleural membrane, 227
pleurisy, 235, 236*f*
pleuritis, 235
pleurocentesis, 231
PMS. *See* premenstrual syndrome
Pneumocystis carinii, in AIDS, 20
pneumonia, 222, 231–235
    bronchial, 233–234
    double, 231
    influenzal, 234–235
    lobar, 231–233
    primary atypical, 234
    resolution, 233

pneumothorax, 230–231
poison ivy, 381–382
poliomyelitis, 332
polycystic kidney(s), 157–159, 159f
polycythemia, 4
    diagnosis of, 99
    primary, 93
    secondary, 93
polydactyly, 47
polydipsia, 259, 274
    in diabetes mellitus, 282
polymorphs, 12
    immune response and, 12
polyp(s), colonic, 183–184
    in ulcerative colitis, 181, 182f
polyuria, 258
    in diabetes mellitus, 282
portal cirrhosis of liver, 199–203
portal vein, 199
potassium, 67
Pott's disease, 355
preeclampsia, 307
pregnancy
    abnormalities of, 305–307
    and alcohol, 78–79
    ectopic, 305, 305f
pregnancy-induced hypertension, 307
premature ventricular contraction(s),
    124
premenstrual syndrome, 303–304
prepuce, 307
primary atypical pneumonia, 234
proctoscope, 187
proerythroblast(s), 86f, 87
progesterone, actions of, 295
prognosis, 8
progression, of carcinogenesis, 32, 33f
promotion, of carcinogenesis, 32, 33f
prostate gland, 307, 309f
    carcinoma of, 311–313
        metastasis, 312, 312f
    diseases of, 310–313
prostatitis, 310–311
protein(s), synthesis, in liver, 194–195
protein-sparing effect, 282
prothrombin, 66, 195
pruritus, 376
pseudohermaphroditism, 56, 58f
psoriasis, 387–388, 388f, 399

psychogenic factor(s)
    in asthma, 226
    in ulcerative colitis, 181
psychoneurotic disorders. See also
        anorexia nervosa
    malnutrition in, 65f
pubic lice, 379
puerperal sepsis, 297–298
puerperium, 297–298
pulmonary circulation, 105–106,
        107f–108f, 130, 130f, 218
pulmonary edema, 112
pulmonary embolism, 134, 135f
pulmonary hypertension, 112
pulmonary stenosis, 114
pulse, regulation of, 107–108
purpura, 94, 137
pustules, 376
PVCs. See premature ventricular contrac-
        tion(s)
pyelitis, 155
pyelonephritis, 153–154, 154f
pyloric sphincter, 168
pyloric stenosis, 59
pyogenic bacteria, 154, 223
pyosalpinx, 296
pyridoxine, 409
pyuria, 154, 162R

R

rabies, 333–334, 334f
radiation, cancer caused by, 33–34, 34f
radical mastectomy, 301
rales, 228
range of motion, joint, 352
rapid plasma reagin test, 317, 319
rash, of Lyme disease, 377
Raynaud's disease, 137–138
RDA. See recommended dietary al-
        lowances
reagin(s), 220–221, 225
recessive disorders, transmission of,
        50f
recessive gene(s), 47
recommended dietary allowances, 410
rectum, carcinoma of, 183–186
red blood cell count, 99
red blood cells, excessive, 93

referred pain, 173
reflex arc, 324, 326*f*
reflux, esophageal, 171
regional enteritis, 180–181, 396
regurgitation, 186
relapse, 8
releasing factors, 250
remission, 8
renal carcinoma, 155, 156*f*
renal failure, 152
   acute, 152
   chronic, 153, 153*f*
renal pelvis, 149
renin, 148
repetitive strain injuries, 360
reproductive system
   diseases of, diagnosis of, 319
   female, 292*f*, 292–294
      diseases of, 296–305
      neoplasms of, 298–302
      physiology of, 294–296
   male
      anatomy of, 307, 308*f*–309*f*
      diseases of, 310–314
      physiology of, 307–310
residual volume, 242*f*
respiratory center, 217
respiratory disease(s), 215–245
   diagnosis of, 242
respiratory epithelium, 218
respiratory system
   functions of, 216–219
   and stress, 398
   structure of, 216–219
rest, for elderly, 402
resuscitation, 124
reticulocyte(s), 86*f*, 87
retrovirus, 20
Reye's syndrome, 335
rhabdomyosarcoma, 368
rheumatic heart disease, 120–121
rheumatoid arthritis, 361–363
   diagnosis of, 368
rheumatoid factor, 362
Rh factor, 27
   newborn, and anemia, 89
Rh incompatibility, 27, 89–92, 90*f*–91*f*
rhodopsin, 65
riboflavin, 409

rickets, 66, 355–356
right lymphatic duct, 16*f*
rigidity, in Parkinson's disease, 337
ringworm, 379
RNA, 6
RPR test. *See* rapid plasma reagin test

S

Sabin vaccine, 332
salivation, 168
Salk vaccine, 332
Salmonella, food poisoning, 181–183
salpingitis, 296–297
salpinx, 296
sarcoma, 36
   versus carcinoma, 38*f*
satiety center, 72
scabies, 380
sclerosing solution, 140
sclerotherapy
   compression, 139
   endoscopic, 140, 201
scrotum, 307
seasonal allergic rhinitis, 220–221
sebaceous cysts, 386–387
sebaceous glands, 375*f*, 376
seborrheic dermatitis, 386
seborrheic keratosis, 387
sebum, 386
seizures, 324, 330
   epileptic, 339–340
self-blood-glucose monitoring, 283
semen analysis, 310
semilunar valves, 104–105
seminal vesicle, 307, 309*f*
seminiferous tubules, 307, 308*f*
seminoma, 313
senility, 399–401
sensory nervous system, 328–329
septal defect(s), 112–113, 114*f*
septic embolism, 134
septicemia, 298
sequela, 9
sequestrum, 354
serotonin, 23, 397
sex chromosome anomalies, 55–56
sex chromosomes, 46
sex glands, 248

sex hormone(s)
   hypersecretion, 286–287
   secretion, abnormalities, 286–287
   therapy, 256
sex-linked inheritance, 51–53, 52*f*
sexual abnormalities, stress-related,
      397–398
sexually transmitted disease, 315–318
   diagnosis of, 319
shingles, 334–335
shock, 142
   anaphylactic, 142, 142*f*
   cardiogenic, 142, 142*f*
   hypovolemic, 142, 142*f*
   neurogenic, 142, 142*f*
   types of, 142, 142*f*
shoes, high heels versus flats, 363
sickle cell anemia, 51, 88–89
SIDS. *See* sudden infant death syndrome
signs, 7–8
Simmond's syndrome, 257*f*, 257–258
sinoatrial node, 107
sinuses, paranasal, 220
skin
   cancer of, 36
   diseases of
      classification of, 376
      diagnostic tests for, 388–389
      hypersensitivity, 380–382
      infectious, 376–380
      neoplastic, 382–386
      stress-related, 398–399
   functions of, 373–374
   metabolic disorders of, 386–388
   structure of, 374–376, 375*f*
skull fracture, 346
sleeping sickness, 331
slipped disk, 364–365, 366*f*
small intestine, 16*f*, 168–169
   mucosal surface of, 169*f*
smoking, cancer caused by, 34*f*, 35
smoking cessation, skin patch for, 408
smooth muscle, 354
snoring, 220
sodium, 67
somatotropin, 251
somnolence, 267
spasmogens, 398
spastic colon, 185–186

specific gravity
   definition of, 151
   urinary, 151, 161
spermatogenesis, 307–308
spider veins, 139
spina bifida, 58, 340–341, 341*f*
spina bifida occulta, 340–341, 341*f*
spinal cord, 324
   injury, 357
spinal nerve(s), 327*f*
spirogram, 242*f*
spirometer, 230
spirometry, 242, 242*f*
spleen, 16*f*
splenectomy, 89
splenomegaly, 89, 199
spontaneous abortion, 306
sprain(s), 360
squamous cell carcinoma, 383–385
staghorn calculus, 156, 157*f*
staphylococci, infection by, 15
stasis, 121, 138
status asthmaticus, 226
stenosis, definition of, 114
sterility, male, evaluation, 310
steroid(s)
   anabolic, 273
   for lupus erythematosus, 19
   muscle-building, 273
stomach, 168
   adenocarcinoma of, 37*f*, 176*f*
   cancer of, 173, 176*f*, 176–178, 177*f*
   diseases of, 173–178
   mucosal lining of, 168, 173
stool
   characteristics, diseases indicated by,
      188
   occult blood in, 188
strabismus, 341
strain(s), 360
strep throat, 221
streptococci
   group A hemolytic, 120
   infection by, 15
   tonsillitis caused by, 221–222
stress, 7, 391–405
   adaptation to, 391–392
   cardiovascular effects of, 397
   effects on body, 392–393

gastrointestinal diseases affected by, 396

respiratory effects of, 398

response to

adrenal cortical hormones in, 393–395, 395*f*

autonomic nervous system in, 393, 394*f*

sexual abnormalities related to, 397–398

skin diseases affected by, 398–399

systemic changes caused by, 399

stress-related disease(s), 396–399

stress ulcers, 396

stretching, benefits of, 400

striae, in Cushing's syndrome, 274

stroke, 343–345

subarachnoid hemorrhage, 346

subcutaneous fatty tissue, 375*f*, 376

subdural hemorrhage, 346

sudden infant death syndrome, 240–241

sunlight, vitamin D production from, 66

sun screens, cancer and, 33

superior vena cava, 131

suppressor T cells, 17*f*, 18

sweat test, 240

symptoms, 7–8

synapse, 328

syncope, 120

syndrome, 8

synovial fluid, 352, 353*f*

synovial membrane, 352, 353*f*

inflammation of, 362

syphilis, 316–317

congenital, 57–58

systemic circulation, 130, 130*f*

systemic lupus erythematosus, 19

systole, 105

systolic pressure, 140

T

T₃. *See* triiodothyronine
T_3. *See* triiodothyronine

T_4. *See* thyroxine

tachycardia, 124, 264

tanning spas, cancer and, 33

Tay Sachs disease, 51

tendon(s), 352–354

tennis elbow, 366

teratoma(s), 42*f*, 299, 300*f*, 313

terminal disease, 8

testicular tumors, 313

testis/testes, 307, 308*f*–309*f*

diseases of, 313–314

undescended, 314, 314*f*

testosterone, 307–308

tetanus, 332–333, 334*f*

tetanus antitoxin, 333

tetanus toxoid, 333

tetany, in hypoparathyroidism, 280, 280*f*

tetralogy of Fallot, 113–115, 115*f*

thalidomide, 58

thiamine, 409

deficiency, 76. *See also* Wernicke's encephalopathy

thoracic duct, 16*f*

thrombocytopenia, 94

thrombolytic drugs, 110

thrombophlebitis, 138

thrombosis, 132–135, 133*f*–134*f*

cerebral, 344–345

thrombus, formation, 132–135, 133*f*–134*f*

in valvular heart disease, 118

thymus gland, 16*f*–17*f*

in myasthenia gravis, 368

thyroid function tests, 260–261, 287

thyroid gland

diseases of, 262–272

function, 260–261

assessment of, 287

structure of, 260, 260*f*

thyroid hormone(s), 260

effects of, 261

regulation of, 262

thyroid-stimulating hormone, 252, 262

assay, 287

deficiency, 254

thyrotropin, 252

in response to stress, 394

thyroxine, 259–260

circulating level, control of, 262, 263*f*

effects of, 261, 262*f*

therapy, 256

TIA. *See* transient ischemic attacks
tidal volume, 242*f*
tissue, vascular changes in, 12
tissue plasminogen activator, 110
tissue repair, 12–15
T lymphocytes, 17*f*, 17–19
tolerance, 19
tonsillitis, 221–222
tonsils, 16*f*, 221, 221*f*
total lung capacity, 242*f*
toxemia of pregnancy, 306*f*, 306–307
toxic shock syndrome, 303
toxins, 15
toxoids, 22
TPA. *See* tissue plasminogen activator
trachea, 216
tracheobronchitis, 223
tracheotomy, 25, 226
transient ischemic attacks, 345
trauma
    inflammation due to, 12*f*
    response to, 4
tremor(s)
    in hyperthyroidism, 264
    in Parkinson's disease, 337
Treponema pallidum, 316
Treponema pallidum immobilization test,
    317
trichomonas, vaginitis, 297
triglycerides, dietary, 410–411
triiodothyronine, 260
trisomy 21, 53. *See also* Down's syn-
    drome
tropic hormone(s), 251
trypsin, 208
TSH. *See* thyroid-stimulating hormone
TSS. *See* toxic shock syndrome
tubercle, 238
tubercle bacilli, 237
tuberculin test, 237–238
tuberculosis, 236–238, 394
    acute miliary, 238
    asymptomatic, 237
    of bone, 355
    chronic fibrocaseous, 238
    increased incidence of, causes of, 236,
        237*f*
    of kidney, 238–239
    transmission of, 236–237

tumor(s)
    benign, 40–42, 42*f*
        versus malignant, 42
    formation, 31–32
    grading, 39
    malignant, 32–40
        versus benign, 42
Turner's syndrome, 55, 56*f*
Tzanck smear, 318

U

ulcer(s)
    duodenal, 175
    gastric, 175
    peptic, 173–175, 174*f*, 178*f*, 188
    perforation of, 176
    stress, 396
    treatment of, 176
ulcerative colitis, 396
    and cancer of colon, 183
    chronic, 181, 182*f*
ultrasound
    of liver and biliary system, 211
    pelvic, 319
ultrasound arteriography, 143
umbilical arteries, 296
upper respiratory disease(s), 219–222
urea, 148–149, 152–153, 195
uremia, 152
ureter(s), 149, 150*f*
    prolapse, 157
ureterocele, 157
urethra, 149, 150*f*
    diseases of, 159–160
    male, 307, 309*f*
urethritis, 160
uric acid, deposits, in gout, 364
urinalysis, 161
urinary bladder. *See* bladder, urinary
urinary calculi, 155–157, 157*f*
urinary meatus, female, 293*f*, 294
urinary system, 149, 150*f*
    in elderly, 400
urine
    color, 161
    formation, 148–149
    glucose in, 162

pH, 161
    specific gravity, 151, 161
urticaria, 380
uterus, 292, 292f
    fibroid tumors of, 298–299, 299f
    proliferative phase, 294
    secretory phase, 295

V

vaccination, 22–23
vagina, 292, 292f
    adenocarcinoma of, 300–301
vaginal opening, 293f, 294
vaginitis, 297
vagus nerve, effects on heart, 107–108
varicose vein(s), 138–140, 139f
    and obesity, 72–73
vascular changes, in inflammation, 13, 13f
vascular disease, diagnosis of, 142–143
vas deferens, 307, 308f, 308, 309f
vasopressin, 258
vasopressin injection test, 287
VDRL test, 317, 319
vegetation(s), valvular
    in infectious endocarditis, 123, 123f
    in rheumatic fever, 121, 121f
vein(s), 131
    diseases of, 138–140
    stripping, 139
Venereal Disease Research Laboratory
        test, 317, 319
venereal wart(s), 378
ventricle(s)
    cardiac, 104–105
        dilated, 111–112
        hypertrophy, 112–113
    cerebral, 325–326
ventricular fibrillation, 124
ventricular septal defect, 112, 114f
venule(s), 131
verruca vulgaris, 378
vertebrae, fractured, 357, 358f
vertebral column, 364, 365f
very low density lipoprotein(s), 412
vesicles, 376
villi
    chorionic, 295–296
    intestinal, 169, 169f

viral infection(s), of skin, 377–378
virilism, adrenal, 274, 276, 277f
viruses, 6
    cancer caused by, 34f, 35
vital capacity, 242f
vitamin(s)
    deficiency, 65–67
        effects of, 66f
    functions of, 409–410
    recommended dietary allowances, 410
    supplements, 410
vitamin A
    deficiency, 65–66, 66t
        geographical distribution of, 65
    hypervitaminosis, 410
    recommended dietary allowances, 410
vitamin B, 409–410
vitamin B_{12}, 409
    malabsorption, in pernicious anemia, 64
vitamin C, 409
    deficiency, 66t, 66–67
vitamin D, 409
    deficiency, 66, 66t
        bone disorders in, 355–356
    production of, 66
vitamin E, 409
vitamin K, 179
    deficiency, 66, 66t
vitiligo, 374
VLDL. *See* very low density lipoprotein(s)
volvulus, 184, 185f
vomiting, 186
VSD. *See* ventricular septal defect
vulva, 293f, 294

W

wart(s), 41, 378
    genital (venereal), 318, 378
    plantar, 378
weight loss, in diabetes mellitus, 283
weight reduction, 74–75
wellness, 407–408
Wernicke's encephalopathy, 76–77
wheals, 380
wheezing, 225
white blood cell count
    differential, 99
    in infection, 15
    total, 99

white blood cells
   chemotaxis and, 13
   diseases of, 95–98
white matter, 325
Wilms' tumor, 155
wound healing, 14*f*, 15
   fibroblasts in, 14*f*

X

X chromosome, 46

Y

Y chromosome, 46